The Use of Robotic Technology in Female Pelvic Floor Reconstruction

Jennifer T. Anger • Karyn S. Eilber
Editors

The Use of Robotic Technology in Female Pelvic Floor Reconstruction

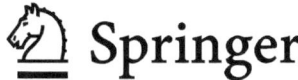 Springer

Editors
Jennifer T. Anger
Department of Surgery, Division
   of Urology
Cedars-Sinai Medical Center
Beverly Hills, CA, USA

Karyn S. Eilber
Department of Surgery, Division of
   Urology
Cedars-Sinai Medical Center
Beverly Hills, CA, USA

ISBN 978-3-319-59610-5   ISBN 978-3-319-59611-2   (eBook)
DOI 10.1007/978-3-319-59611-2

Library of Congress Control Number: 2017946483

Printed on acid-free paper

This Springer imprint is published by Springer Nature
The registered company is Springer International Publishing AG
The registered company address is: Gewerbestrasse 11, 6330 Cham, Switzerland

Foreword

In the last decade surgeons have advanced minimally invasive approaches to abdominal and pelvic surgery, utilizing both standard laparoscopy and robotic technology to improve the scope of possibilities. The rapid adoption of robotic techniques has afforded the female pelvic surgeon a broader armamentarium to pelvic floor reconstruction, with a specific aim of offering our patient population a more durable and efficacious approach to pelvic floor repairs.

This comprehensive textbook of robotic technology applied to female pelvic reconstruction is the first of its kind and will be a valuable educational tool for surgeons. Numerous prolific female pelvic surgeons with both urological and gynecological backgrounds have contributed to this text, covering all aspects of patient selection, optimization of robotic techniques, and pitfalls. Additionally, options for management of the uterus at the time of prolapse repair will be discussed. This topic has become more critical as more of our patients inquire about less invasive approaches.

This surgical textbook encompasses the spectrum of pelvic floor disease and a unique approach to reconstructive techniques. It should serve as an educational tool for the surgeon-in-training as well as the experienced female pelvic surgeon seeking to expand his/her armamentarium for reconstruction.

NYU Langone Medical Center   Nirit Rosenblum, M.D.
New York, NY, USA

Preface

Welcome to the textbook, *The Use of Robotic Technology in Female Pelvic Floor Reconstruction*. The fields of urology and urogynecology, now collectively termed Female Pelvic Medicine and Reconstructive Surgery, have rapidly evolved over time. Surgeons adopt new technology with the ultimate goal of providing better care for patients. Robotic surgery is a technological advancement that provides durability through a minimally invasive approach. Outcomes are comparable to laparoscopic surgery. Since robotic technology allows surgeons without laparoscopic training to perform good laparoscopy, we anticipate that the use of the robot in FPMRS will only increase.

This textbook is designed to provide guidance for surgeons wishing to perform the most common robotic procedures in FPMRS. We first seek to teach robotic surgery to readers with a background in FPMRS but not in robotics. We were once in that place, experiencing the frustrations of a beginner learning a new technology, despite fellowship training and expertise with other approaches. We also wish to reach out to non-FPMRS surgeons, specifically urologists adept at robotic prostatectomy, who may be able to technically perform the steps of a robotic ASC, yet may not know certain nuances. Such nuances, which include when to place a prophylactic sling and when to perform a concomitant posterior vaginal wall repair, have a significant impact on postoperative outcomes. And lastly, we seek to reach out to anyone in training, either before, during, or after residency, who seek to learn more about robotic technology in FPMRS.

We wish to thank each author in this textbook, each of whom has specific expertise in the field and provides a wealth of information. Dr. Amy Rosenman, Past President of the American Urogynecologic Society, has years of experience treating prolapse bother surgically and nonsurgically and provides an excellent review on patient candidacy for surgery. Drs. Una Lee and Arianna Smith each provide detailed explanations addressing concomitant surgeries and when they should and should not be performed. Thank you to Drs. Kim Kenton, M. Jonathon Solnik, and Christopher Tarnay, all gynecologists by training, not only for your chapters, but especially for your willingness to train us (urologists) and make us proficient in robotic hysterectomy. Drs. David Magner and Beth Moore have taught us a great deal about the role of robotic technology in combined rectal and vaginal prolapse. Dr. Bilal Chughtai provides a comprehensive synthesis of the literature addressing uterine sparing approaches robotically. And lastly, our own colleagues at Cedars-Sinai Medical Center, Drs. Hyung Kim, Christopher Dru, and Devin

Patel, who demonstrate how to apply robotic technology to robotic reconstructive procedures other than sacrocolpopexy.

Thank you to Springer Publishing Company for the support and inspiration to write this book, and a special thanks to Miss Elise Paxson, who has helped us so patiently in putting all the pieces of this book together. We are also grateful to each other for patiently assisting as we each climbed, and ultimately passed, our individual learning curves in robotic surgery.

We dedicate this textbook to the Anger family (Lowell, Arielle, Amanda, and Joshua) and the Eilber family (Fritz, Dylan, Parker, and Alexandra), who understand the sacrifices that the two of us make on a daily basis to be wives, mothers, and surgeons. We are indebted, grateful, and, because of your support, tireless.

Beverly Hills, CA, USA   Jennifer T. Anger, M.D., M.P.H.
                                                                          Karyn S. Eilber, M.D.

Contents

Contributors

A. Lenore Ackerman, M.D., Ph.D. Department of Surgery, Department of Urology, Cedars-Sinai Medical Center, Beverly Hills, CA, USA

Sarah A. Adelstein, M.D. Section of Urology and Renal Transplantation, Virginia Mason, Seattle, WA, USA

Jennifer T. Anger, M.D., M.P.H. Department of Surgery, Division of Urology, Cedars-Sinai Medical Center, Beverly Hills, CA, USA

Katarzyna Bochenska, M.D. Division of Female Pelvic Medicine and Reconstructive Surgery, Department of Obstetrics and Gynecology, Northwestern University, Prentice Women's Hospital, Chicago, IL, USA

Bilal Chughtai, M.D. Department of Urology, Weill Cornell Medicine/New-York Presbyterian, New York, NY, USA

Sarah Collins, M.D. Division of Female Pelvic Medicine and Reconstructive Surgery, Department of Obstetrics and Gynecology, Northwestern University, Prentice Women's Hospital, Chicago, Illinois, USA

Christopher J. Dru, M.D. Department of Surgery, Division of Urology, Cedars-Sinai Medical Center, Los Angeles, CA, USA

Karyn S. Eilber, M.D. Department of Surgery, Division of Urology, Cedars-Sinai Medical Center, Beverly Hills, CA, USA

Juzar Jamnagerwalla, M.D. Department of Surgery, Division of Urology, Cedars-Sinai Medical Center, Beverly Hills, CA, USA

Hyung L. Kim, M.D. Department of Surgery, Division of Urology, Cedars-Sinai Medical Center, Los Angeles, CA, USA

Kathleen C. Kobashi, M.D., F.A.C.S. Virginia Mason Medical Center, Seattle, WA, USA

Una J. Lee, M.D. Section of Urology and Renal Transplantation, Virginia Mason, Seattle, WA, USA

Lea Luketic, M.Sc., M.D. Department of Obstetrics and Gynecology, Mount Sinai Hospital, Toronto, ON, Canada

David P. Magner, M.D., F.A.C.S. Department of Surgery, Division of Colorectal Surgery, Cedars-Sinai Medical Center, Los Angeles, CA, USA

Beth A. Moore, M.D., F.A.C.S., F.A.S.C.R.S. Department of Surgery, Division of Colorectal Surgery, Cedars-Sinai Medical Center, Los Angeles, CA, USA

Janine L. Oliver, M.D. Division of Urology, Department of Surgery, University of Colorado Hospital, Aurora, CO, USA

Devin Patel, M.D., M.B.A. Department of Surgery, Division of Urology, Cedars Sinai Medical Center, Los Angeles, CA, USA

Amy E. Rosenman, M.D. David Geffen School of Medicine, University of California at Los Angeles, Santa Monica, CA, USA

Emily Siegel, M.D. Department of Surgery, Division of Colorectal Surgery, Cedars Sinai Medical Center, Los Angeles, CA, USA

Ariana L. Smith, M.D. Department of Surgery, Perelman School of Medicine, University of Pennsylvania Health System, Philadelphia, PA, USA

M. Jonathon Solnik, M.D., F.A.C.O.G., F.A.C.S. University of Toronto Faculty of Medicine, Mount Sinai Hospital, Toronto, ON, Canada

Christopher M. Tarnay, M.D. Department of Obstetrics & Gynecology; Urology, Ronald Reagan UCLA Medical Center, Los Angeles, CA, USA

Dominique Thomas, B.S. Department of Urology, Weill Cornell Medicine/New-York Presbyterian, New York, NY, USA

Adam Truong, M.D. Department of Surgery, Division of Colorectal Surgery, Cedars-Sinai Medical Center, Los Angeles, CA, USA

Steven J. Weissbart, M.D. Department of Urology, Stony Brook University, Stony Brook, NY, USA

Jessica S. Zigman, M.D. Female Pelvic Medicine and Reconstructive Surgery Fellow, Harbor UCLA Medical Center, Torrance, CA, USA

Abbreviations

ACCESS	Abdominal colpopexy: comparison of endoscopic surgical strategies
AH	Abdominal hysterectomy
ASC	Abdominal sacral colpopexy or abdominal sacrocolpopexy
ASH	Abdominal sacrohysteropexy
AUB	Abnormal uterine bleeding
BMI	Body mass index
BS	Bilateral salpingectomy
CARE	Colpopexy and urinary reduction efforts
CRADI	Colorectal-Anal Distress Inventory
EEA	End-to-end anastomosis
EBL	Estimated blood loss
EQ5D	EuroQol five dimensions questionnaire
FDG	Fluorodeoxyglucose
FSFI	Female Sexual Function Index
HLRCC	Hereditary leiomyomatosis and renal cell cancer
HNPCC	Hereditary nonpolyposis colorectal cancer
HPF	High-power field
HPV	Human papillomavirus
ICIQ-VS	International Consultation on Incontinence Questionnaire of vaginal symptoms
ICS	International Continence Society
ISD	Intrinsic sphincter deficiency
IVF	In vitro fertilization
LASC	Laparoscopic sacrocolpopexy
LDH	Lactate dehydrogenase
LMH	Laparoscopic mesh sacrohysteropexy
LSC	Laparoscopic sacrocolpopexy
LSH	Laparoscopic suture sacrohysteropexy
MAUDE	Manufacturer and User Facility Device Experience database
MIS	Minimally invasive surgery
MRI	Magnetic resonance imaging
MTR	Microscopic tubal reanastomosis
NNT	Number needed to treat
OPUS	Outcomes following vaginal prolapse repair and midurethral sling

OR	Odds ratio
PCOS	Polycystic ovarian syndrome
PEG	Polyethylene glycol
PET	Positron emission tomography
PFD	Pelvic floor disorder
PFDI	Pelvic Floor Distress Inventory
PFDN	PELVIC Floor Disorders Network
POP	Pelvic organ prolapse
POP-Q	Pelvic organ prolapse quantification
POPDI-6	Pelvic Organ Prolapse Distress Inventory 6
PTFE	Polytetrafluoroethylene
QOL	Quality of life
RASC	Robotic-assisted sacrocolpopexy
RALH	Robotic-assisted laparoscopic hysterectomy
RALM	Robotic-assisted laparoscopic myomectomy
RALS	Robotic-assisted laparoscopic sacrohysteropexy
RASC	Robotic-assisted sacrocolpopexy
RCC	Renal cell carcinoma
SRH	Supracervical robotic hysterectomy
SSLF	Sacrospinous ligament fixation
SUI	Stress urinary incontinence
TLH	Total laparoscopic hysterectomy
TRH	Total robotic hysterectomy
TOMUS	Trial of midurethral slings
ULMS	Uterine leiomyosarcoma
US FDA	US Food and Drug Administration
USLS	Uterosacral ligament suspension
VCUG	Voiding cystourethrogram
VVF	Vesicovaginal fistula

Jennifer T. Anger and Karyn S. Eilber

Approximately one in five women undergoes surgery for prolapse or incontinence in her lifetime [1]. Of these, up to 30% require a re-operation for recurrence of their prolapse or incontinence symptoms [2]. It has been estimated that one in nine women will undergo a hysterectomy in her lifetime, and up to 10% of these women will require surgery for symptomatic vaginal vault prolapse [2, 3]. The search for the ideal repair for vaginal vault prolapse has led to the invention of several approaches to this problem [4].

The transabdominal sacrocolpopexy is considered the gold standard in the surgical management of vaginal vault prolapse, with long-term success rates of up to 100% [5]. Randomized comparative effectiveness trials and systematic literature reviews have demonstrated the anatomic superiority of sacrocolpopexy to vaginal vault suspension [6–8]. The sacrocolpopexy involves an attachment of a Y-shaped surgical mesh to the vaginal apex and anterior and posterior vaginal walls. The tail end of the mesh is sutured to the anterior longitudinal ligament overlying the sacral promontory.

Although the most successful operation for vaginal vault prolapse, the open approach to sacrocolpopexy requires an abdominal incision. In an effort to develop minimally invasive alternatives to open sacrocolpopexy, vaginal approaches that utilize synthetic mesh were developed. The placement of mesh vaginally is theoretically advantageous. However, vaginal approaches to prolapse have a lower cure rate than sacrocolpopexy [6] and are associated with significant complications. The frequency and severity of such complications led to the publication by the U.S. Food and Drug Administration (FDA) of the following warning to healthcare providers on October 20, 2008 [9]: "This is to alert you to complications associated with transvaginal placement of surgical mesh to treat Pelvic Organ Prolapse (POP) and Stress Urinary Incontinence (SUI). Although rare, these complications can have serious consequences. Over the past 3 years, FDA has received over 1000 reports from nine surgical mesh manufacturers of complications that were associated with surgical mesh devices used to repair POP and SUI.... The most frequent complications included erosion through vaginal epithelium, infection, pain, urinary problems, and recurrence of prolapse and/or incontinence. There were also reports of

J.T. Anger, M.D., M.P.H. (✉) • K.S. Eilber, M.D.
Department of Surgery, Division of Urology,
Cedars-Sinai Medical Center, 99 North La Cienega
Boulevard, Suite 307, Beverly Hills, CA, USA
e-mail: Jennifer.Anger@cshs.org

bowel, bladder, and blood vessel perforation during insertion." As the number of vaginal mesh-related cases rose to over 3874, the FDA communicated a second safety notification to providers on July 13, 2011 [10]. Ultimately, the FDA gave an order to reclassify transvaginal mesh kits from class II (which generally includes moderate-risk devices) to class III (which generally includes high-risk devices). The FDA also issued a second order that requires manufacturers to submit a premarket approval (PMA) application to support the safety and effectiveness of transvaginal mesh [11].

The high complication rate of vaginally placed mesh led many pelvic surgeons to return to the gold standard technique for vaginal vault prolapse—the abdominal sacrocolpopexy. During the same time period that transvaginal mesh became controversial, robotic surgery gained rapid popularity in the world of urology. Specifically, the number of robot-assisted radical prostatectomies performed worldwide nearly tripled between 2007 and 2010, from 80,000 to 205,000 [12]. Between 2007 and 2009, the number of da Vinci systems installed in U.S. hospitals grew by approximately 75%, from almost 800 to around 1400. Soon after radical prostatectomy, robotic surgery began to diffuse across many other surgical specialties. The rapid innovation of robotic surgery, combined with the negative media attention surrounding transvaginal mesh, contributed to the rapid adoption of robotic-assisted sacrocolpopexy. In fact, the rate of sacrocolpopexy procedures almost doubled yearly from 2008 to 2011 among Medicare beneficiaries [13].

For the skilled laparoscopic surgeon, laparoscopy offers a minimally invasive alternative to open sacrocolpopexy. However, suturing the mesh to the vagina laparoscopically is tedious, and access to the deep pelvis is often difficult. In operations where a pure laparoscopic approach is feasible, such as in appendectomy and cholecystectomy, the use of robotic assistance may not be justifiable financially. However, the sacrocolpopexy is an operation that benefits greatly from robotic assistance. The use of robotic technology has made laparoscopic sacrocolpopexy a more feasible procedure for many pelvic surgeons, not just expert laparoscopists. The improved dexterity of the robot and precision of instruments allow suturing of mesh to the vagina to be accomplished with ease. Further, the three-dimensional imaging of the robotic camera provides close visualization of the vessels overlying the sacral promontory and may allow for better preservation of these vessels and less blood loss.

Like many techniques in pelvic surgery, trends in the management of vaginal vault prolapse have continued to evolve. Unfortunately, such trends are not supported by level I data, specifically that provided by randomized clinical trials. Although robotic technology is new and rapidly spreading throughout the urologic and gynecologic communities, there have been no randomized trials comparing outcomes of robotic versus open sacrocolpopexy. Retrospective series indicate comparable efficacy with respect to cure of prolapse. However, to date, it is unknown how robotic surgery compares to open techniques with respect to patient safety, pain, and ability to return to normal activities.

The use of the robot in laparoscopic surgery is costly. The costs of purchasing a robot have been estimated at $1.5 million dollars with annual maintenance costs of $112,000 [14]. In addition, additional costs exist for the robotic equipment utilized with each case. It is arguable that the maintenance and operative equipment costs may overshadow any potential savings in length of hospital stay and patient convalescence [15]. However, we have shown in a randomized trial that, when costs of robot purchase and maintenance were excluded, there was no statistical difference in initial day of surgery costs of robotic compared with laparoscopic sacrocolpopexy [16, 17]. If robotic sacrocolpopexy can provide better immediate quality of life, less pain, and faster recovery compared to open techniques and can allow good laparoscopy to be performed by many pelvic surgeons (not just expert laparoscopists), the investment in robotic techniques may very well be cost-effective when a societal perspective is taken.

In this textbook, we seek to present concepts important to the pelvic surgeon with interest in robotic-assisted sacrocolpopexy (RASC). We will review patient candidacy and alternatives, choice of concomitant vaginal procedures, and management of concomitant stress urinary incontinence (symptomatic and occult). We will also provide detailed descriptions of the set up and steps of RASC. Several chapters will address uterine prolapse and management of the ovaries and fallopian tubes, as well as controversies surrounding uterine morcellation. We will also address robotic management of enterocele and rectal prolapse, which often occur simultaneously with vaginal prolapse. Other pelvic procedures that can successfully be performed robotically, including vesicovaginal fistula repair and robotic-assisted ureteral reimplantation, will be reviewed in detail. Lastly, we will review complications unique to robotic surgery and their management.

References

1. Wu JM, Matthews CA, Conover MM, Pate V, Funk MJ. Lifetime risk of stress incontinence or pelvic organ prolapse surgery. Obstet Gynecol. 2014;123(6):1201.
2. Olsen AL, Smith VJ, Bergstrom JO, Colling JC, Clark AL. Epidemiology of surgically managed pelvic organ prolapse and urinary incontinence. Obstet Gynecol. 1997;89(4):501–6.
3. Marchionni M, Bracco G, Checcucci V, Carabaneanu A, Coccia EM, Mecacci F, Scarselli G. True incidence of vaginal vault prolapse. Thirteen years of experience. J Reprod Med. 1999;44(8):679–84.
4. Elliott DS, Krambeck AE, Chow GK. Long-term results of robotic assisted laparoscopic sacrocolpopexy for the treatment of high grade vaginal vault prolapse. J Urol. 2006;176(2):655–9.
5. Nygaard IE, McCreery R, Brubaker L, Connolly A, Cundiff G, Weber AM, et al. Abdominal sacrocolpopexy: a comprehensive review. Obstet Gynecol. 2004;104(4):805–23.
6. Benson JT, Lucente V, McClellan E. Vaginal versus abdominal reconstructive surgery for the treatment of pelvic support defects: a prospective randomized study with long-term outcome evaluation. Am J Obstet Gynecol. 1996;175(6):1418–22.
7. Maher C, Baessler K, Glazener CM, Adams EJ, Hagen S. Surgical management of pelvic organ prolapse in women: a short version Cochrane review. Neurourol Urodyn. 2008;27(1):3–12.
8. Siddiqui NY, Grimes CL, Casiano ER, et al. Mesh sacrocolpopexy compared with native tissue vaginal repair: a systematic review and meta-analysis. Obstet Gynecol. 2015;125(1):44.
9. FDA public health notification: serious complications associated with transvaginal placement of surgical mesh in repair of pelvic organ prolapse and stress urinary incontinence. 2008. http://www.fda.gov/MedicalDevices/Safety/AlertsandNotices/PublicHealthNotifications/ucm061976.htm. Accessed 5 April 2009.
10. UPDATE on serious complications associated with transvaginal placement of surgical mesh for pelvic organ prolapse: FDA safety communication. 2011. http://www.fda.gov/MedicalDevices/Safety/AlertsandNotices/ucm262435.htm. Accessed 13 July 2011.
11. FDA strengthens requirements for surgical mesh for the transvaginal repair of pelvic organ prolapse to address safety risks. 2016. http://www.fda.gov/NewsEvents/Newsroom/PressAnnouncements/ucm479732.htm. Accessed 4 Jan 2016.
12. Barbash GI, Glied SA. New technology and health care costs—the case of robot-assisted surgery. New Engl J Med. 2010;363(8):701–4.
13. Wang LC, Al Awamlh BAH, Hu JC, Hu JC, Laudano MA, Davison WL, et al. Trends in mesh use for pelvic organ prolapse repair from the Medicare database. Urology. 2015;86(5):885–91.
14. Steinberg PL, Merguerian PA, Bihrle W, Heaney JA, Seinge JD. Vinci robot system can make sense for a mature laparoscopic prostatectomy program. JSLS. 2008;12(1):9.
15. Lotan Y, Cadeddu JA, Gettman MT. The new economics of radical prostatectomy: cost comparison of open, laparoscopic and robot assisted techniques. J Urol. 2004;172(4):1431–5.
16. Anger JT, Mueller ER, Tarnay C, et al. Robotic compared with laparoscopic sacrocolpopexy: a randomized controlled trial. Obstet Gynecol. 2014;123(1):5.
17. Anger JT, Mueller ER, Tarnay C, et al. Erratum: robotic compared with laparoscopic sacrocolpopexy: a randomized controlled trial. Obstet Gynecol. 2014;124(1):165.

Jessica S. Zigman and Amy E. Rosenman

Introduction

When analyzing prevalence of pelvic organ prolapse (POP), anterior vaginal wall prolapse is the most common type, but loss of apical support is usually present in women with prolapse that extends beyond the hymen [1, 2]. Adequate support for the vaginal apex is an essential component of a durable surgical repair for women with advanced prolapse [3, 4]. Anterior and posterior wall repair may fail without the support of the vaginal apex at the time of surgical correction of prolapse [5, 6].

History of Sacrocolpopexy

The evolution of what has become the robotic-assisted laparoscopic sacrocolpopexy (RASC) dates back to 1957, when Arthure and Savage attempted to prevent recurrent enteroceles that formed after standard apical prolapse procedures by anchoring the posterior uterine fundus to the sacral anterior longitudinal ligament [7]. The procedure further evolved with the addition of concomitant hysterectomy and an intervening graft between the vagina and sacrum to overcome excessive tension [8]. Birnbaum felt that the sacral promontory was too anterior for mesh placement, given that the upper vagina is normally directed into the hollow of the sacrum, and instead placed the mesh at the level of S3–S4 to recreate the natural angle [9]. Due to the increased risk of hemorrhage in the pre-sacral space at the S3–S4 site, Sutton advocated anchoring the graft higher, at the S1–S2 level, where the middle sacral artery could be visualized and avoided.

The procedure was further modified by extending the graft along the full length of the rectovaginal septum to decrease graft detachment and improve posterior vaginal wall support [10]. Addison et al. initially used a folded, conical graft configuration to maximize the surface area for mesh attachment, but due to increased risk of mesh erosion, the approach was changed to two separate graft strips sutured with monofilament sutures. This approach also allowed the surgeon to exert differential tension on the anterior and posterior grafts, thereby potentially decreasing urinary incontinence caused by an overcorrected urethrovesical angle [11]. Several surgeons used autologous or allogenic grafts in attempts to decrease mesh erosion, but better

J.S. Zigman, M.D.
Female Pelvic Medicine and Reconstructive Surgery Fellow, Harbor UCLA Medical Center, Torrance, CA, USA

A.E. Rosenman, M.D. (✉)
David Geffen School of Medicine, University of California at Los Angeles, Santa Monica, CA, USA
e-mail: Arosenman@Mednet.ucla.edu

© Springer International Publishing AG 2018
J.T. Anger, K.S. Eilber (eds.), *The Use of Robotic Technology in Female Pelvic Floor Reconstruction*, DOI 10.1007/978-3-319-59611-2_2

anatomic cure rates have been found with nonabsorbable synthetic mesh [12–16].

This procedure has been performed since 1957 when it was first described by Arthure and Savage and has been modified in technique by changing graft material and altering the approach from abdominal to laparoscopic, with and without robotic assistance [8, 17]. A review of the abdominal sacrocolpopexy literature found the surgical procedure to be a reliable procedure that effectively resolves vaginal vault prolapse [12]. In a retrospective cohort study comparing robotic to abdominal sacrocolpopexy with placement of permanent mesh, RASC demonstrated similar short-term vaginal vault support compared with abdominal sacrocolpopexy (slight improvement on Pelvic Organ Prolapse Quantification System (POP-Q) (Table 2.1) C point, −9 cm compared with −8 cm, $p = 0.008$), with longer operative time (328 ± 55 min compared with 223 ± 61 min, $p < 0.001$), less blood loss (103 ± 96 mL compared with 255 ± 155 mL, $p < 0.001$), and shorter length of stay (1.3 ± 1.8 days compared with 2.7 ± 1.4 days, $p < 0.001$) [18]. Long-term data of surgical outcomes of women who underwent open sacrocolpopexy were compared both by objective measure of POP-Q and by validated patient questionnaires [19].

Patient Selection

Who Is a Candidate for Robotic Surgery?

Patient selection for RASC has not been well-studied. Selection depends on many factors, including the surgeon's level of expertise with this surgical technique, resources available at the hospital or surgery center, and patient factors. These include the need for concomitant procedures, age, functional status, body mass index (BMI), previous prolapse or incontinence surgery, and comorbidities that may limit the duration of the anesthesia [14] (Table 2.2). In our opinion, criteria from the Abdominal Colpopexy: Comparison of Endoscopic Surgical Strategies (ACCESS) study should be used for patient selection. Patients must have symptomatic stage II–IV pelvic organ prolapse according to the POP-Q system with significant apical descent, defined as prolapse of the vaginal apex or cervix to at least halfway into the vaginal canal (POP-Q point C ≥ TVL/2) as well as vaginal bulge symptoms [20].

Table 2.1 Pelvic organ prolapse quantification (POP-Q)

Aa	Ba	C
GH	PB	TVL
Ap	Bp	D

Stage 0: no prolapse is demonstrated. Aa, Ba, Ap, Bp = −3 and C or D ≤ −(TVL-2) cm

Stage 1: The most distal portion of the prolapse is more than 1 cm above the level of the hymen

Stage 2: The most distal portion of the prolapse is 1 cm or less proximal or distal to the hymenal plane

Stage 3: The most distal portion of the prolapse protrudes more than 1 cm below the hymen but protrudes no farther than 2 cm less than the total vaginal length

Stage 4: Most distal edge of prolapse if ≥ + (TVL-2) cm

Aa point A anterior, *Ap* point A posterior, *Ba* point B anterior, *Bp* point B posterior, *C* cervix or vaginal cuff, *D* posterior fornix (if cervix is present), *GH* genital hiatus, *PB* perineal body, *TVL* total vaginal length

Table 2.2 Consideration for robotic surgery

Considerations
BMI
Comorbidities
Previous abdominal/pelvic procedures: consider extra-peritoneal
Ability to obtain informed consent for a procedure that involved surgery, mesh, morcellation
Dedicated operating room for robotics
Cost of robotic system
Robotic instrumentation and maintenance

Table 2.3 Benefits of laparoscopic and robotic surgery compared to abdominal surgery

Benefits of laparoscopic/robotic surgery
Reduced postoperative pain
Improved cosmesis (smaller incisions)
Shorter hospital stays
Faster postoperative recovery
Potentially lower costs (laparoscopic)
Improved patient satisfaction
Improved visualization for deep pelvic dissections

Benefits of Laparoscopy

Benefits of minimally invasive abdominal surgery performed laparoscopically consist of reduced postoperative pain, improved cosmesis due to smaller incisions, shorter hospital stays, faster postoperative recovery, potentially lower costs, and improved patient satisfaction [21] (Table 2.3). Laparoscopic surgery may be beneficial for obese patients compared to an open procedure where the pelvis may be deep and more difficult to visualize. For deep pelvic dissections required during a sacrocolpopexy, laparoscopy allows for a two-dimensional view of the field that can be magnified.

Laparoscopic Versus Robotic Approach in Gynecologic Surgery

In a recent meta-analysis comparing the outcomes of laparoscopic sacrocolpopexy (LSC) and RASC, data on 264 RASC and 267 LSC procedures were collected from seven studies. Pan et al. reported similarities in estimated blood loss (114.4 vs. 160.1 mL; $p = 0.36$) and incidence of intraoperative/postoperative complications ($p = 0.85$ vs. $p = 0.92$). RASC was found to be more costly ($p < 0.01$) and had a higher mean operative time (245.9 vs. 205.9 min; $p < 0.001$) [22].

In an effort to compare LSC and RASC for vaginal apex prolapse, a blinded randomized trial included participants with stage 2–4 posthysterectomy vaginal prolapse. One year after prolapse repair, both groups demonstrated significant improvement in vaginal support and functional outcomes, but RASC had a longer operating time, increased pain postoperatively, and a higher surgical cost [23]. Anger et al. randomized 78 women to laparoscopic ($N = 38$) and robotic ($N = 40$) sacrocolpopexies. The initial day of surgery hospital costs for RASC were $2419 higher when robotic costs were included ($13,992 compared with $11,573; $p = 0.001$), and over 6 weeks, hospital costs were $3104 higher for RASC when robotic costs were included ($15,274 compared with $12,170; $p < 0.001$). Both the initial and 6-week costs remain significantly higher for robotic sacrocolpopexy when robotic costs were included [24].

In a retrospective cohort study comparing abdominal sacrocolpopexy with RASC, there was similar short-term vaginal vault support but the latter had a longer operative time, less blood loss, and a shorter length of stay [18]. A cost minimization study was performed comparing open with RASC and found the robotic approach to be equal or less costly than the open approach depending on the institutional robotic case volume [25]. Although laparoscopic sacrocolpopexy has been shown to be equivalent or better in some aspects mentioned, the skills required are not easily acquired and the learning curve is long. It is technically challenging to place the large number of sutures necessary without wristed instruments, and the physical cost to the surgeon has not yet been studied in wear and tear on the neuromuscular skeletal system. Interestingly, the learning curve for RASC is shorter than LSC even though it is considered a complex robotic surgery.

Anesthetic Concerns

Despite the advantages of laparoscopic or robotic gynecologic surgery, there are concerns from the other side of the surgical curtain. Concerns from anesthesia providers range from positioning of

Fig. 2.1 Access to the
patient is limited for the
anesthesiology team
during robotic surgery
(© 2016, Intuitive
Surgical, Inc)

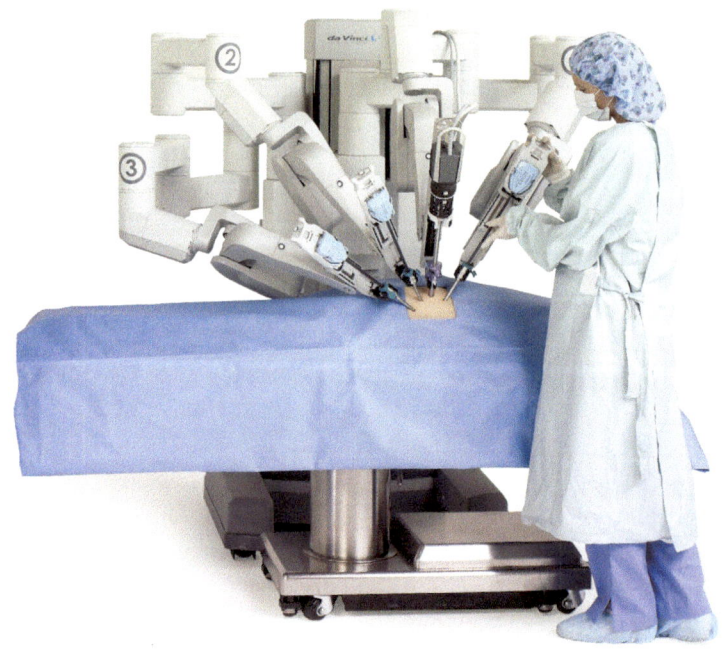

Table 2.4 Concerns from the anesthesiology providers

Physiological effects of pneumoperitoneum in the Trendelenburg position
Restricted access to the patient due to the mass of the equipment set over the patient, tucked arms, docked robot
Patient obesity (see Table 2.5)
Prolonged lithotomy position

the patient to physiologic changes. From the beginning of the surgical procedure, the anesthesiology team has restricted access to the patient due to the mass of the equipment set over the patient (Fig. 2.1). During robotic surgery, access is even further restricted by docking the robot, as the patient cannot be moved after this point. Furthermore, the arms are completely tucked and often wrapped or padded, limiting access for intraoperative blood draws or placement of an arterial catheter or additional venous access during the procedure (Table 2.4).

Pneumoperitoneum and Trendelenburg Position

Prevention and treatment of complications due to induced pneumoperitoneum, prolonged lithotomy position, and steep Trendelenburg positions have been explored. Although apparently well-tolerated by most patients, the combined effect of the steep Trendelenburg position, which is about 40°, and carbon dioxide pneumoperitoneum during these long procedures, has not been completely defined. In one observational study of robotic endoscopic radical prostatectomy, Trendelenburg position combined with a carbon dioxide pneumoperitoneum significantly influenced cardiovascular, cerebrovascular, and respiratory homeostasis, but variables remained within a clinically acceptable range.

Mean arterial pressure is increased by increased cardiac output, systemic vascular resistance, or both. These changes have been demonstrated by an increased intra-abdominal pressure compressing the aorta and increasing the afterload, possibly further enhanced by humoral factors during laparoscopic surgery [26]. Also, transesophageal Doppler measurements have shown a significant increase in stroke volume when patients are placed in steep Trendelenburg position [27]. Furthermore, regional cerebral oxygenation was well-preserved and the cerebral perfusion pressure remained above the lower limit of the cerebral autoregulation [28, 29].

Cardiovascular Considerations

The assessment of a patient's cardiac risk in the perioperative period is made during the history, physical examination, and electrocardiogram. Depending on a patient's cardiac risk, the surgeon should decide if surgery should proceed without further cardiovascular testing, or be postponed for further testing such as stress testing, echocardiography, or 24 h ambulatory monitoring. The planned surgery may have to be changed to a lesser risk surgery, or conservative management may be chosen instead of surgical treatment. In patients assessed to be at increased cardiovascular risk, a referral to a cardiologist for further evaluation may be indicated preoperatively [30].

A history of ischemic heart disease, congestive heart failure, cerebral vascular disease, renal dysfunction, and preoperative insulin treatment all increase the risk of cardiac complications. Studies have shown a 10–30% reduction in cardiac output in Trendelenburg. Parameters including heart rate, arterial pressure, stroke volume, carbon dioxide elimination, and total respiratory compliance have been measured. Using these values, mean arterial pressure, total peripheral resistance, stroke index, and cardiac index were calculated. At maximum hemodynamic strain, stroke index and cardiac index were reduced by 42%, without significant changes in heart rate and mean arterial pressure. Total peripheral resistance was increased by 50–100% [31].

The Trendelenburg position in awake and anesthetized patients increases pulmonary arterial pressures, central venous pressure, and pulmonary capillary wedge pressure. The cardiac index, a parameter that relates the cardiac output from left ventricle in 1 min to body surface, decreased with anesthesia induction and then again further during laparoscopy. Soon after deflation after laparoscopy, the cardiac index returns to pre-insufflation values [32].

Obese Patients

Concerns have been raised about the applicability of robotic and laparoscopic surgery in the obese patient (Table 2.5). Arterial oxygenation and alveolar-arterial difference in oxygen tension are significantly impaired in obese patients. One study looking at the issues of obesity in a surgical population compared 15 overweight and 15 nonobese patients undergoing robot-assisted radical prostatectomy under general anesthesia. This procedure is similar to a RASC in length and in Trendelenburg positioning of the patient. The alveolar-arterial difference in oxygen tension is a measure of the difference between the alveolar concentration of oxygen and the arterial concentration of oxygen and is used in diagnosing the source of hypoxemia. This small study demonstrated that overweight (BMI of 25–29.9 kg m^2) patients had impaired arterial oxygenation with a higher alveolar-arte-

Table 2.5 Considerations in obese patients

Arterial oxygenation and A(a) DO2 are significantly impaired in overweight patients under general anesthesia in Trendelenburg position
Pneumoperitoneum may transiently reduce impairment in arterial oxygenation and decrease A(a) DO2
Higher expiratory airway pressures
Increased open conversion rates
Increased airway pressures after placing a morbidly obese patient in the lithotomy and steep Trendelenburg positions, possibility of aborting or converting to an open procedure
Hemodynamic parameters are not affected by BMI

rial difference in oxygen tension levels after induction of anesthesia and Trendelenburg positioning. In these overweight patients, pneumoperitoneum reduced the impairment of arterial oxygenation as well [33].

In a study to determine the impact of BMI on perioperative functional and oncological outcomes in patients undergoing robotic laparoscopic radical prostatectomy, 945 patients were stratified by BMI: normal weight (BMI < 25 kg/m^2), overweight (BMI = 25 to <30 kg/m^2), and obese (BMI ≥ 30 kg/m^2). Obese patients experienced increased open conversion rates (2.3%) compared with nonobese patients (0.9%), with over 80% of these open conversion cases due to higher expiratory airway pressures while in Trendelenburg [34].

Hemodynamic parameters have not been shown to be affected by BMI in laparoscopic or robotic surgeries [33, 35]. A recent retrospective study on obese patients (BMI of 30 kg/m^2) followed 1032 patients who underwent robotic gynecological surgery at two institutions between 2006 and 2012 and found that 14% had any complication, but only 3% of patients had a pulmonary complication. The degree of obesity did not predict complications or success of robotic surgery. Age was significantly associated with a higher risk of pulmonary complications ($p = 0.01$). Older age ($p = 0.0001$), higher estimated blood loss ($p < 0.0001$), and longer case length ($p = 0.004$) were associated with a higher rate of all-cause complications. The authors concluded that the vast majority of obese patients can tolerate robotic gynecological surgery with low complication rates and even lower rates of pulmonary complications [36]. In a subgroup analysis, there was no clinical difference between patients who underwent robotic gynecologic surgery for oncologic versus benign indications [37].

Alternative Surgical Strategies

When considering candidacy for RASC, it is important to understand the other surgical options available for apical POP repair, as there are sev-

eral good options for surgical correction of apical prolapse with relatively high success rates.

Transvaginal Approaches

Sacrospinous Ligament Fixation

Sacrospinous ligament fixation (SSLF) is one of the most frequently performed and well-studied of the hysteropexy/colpopexy techniques. This procedure involves performing an extraperitoneal dissection until the sacrospinous ligament is identified and exposed. The right sacrospinous ligament is often used due to the left side's proximity to the rectum. With the use of a reusable ligature carrier or a suture delivery device, the sacrospinous ligament is attached to the posterior cervix, vagina, or possibly the uterosacral ligament using a permanent monofilament suture, delayed absorbable sutures, or a combination of both (Fig. 2.2).

The safety profile, as well as the success of this procedure, has been extensively studied and described in detail in the literature. Generally, there is a low recurrence rate [38], shorter recovery times, less morbidity, shorter operating times, less pain, and a shorter hospital stay when a SSLF is performed without a hysterectomy [39]. In one randomized controlled trial, 71 women either underwent a SSLF without a hysterectomy or vaginal hysterectomy and uterosacral ligament suspension (USLS). There were no differences in quality of life, prolapse or incontinence symptoms, or reoperation rates at 1 year. Although subjectively, prolapse symptoms were the same 1 year postoperatively, 27% of the SSLF group had stage II or greater prolapse on the POP-Q (Table 2.6) compared to only 11% in the vaginal hysterectomy with USLS group. SSLF was associated with shorter hospitalization, shorter recovery with more rapid return to work, and a significantly longer mean total vaginal length of 8.8 versus 7.3 cm than the hysterectomy with apical suspension group ($p < 0.01$) [40]. Most recently, SSLF was reported to be non-inferior to vaginal hysterectomy with suspension of the uterosacral ligaments for symptomatic recurrent prolapse of the apical compartment. Although the

Fig. 2.2 Placement of suture with a suture delivery device through the sacrospinous ligament (Image used with permission from Boston Scientific, 2017)

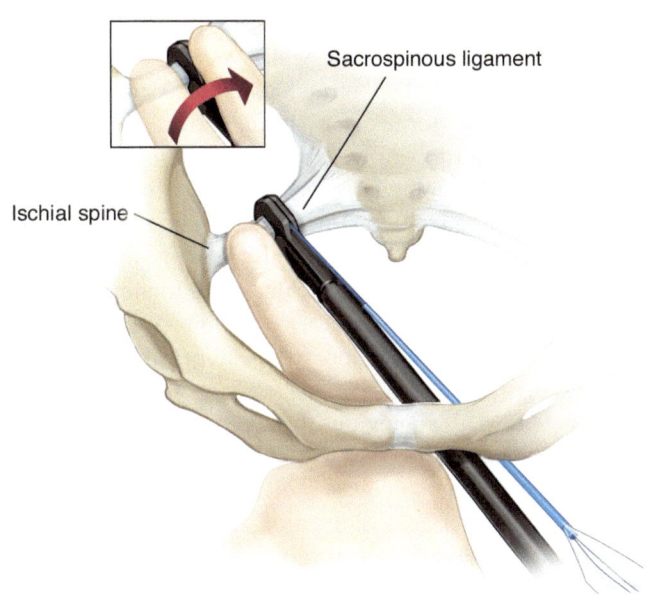

Sacrospinous ligament

Ischial spine

Table 2.6 Relative contraindications to laparoscopic or robotic surgery

Relative contraindications
BMI
Patient preference for Pfannenstiel/previous Pfannenstiel
Pelvic/abdominal radiation therapy
Immunosuppression: chemotherapy, chronic steroid use, immunosuppressive medications
Connective tissue disorders causing poor wound healing
Severe intra-abdominal adhesions
Compromised pulmonary status
Inability to tolerate positioning
Prior upper limb neural injury during surgery

main outcome was POP recurrence at Stage II or higher of the apical compartment, this study also reported no significant differences between anatomical recurrences, functional outcomes, or quality of life [41].

Because this procedure is short in duration, has minimal blood loss, and does not require entering the posterior cul de sac, patients with comorbidities that do not allow for long procedures or patients who have scarring in the cul de sac due to previous surgeries, endometriosis, or pelvic inflammatory disease, may be good candidates.

Uterosacral Ligament Suspension

This technique involves entering the peritoneal cavity through the vagina at the location of the vaginal cuff in a post-hysterectomy patient, through a posterior colpotomy in a uterine-sparing procedure, or through the open cuff at the time of a vaginal hysterectomy. One to three delayed absorbable sutures and/or permanent sutures are placed through each uterosacral ligament at or above the ischial spine. The sutures are then attached either extra-peritoneally or intra-peritoneally to the cervix or vaginal apex. This procedure is done extra-peritoneally when the surgeon choses to avoid the posterior cul de sac due to a previous history of pelvic surgery, endometriosis, pelvic inflammatory disease, or other known pelvic scarring.

One retrospective study compared 100 cases of USLS to 100 cases of USLS at the time of a vaginal hysterectomy and found similar objective results at the postoperative mark of 1.5 years. Objective apical support was 96.4%, with no difference between hysteropexy and cuff suspension (96.0% vs. 96.8%, $p = 0.90$), cystocele (86.8% vs.

93.8%, $p = 0.31$), or rectocele (97.8% vs. 100%, $p = 0.16$) at 2 years after surgery [42].

Using the POP-Q D point, which is the point of the posterior fornix, has been shown to correlate with postoperative apical support, and a clinically meaningful relationship exists between the preoperative D point and anatomic apical success. D points are only present in patients who have a uterus. Richter et al. found that a more negative preoperative D point was significantly related to improved postoperative apical support ($p = 0.0005$). This study excluded women who had a previous hysterectomy, as they did not have a preoperative D point [43]. In our experience, the outcomes are similar except when there is cervical elongation (more than 4 cm) and/or when there is a very large anterior compartment defect, in which case it is difficult to adequately elevate and support the anterior wall with the cervix in place, or even with sufficient elevation of the apex or anterior wall, the elongated cervix may cause the patient bulge symptoms.

Manchester Procedure

Originally described in 1888, the Manchester procedure involved amputation of the cervix, colporrhaphy, and attachment of the cervical stump to the transposed contralateral uterosacral-cardinal ligament complex [44]. Since then, modifications have been made, involving plication of the uterosacral ligaments instead of cutting and transposing the ligaments [45].

In a study comparing the modified Manchester to vaginal hysterectomy with uterosacral ligament suspension outcomes, 98 patients returned for a 1 year follow-up (51 in modified Manchester group and 48 in TVH with USLS group) and were included in this comparison. There were similar anterior and posterior compartment prolapse recurrences (POP stage greater than or equal to stage II) of about 50%, but no apical recurrence for the modified Manchester group. In the modified Manchester group, there was no apical recurrence versus two patients with objective apical recurrence in

the vaginal hysterectomy group. Despite more apical recurrence objectively, there was no difference in the pre- and postoperative subjective scores between groups [46]. This procedure is less commonly performed because cervical amputation has been associated with hematometra, which is retention of blood in the uterine cavity caused by obstruction to uterine flow at the level of the uterus, cervix, or vagina, infection in the uterus, infertility, miscarriage, and preterm delivery [47].

Colpocleisis

Colpocleisis is a surgical technique for POP that can be uterine-sparing, with the benefits of short operating room time, low morbidity and reoperation rates, high satisfaction rates, and improved body image. The LeFort colpocleisis leaves the uterus in situ while the total colpocleisis is performed on patients without a uterus. During both procedures, the vagina is sutured closed and the operation is, therefore, only appropriate for patients who do not wish to have vaginal intercourse. High satisfaction and low regret seen 24 weeks after surgery provide reassurance that colpocleisis is an excellent option for appropriate patients who do not desire the option of sexual intercourse [22].

Although there are no studies comparing obliterative procedures in these groups, there are many reasons to perform a concomitant TVH in appropriate patients who have risk factors for cervical cancer, such as current or recent high risk human papillomavirus infection or cervical intraepithelial neoplasia, or increased risk factors for endometrial cancer such as obesity, tamoxifen use, or Lynch syndrome. Lynch syndrome is also called hereditary nonpolyposis colorectal cancer (HNPCC) and it is an inherited disorder that increases the risk of many types of cancer, including endometrial cancer. It is advised that women who are at average risk of cervical and/or endometrial cancer consider concomitant hysterectomy at the time of colpocleisis so that cervical screening or endometrial sampling is not needed in the future.

Indications for removing the uterus are current tamoxifen therapy, familial cancer syndromes (BRCA 1, BRCA 2, Hereditary Nonpolyposis Colonic Cancer Syndrome), inability to comply with routine gynecologic exams, uterine abnormalities such as fibroids, adenomyosis, abnormal endometrial lining, or abnormal uterine bleeding [48]. If a patient is in reasonable physical health and has an extended life-expectancy, she may benefit from a hysterectomy at the time of colpocleisis. The overall rate of major perioperative and postoperative adverse events in women undergoing colpocleisis is low; however, when a hysterectomy is performed at the same time, the operative times are longer and the blood loss is greater [49].

Special Considerations of the Use of Vaginal Mesh

In 2002, the US Food and Drug Administration (FDA) approved vaginal insertion of mesh for the surgical treatment of pelvic organ prolapse, and in 2008, released a public health notification of risks associated with this use of surgical mesh. Surgical mesh placed through the abdomen for procedures, including sacrocolpopexy, had been performed for decades prior. The FDA public health notification stated that there were serious, but rare, complications associated with transvaginal placement of surgical mesh in repair of POP and stress urinary incontinence [50].

In 2011, prompted by concerns regarding the long-term safety of vaginally placed synthetic mesh, the FDA released an updated communication questioning the effectiveness of vaginal mesh for POP as compared with the non-mesh repair of POP (slings for stress urinary incontinence, with much lower complication rates, were excluded from this warning). The FDA reported a fivefold increase in mesh-related events from January 1, 2008, through December 31, 2010 [51]. The FDA's literature review found that extrusion of mesh through the vagina is the most common and consistently reported mesh-related complication from transvaginal placement of surgical mesh for POP. Shortly thereafter, the American Urogynecologic Society (AUGS) released guidelines for privileging and credentialing of physicians planning to implement or continue using transvaginal mesh for pelvic organ prolapse [52].

In 2015, the FDA issued two orders to manufacturers and the public to strengthen the data requirements for transvaginal surgical mesh for POP. One order reclassifies these medical devices from class II, which generally includes moderate-risk devices, to class III, which includes high-risk devices. The second order requires manufacturers to submit a premarket approval application to support the safety and effectiveness of surgical mesh for the transvaginal repair of POP [53] (Fig. 2.3).

The use of vaginal mesh for uterovaginal prolapse is controversial, and while there are complications noted in the literature, there is also evidence of anatomic success and patient satisfaction. Although many vaginal mesh kits have been voluntarily taken off the market, some are still available [54, 55]. Studies performed earlier continue to be published and there are many more studies in progress that will be published in the future. A recent study by Huang et al. compared 24 patients who had mesh placed at the time of hysterectomy to 78 patients who had uterine-sparing surgery with anterior mesh alone. There were no differences in functional or anatomic outcomes or statistically significant differences in postoperative adverse events [56].

Another study comparing an anterior and apical mesh system in a uterine-sparing procedure to one with concomitant hysterectomy reported anatomic success along with a similar complication rate. There was a trend toward increased mesh extrusion when a hysterectomy was done at the same time, but larger studies are needed to determine the true impact [57]. Cho et al. found a 97.1% anatomic success rate 2 years after transvaginal pelvic floor repairs with an anterior vaginal mesh system. Validated

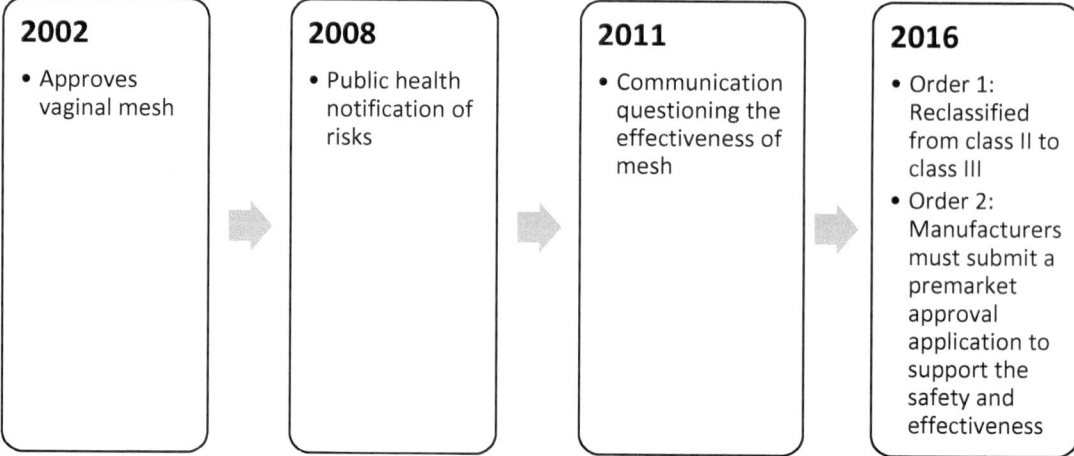

Fig. 2.3 FDA actions regarding vaginal mesh

quality of life scales improved and there was an improvement in all points when comparing the pre- and postoperative POP-Q [58]. A recent multicenter study by Jirschele et al. reported a good safety profile, as well as effective prolapse repair when the procedure was performed on 99 women with an apical polypropylene mesh kit after 12 months of follow-up [59].

Abdominal Approaches

Abdominal Sacrohysteropexy
The earliest abdominal approaches focused on transfixing the uterus to the anterior abdominal wall. However, more recently, an abdominal laparotomy incision has been used to perform a sacrohysteropexy. This procedure can be performed with or without graft material and usually involves securing mesh to both the posterior cervix and through windows made in the broad ligaments to the anterior cervix. The mesh is then attached to the anterior longitudinal ligament that runs over the sacrum. In the past decade, multiple small prospective and retrospective studies show anatomical success and symptomatic improvement for patients [60]. More recently, physicians are moving toward more minimally invasive techniques to accomplish this, techniques which will be reviewed in another chapter of this textbook.

Laparoscopic/Robotic Uterosacral Ligament Suspension
Laparoscopic uterosacral ligament suspension was first described in 1994 and typically is performed with one to two suspension sutures that are placed in each ligament near the level of the ischial spine and then attached to the vaginal apex or cervix [60]. In a study by Krantz et al., the association between intraoperative ($\chi2 = 0.83$, $p = 0.36$), postoperative ($\chi2 = 1.88$, $p = 0.17$), or overall ($\chi2 = 0.53$, $p = 0.47$) complications for those undergoing a laparoscopic ($N = 23$) or transvaginal USLS ($N = 23$) approach was not significant [61].

Laparoscopic Hysteropexy
Different methods of laparoscopic sacrohysteropexy have been described with suture, graft, and mesh and there are currently ongoing studies. In the Oxford laparoscopic sacrohysteropexy technique, the procedure is performed with graft material and involves securing mesh to both the posterior cervix and through the windows made in the broad ligaments, to the anterior cervix. The

arms of the mesh are transfixed anterior to the cervix with three nonabsorbable sutures [62].

One-year follow-up data were analyzed for women randomized to laparoscopic hysteropexy or vaginal hysterectomy with USLS. Outcomes were favorable for the laparoscopic hysteropexy showing faster return to normal activity, decreased estimated blood loss, and pain score 24 h postoperatively [63]. In another study of 140 patients who underwent laparoscopic hystero-pexy for POP, 89% felt their prolapse was "very much" or "much" better and there was a statistically significant improvement in all parameters of POP-Q [64]. In a prospective, controlled study, 34 of the 72 consecutive patients with symptom-atic POP were treated with sacrohysteropexy and the other 38 with hysterectomy followed by sacrocolpopexy with mesh. The authors report safety in sacrohysteropexy for women who request uterine preservation. Whether the uterus was preserved or not, patients had similar results in terms of prolapse resolution, urodynamic out-comes, and improvements in voiding and sexual dysfunctions. In the uterine-sparing surgery, the operating time was shortened and there was less blood loss [65].

Costantini et al. followed 52 patients for 60 ± 34 months who underwent sacrohy-steropexy, 47 laparoscopic, and eight abdominal. The study found that anterior compartment recur-rence (stage ≥ 2) was present in 4 out of 52 patients (7.7%), while posterior compartment prolapse was present in three (5.7%). Sexual activity was maintained in 28 out of 29 patients (95.5%) [66].

Robotic Sacrohysteropexy

In addition to laparoscopic techniques, some sur-geons have made the transition to robotic-assisted laparoscopic approaches. A retrospective cohort study of 168 patients compared three robotic groups, total hysterectomy plus mesh sacrocol-popexy, mesh sacrohysteropexy, and hysterec-tomy plus uterosacral suspension and showed a sixfold increase in POP recurrence in the utero-sacral suspension group. Furthermore, with a median follow-up of 36 months in all surgery groups, there was no difference in the complica-tion rates and functional outcomes, but operation time was longest in the hysterectomy plus sacro-colpopexy group. The authors suggest that the use of mesh, rather than hysterectomy, might be necessary for successful POP surgery [67]. Mourik et al. described the technique of robotic-assisted sacrohysteropexy in a series of 40 patients to emphasize that for those wishing to keep their uterus, success rates remain high. Before operation, overall well-being by validated questionnaires was scored at 67.7% and after sur-gery, this improved to 82.1% ($p = 0.03$) [68]. There is a risk of nerve damage and bleeding dur-ing the dissection to the anterior longitudinal ligament at the sacral promontory.

A Cochrane review concluded that sacrocol-popexy had superior outcomes compared to sacrospinous ligament fixation, uterosacral liga-ment suspension, and vaginal mesh. Due to supe-rior results, this method is gaining popularity, but must be balanced with the increase in operating room time and higher cost of the robotic approach [69]. The popularity of RASC is increasing as transvaginal mesh is becoming less acceptable to patients and offered less often by surgeons. The ability to perform a sacral suspension procedure without a big incision appeals to women and phy-sicians alike. It is a complicated skill set and requires adequate time and volume to learn and maintain these skills.

AUGS released Guidelines for Privileging and Credentialing Physicians for Sacrocolpopexy in 2013 for POP, which provided recommenda-tions to assist health care institutions when con-sidering granting privileges to perform sacrocolpopexy. The guidelines recommend that sacrocolpopexy for POP should be performed by surgeons with board certification or active candi-dacy for board certification in obstetrics and gynecology or urology who also have requisite knowledge, surgical skills, and experience in reconstructive pelvic surgery [70]. The surgeon should be qualified to perform the procedure open as well.

In 2012, a Cochrane review of robotic surgery for benign gynecological disease concluded that current evidence did not support the use of robotic surgery for patients with benign gynecologic disease, specifically for sacrocolpopexy and hysterectomy. The review stated that the current studies fail to show any superiority as compared to laparoscopic surgery [71]. This statement was withdrawn for an updated version of the review that was released in 2014 and included gynecologic oncology procedures. Their view was softened from the previous version with regard to sacrocolpopexy. The RASC was concluded to be a longer procedure with a shorter hospital stay, and the authors suggest further studies are warranted [72].

Conclusion

With some modifications in technique, the sacrocolpopexy has been used to correct prolapse of the vaginal apex since 1957. The operation, which is designed to restore the vagina to its normal position and function by re-suspending the vaginal apex using graft material, can be performed open, laparoscopically, and most recently with robotic-assisted technology. There is no explicit research on the topic, and more studies specifically looking at the best candidates for robotic surgery are needed. Understanding the conservative treatments of pelvic organ prolapse and the other surgical techniques help the surgeon tailor the options for apical support to individual patients.

When choosing RASC, it is important to consider the other options available for apical support, which vary from vaginal approaches to abdominal approaches, and open procedures to minimally invasive surgeries. Furthermore, patient selection should take into consideration advantages and challenges of robotic surgery along with specific patient criteria such as baseline health, cardiovascular status, BMI, and requirements for steep Trendelenburg and dorsal lithotomy patient positioning.

References

1. Swift SE. The distribution of pelvic organ support in a population of female subjects seen for routine gynecologic health care. Am J Obstet Gynecol. 2000;183(2):277–85.
2. DeLancey JO. Fascial and muscular abnormalities in women with urethral hypermobility and anterior vaginal wall prolapse. Am J Obstet Gynecol. 2002;187(1):93–8.
3. Shull BL. Pelvic organ prolapse: anterior, superior, and posterior vaginal segment defects. Am J Obstet Gynecol. 1999;181(1):6–11.
4. Toozs-Hobson P, Boos K, Cardozo L. Management of vaginal vault prolapse. Br J Obstet Gynaecol. 1998;105(1):13–7.
5. Rooney K, Kenton K, Mueller ER, FitzGerald MP, Brubaker L. Advanced anterior vaginal wall prolapse is highly correlated with apical prolapse. Am J Obstet Gynecol. 2006;195(6):1837–40.
6. Hsu Y, Chen L, Summers A, Ashton-Miller JA, DeLancey JO. Anterior vaginal wall length and degree of anterior compartment prolapse seen on dynamic MRI. Int Urogynecol J Pelvic Floor Dysfunct. 2008;19(1):137–42.
7. Arthure HG, Savage D. Uterine prolapse and prolapse of the vaginal vault treated by sacral hysteropexy. J Obstet Gynaecol Br Emp. 1957;64(3):355–60.
8. Lane FE. Repair of posthysterectomy vaginal-vault prolapse. Obstet Gynecol. 1962;20:72–7.
9. Birnbaum SJ. Rational therapy for the prolapsed vagina. Am J Obstet Gynecol. 1973;115(3):411–9.
10. Snyder TE, Krantz KE. Abdominal-retroperitoneal sacral colpopexy for the correction of vaginal prolapse. Obstet Gynecol. 1991;77(6):944–9.
11. Addison WA, Cundiff GW, Bump RC, Harris RL. Sacral colpopexy is the preferred treatment for vaginal vault prolapse. J Gynecol Technol. 1996;2:69–74.
12. Nygaard IE, McCreery R, Brubaker L, Connolly A, Cundiff G, Weber AM, et al. Abdominal sacrocolpopexy: a comprehensive review. Obstet Gynecol. 2004;104(4):805–23.
13. Ridgeway B, Chen CC, Paraiso MF. The use of synthetic mesh in pelvic reconstructive surgery. Clin Obstet Gynecol. 2008;51(1):136–52.
14. McDermott CD, Hale DS. Abdominal, laparoscopic, and robotic surgery for pelvic organ prolapse. Obstet Gynecol Clin N Am. 2009;36(3):585–614.
15. Barbolt TA. Biology of polypropylene/polyglactin 910 grafts. Int Urogynecol J Pelvic Floor Dysfunct. 2006;17(Suppl 1):S26–30.
16. Ostergard DR. Polypropylene vaginal mesh grafts in gynecology. Obstet Gynecol. 2010;116(4):962–6.

17. Barbalat Y, Tunuguntla HS. Surgery for pelvic organ prolapse: a historical perspective. Curr Urol Rep. 2012;13(3):256–61.

18. Geller EJ, Siddiqui NY, JM W, Visco AG. Short-term outcomes of robotic sacrocolpopexy compared with abdominal sacrocolpopexy. Obstet Gynecol. 2008;112(6):1201–6.

19. Siddiqui NY, Geller EJ, Visco AG. Symptomatic and anatomic 1-year outcomes after robotic and abdominal sacrocolpopexy. Am J Obstet Gynecol. 2012;206(5):435.

20. Anger JT, Mueller ER, Tarnay C, Smith B, Stroupe K, Rosenman A, et al. Robotic compared with laparoscopic sacrocolpopexy: a randomized controlled trial. Obstet Gynecol. 2014;123(1):5–12.

21. Fuchs KH. Minimally invasive surgery. Endoscopy. 2002;34(2):154–9.

22. Crisp CC, Book NM, Cunkelman JA, Tieu AL, Pauls RN. Body image, regret, and satisfaction 24 weeks after colpocleisis: a multicenter study. Female Pelvic Med Reconstr Surg.s 2015. PMID: 26571434.

23. Paraiso MF, Jelovsek JE, Frick A, Chen CC, Barber MD. Laparoscopic compared with robotic sacrocolpopexy for vaginal prolapse: a randomized controlled trial. Obstet Gynecol. 2011;118(5):1005–13.

24. Anger JTMER, Tarnay C, Smith B, Stroupe K, Rosenman A, Brubaker L, et al. Robotic compared with laparoscopic sacrocolpopexy: a randomized controlled tria [Erratum]. Obstet Gynecol. 2014;124(1):165.

25. Elliott CS, Hsieh MH, Sokol ER, Comiter CV, Payne CK, Chen B. Robot-assisted versus open sacrocolpopexy: a cost-minimization analysis. J Urol. 2012;187(2):638–43.

26. O'Malley C, Cunningham AJ. Physiologic changes during laparoscopy. Anesthesiol Clin North Am. 2001;19(1):1–19.

27. Falabella A, Moore-Jeffries E, Sullivan MJ, Nelson R, Lew M. Cardiac function during steep Trendelenburg position and CO2 pneumoperitoneum for robotic-assisted prostatectomy: a transoesophageal Doppler probe study. Int J Med Robot. 2007;3(4):312–5.

28. Kalmar AF, Foubert L, Hendrickx JF, Mottrie A, Absalom A, Mortier EP, et al. Influence of steep Trendelenburg position and CO(2) pneumoperitoneum on cardiovascular, cerebrovascular, and respiratory homeostasis during robotic prostatectomy. Br J Anaesth. 2010;104(4):433–9.

29. Gainsburg DM. Anesthetic concerns for robotic-assisted laparoscopic radical prostatectomy. Minerva Anestesiol. 2012;78(5):596–604.

30. Fleisher LA, Fleischmann KE, Auerbach AD, Barnason SA, Beckman JA, Bozkurt B, et al. ACC/AHA guideline on perioperative cardiovascular eval-uation and management of patients undergoing non-cardiac surgery: a report of the American College of Cardiology/American Heart Association Task Force on practice guidelines. J Am Coll Cardiol. 2014;64(22):e77–137.

31. Johannsen G, Andersen M, Juhl B. The effect of general anaesthesia on the haemodynamic events during laparoscopy with CO2-insufflation. Acta Anaesthesiol Scand. 1989;33(2):132–6.

32. Hirvonen EA, Nuutinen LS, Kauko M. Hemodynamic changes due to Trendelenburg positioning and pneumoperitoneum during laparoscopic hysterectomy. Acta Anaesthesiol Scand. 1995;39(7):949–55.

33. Meininger D, Zwissler B, Byhahn C, Probst M, Westphal K, Bremerich DH. Impact of overweight and pneumoperitoneum on hemodynamics and oxygenation during prolonged laparoscopic surgery. World J Surg. 2006;30(4):520–6.

34. Wiltz AL, Shikanov S, Eggener SE, Katz MH, Thong AE, Steinberg GD, et al. Robotic radical prostatectomy in overweight and obese patients: oncological and validated-functional outcomes. Urology. 2009;73(2):316–22.

35. Sullivan MJ, Frost EA, Lew MW. Anesthetic care of the patient for robotic surgery. Middle East J Anaesthesiol. 2008;19(5):967–82.

36. Wysham WZ, Kim KH, Roberts JM, Sullivan SA, Campbell SB, Roque DR, et al. Obesity and perioperative pulmonary complications in robotic gynecologic surgery. Am J Obstet Gynecol. 2015;213(1):33–7.

37. Gkegkes ID, Iavazzo C, Iavazzo PE. Perioperative pulmonary complications in obese patients undergoing robotic procedures for gynecological cancers. Am J Obstet Gynecol. 2016;214(2):296.

38. Hefni MA, El-Toukhy TA. Long-term outcome of vaginal sacrospinous colpopexy for marked uterovaginal and vault prolapse. Eur J Obstet Gynecol Reprod Biol. 2006;127(2):257–63.

39. Maher CF, Cary MP, Slack MC, Murray CJ, Milligan M, Schluter P. Uterine preservation or hysterectomy at sacrospinous colpopexy for uterovaginal prolapse? Int Urogynecol J Pelvic Floor Dysfunct. 2001;12(6):381–4.

40. Dietz V, van der Vaart CH, van der Graaf Y, Heintz P, Schraffordt Koops SE. One-year follow-up after sacrospinous hysteropexy and vaginal hysterectomy for uterine descent: a randomized study. Int Urogynecol J. 2010;21(2):209–16.

41. Detollenaere RJ, den BJ, Stekelenburg J, IntHout J, Vierhout ME, Kluivers KB, et al. Sacrospinous hysteropexy versus vaginal hysterectomy with suspension of the uterosacral ligaments in women with uterine prolapse stage 2 or higher: multicentre randomised non-inferiority trial. BMJ. 2015;351:h3717.

42. Romanzi LJ, Tyagi R. Hysteropexy compared to hysterectomy for uterine prolapse surgery: does durability differ? Int Urogynecol J. 2012;23(5):625–31.

43. Richter LA, Park AJ, Boileau JE, Janni M, Desale S, Iglesia CB. Does pelvic organ prolapse quantification examination d point predict uterosacral ligament suspension outcomes? Female Pelvic Med Reconstr Surg. 2016;22(3):146–50.

44. Tipton RH, Atkin PF. Uterine disease after the Manchester repair operation. J Obstet Gynaecol Br Commonw. 1970;77(9):852–3.

45. Khunda A, Vashisht A, Cutner A. New procedures for uterine prolapse. Best Pract Res Clin Obstet Gynaecol. 2013;27(3):363–79.

46. de Boer TA, Milani AL, Kluivers KB, Withagen MI, Vierhout ME. The effectiveness of surgical correction of uterine prolapse: cervical amputation with uterosacral ligament plication (modified Manchester) versus vaginal hysterectomy with high uterosacral ligament plication. Int Urogynecol J Pelvic Floor Dysfunct. 2009;20(11):1313–9.

47. Ridgeway BM. Does prolapse equal hysterectomy? The role of uterine conservation in women with uterovaginal prolapse. Am J Obstet Gynecol. 2015;213(6):802–9.

48. Kow N, Goldman HB, Ridgeway B. Management options for women with uterine prolapse interested in uterine preservation. Curr Urol Rep. 2013;14(5):395–402.

49. Hill AJ, Walters MD, Unger CA. Perioperative adverse events associated with colpocleisis for uterovaginal and posthysterectomy vaginal vault prolapse. Am J Obstet Gynecol. 2015. PMID: 26529371.

50. U.S. Food and Drug Administration. FDA Public Health Notification: serious complications associated with transvaginal placement of surgical mesh in repair of pelvic organ prolapse and stress urinary incontinence; 2008.

51. U.S. Food and Drug Administration. UPDATE on serious complications associated with transvaginal placement of surgical mesh for pelvic organ prolapse: FDA Safety Communication; 2011.

52. Guidelines for providing privileges and credentials to physicians for transvaginal placement of surgical mesh for pelvic organ prolapse. Female Pelvic Med Reconstr Surg. 2012;18(4):194–7.

53. Obstetrical and gynecological devices; reclassification of surgical mesh for transvaginal pelvic organ prolapse repair; final order. Fed Regist 2016;81(2):353–61.

54. AstoraHealth.com. Astora Women's Health: Physicians, Hospitals, Centers, Investigators FAQs; 2016.

55. Kozal S, Ripert T, Bayoud Y, Menard J, Nicolacopoulos I, Bednarzyck L. Morbidity and functional mid-term outcomes using Prolift pelvic floor repair systems. Can Urol Assoc J. 2014;8(9–10):E605–9.

56. Huang LY, Chu LC, Chiang HJ, Chuang FC, Kung FT, Huang KH. Medium-term comparison of uterus preservation versus hysterectomy in pelvic organ prolapse treatment with Prolift mesh. Int Urogynecol J. 2015;26(7):1013–20.

57. Stanford EJ, Moore RD, Roovers JP, VanDrie DM, Giudice TP, Lukban JC, et al. Elevate and uterine preservation: two-year results. Female Pelvic Med Reconstr Surg. 2015;21(4):205–10.

58. Cho MK, Kim CH, Kang WD, Kim JW, Kim SM, Kim YH. Anatomic and functional outcomes with the prolift procedure in elderly women with advanced pelvic organ prolapse who desire uterine preservation. J Minim Invasive Gynecol. 2012;19(3):307–12.

59. Jirschele K, Seitz M, Zhou Y, Rosenblatt P, Culligan P, Sand P. A multicenter, prospective trial to evaluate mesh-augmented sacrospinous hysteropexy for uterovaginal prolapse. Int Urogynecol J. 2015;26(5):743–8.

60. Gutman R, Maher C. Uterine-preserving POP surgery. Int Urogynecol J. 2013;24(11):1803–13.

61. Krantz TE, McKuen MJ, Medina C. Uterosacral ligament suspension complications between laparoscopic and transvaginal approaches. J Minim Invasive Gynecol. 2015;22(6S):S65.

62. Rahmanou P, Price N, Jackson S. Laparoscopic hysteropexy: a novel technique for uterine preservation surgery. Int Urogynecol J. 2014;25(1):139–40.

63. Rahmanou P, Price N, Jackson SR. Laparoscopic hysteropexy versus vaginal hysterectomy for the treatment of uterovaginal prolapse: a prospective randomized pilot study. Int Urogynecol J. 2015;26(11):1687–94.

64. Rahmanou P, White B, Price N, Jackson S. Laparoscopic hysteropexy: 1- to 4-year follow-up of women postoperatively. Int Urogynecol J. 2014;25(1):131–8.

65. Costantini E, Mearini L, Bini V, Zucchi A, Mearini E, Porena M. Uterus preservation in surgical correction of urogenital prolapse. Eur Urol. 2005;48(4):642–9.

66. Costantini E, Lazzeri M, Zucchi A, Bini V, Mearini L, Porena M. Five-year outcome of uterus sparing surgery for pelvic organ prolapse repair: a single-center experience. Int Urogynecol J. 2011;22(3):287–92.

67. Jeon MJ, Jung HJ, Choi HJ, Kim SK, Bai SW. Is hysterectomy or the use of graft necessary for the reconstructive surgery for uterine prolapse? Int Urogynecol J Pelvic Floor Dysfunct. 2008;19(3):351–5.

68. Mourik SL, Martens JE, Aktas M. Uterine preservation in pelvic organ prolapse using robot assisted laparoscopic sacrohysteropexy: quality of life and technique. Eur J Obstet Gynecol Reprod Biol. 2012;165(1):122–7.

69. Maher C, Feiner B, Baessler K, Schmid C. Surgical management of pelvic organ prolapse in women. Cochrane Database Syst Rev. 2013;(4):CD004014.

70. Guidelines for privileging and credentialing physicians for sacrocolpopexy for pelvic organ prolapse. Female Pelvic Med Reconstr Surg. 2013;19(2):62–5.

71. Liu H, Lu D, Shi G, Song H, Wang L. WITHDRAWN: robotic surgery for benign gynaecological disease. Cochrane Database Syst Rev. 2014;(12):CD008978.

72. Liu H, Lawrie TA, Lu D, Song H, Wang L, Shi G. Robot-assisted surgery in gynaecology. Cochrane Database Syst Rev. 2014;(12):CD011422.

Selection of Concomitant Vaginal Procedures

Sarah A. Adelstein and Una J. Lee

Introduction

The abdominal approach to vaginal vault prolapse repair, abdominal sacral colpopexy (ASC), was first introduced by Lane et al. in 1962 [1]. The procedure has since evolved in terms of the introduction of graft to decrease vaginal tension, choice of graft material, retroperitonealization of synthetic graft, extent of graft attachment to vagina and sacrum, and choice of suture material. ASC is associated with superior anatomic outcomes compared to vaginal repair of pelvic organ prolapse (POP), as well as lower recurrence and reoperation rates, longer time to recurrence, and lower rate of dyspareunia; thus, sacrocolpopexy is widely acknowledged as the gold standard procedure for vaginal vault prolapse. However, it has a longer procedure time; longer recovery time; higher cost compared to vaginal surgery; and a different risk profile of surgical complications related to the intra-abdominal exposure, anatomy, and graft material [2, 3]. Most recently, the rise of robotic technology has allowed the adaptation of

a minimally invasive robotic-assisted laparoscopic approach to the sacrocolpopexy (RASC). This technique has been adopted by surgeons almost more rapidly than the literature has materialized to support its optimal implementation [4]. Theoretically, RASC achieves the benefits of open sacrocolpopexy results while mitigating its risks and morbidity.

POP is a complex pelvic floor disorder with apical, anterior, and posterior vaginal defects which result in varying degrees of anatomic loss of support and related symptoms. Despite advances in technique, technology, and evidence, some surgeons would argue that ASC or RASC may or may not adequately address multi-compartment prolapse. Concomitant anterior or posterior colporrhaphy at the time of vault suspension can be employed by pelvic floor surgeons. However, the data for or against concomitant vaginal repair is limited, and the choice is often driven by surgeon preferences and patient-specific anatomy. The objective of this chapter is to review and discuss the available literature on this topic. Since the data and direct evidence on factors impacting selection of concomitant vaginal surgery at the time of RASC is limited, we will also review some of the pre-robotic ASC data that support our discussion of the theory behind multi-compartment defects and levels of support and outcomes of sacrocolpopexy by compartment.

S.A. Adelstein, M.D. • U.J. Lee, M.D. (✉)
Section of Urology and Renal Transplantation, Virginia Mason, 1100 9th Avenue, C7-URO, Seattle, Washington, USA
e-mail: Una.Lee@VirginiaMason.org

© Springer International Publishing AG 2018
J.T. Anger, K.S. Eilber (eds.), *The Use of Robotic Technology in Female Pelvic Floor Reconstruction*, DOI 10.1007/978-3-319-59611-2_3

Background

Weakness in the musculofascial support of the pelvic floor related to age, estrogen status, parity, and other factors is manifested by POP. A useful paradigm for conceptualizing the complex anatomic weaknesses that may occur is the three vaginal compartments: the anterior, apical, and posterior compartment defects which can be described as cystocele, vault prolapse or enterocele, and rectocele and/or perineal descent, respectively. Pelvic reconstruction for prolapse must often address defects in multiple compartments. Apical support is a vital part of restoring pelvic floor anatomy, which contributes to the key role that sacrocolpopexy plays in surgical reconstructive options.

POP may occur in up to 50% of parous women, and one in every 12 American women may require reconstructive surgery for prolapse by age 80 [5]. In order to treat patients with safe, effective, and durable procedures, pelvic floor surgeons must carefully select a repair technique to minimize the need for repeat procedures. Historically, based on 1997 data, the recurrence rate after POP repair is reported as high as 30% with prolapse persistence or recurrence rates at 1 year up to 60% [6]. However, this data was based on strict anatomic outcomes. Re-analysis using varying definitions of success demonstrates that there is a great deal of variability related to prolapse surgical outcomes [7].

A variety of urinary, bowel, and sexual symptoms may be associated with POP [3] and should be taken into account when selecting concomitant procedures. Indeed, recent evidence has emphasized the importance of patient-driven and composite outcomes measures as the appropriate end point for prolapse surgery [8, 9]. Contemporary systematic reviews of ASC and laparoscopic sacrocolpopexy (LASC) using composite outcomes measures report median reoperation rates for prolapse at 1.2–4.4% (ranges 0–31%) with less than 4 years of follow-up [10–12].

Advanced POP results from multicompartment defects. DeLancey first described anatomic findings of POP from cadaveric studies in 1992. He described three levels of support (Fig. 3.1) [13]. The upper third of the vagina is suspended from the pelvic wall by the vertical fibers of the paracolpium, including the cardinal ligament and the uterosacral ligaments. He coined the term Level I support and hypothesized that Level I forms the critical factor that differentiates vaginal eversion (high-grade prolapse) from isolated cystocele, rectocele, or enterocele. The middle third of the vagina (Level II) is supported by lateral paracolpium attachments to the arcus tendineus and the levator ani fascia and is the location of defects causing isolated cystocele and rectocele. Finally, Level III, the lower third of vaginal support, contains the perineal body, perineal membrane, and levator ani muscles that prevent perineal descent. By integrating these concepts, the surgeon can appreciate that isolated vault suspension may contribute to, or even independently achieve, reduction of cystocele that prolapses beyond the hymen (Fig. 3.2).

While most surgeons would agree that all compartments need to be addressed in some way to achieve successful reconstruction, they may differ on whether concomitant vaginal repair in women undergoing abdominal apical suspension is necessary. Some advocate restoring topography

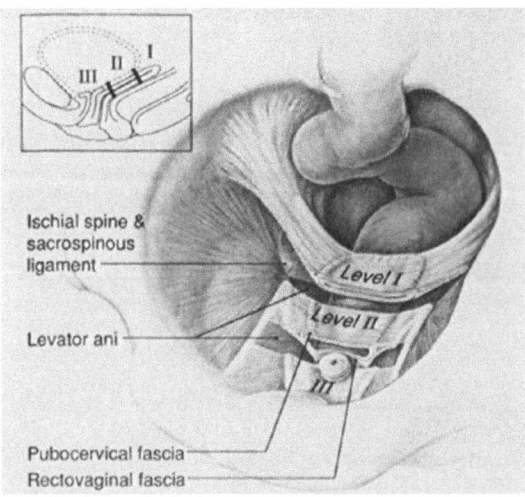

Fig. 3.1 DeLancey's levels of vaginal support. Reprinted from American Journal of Obstetrics and Gynecology, Vol. 166 No. 6 (1), John O.L. DeLancey, Anatomic aspect of vaginal eversion, page 1719, Copyright (1992), with permission from Elsevier

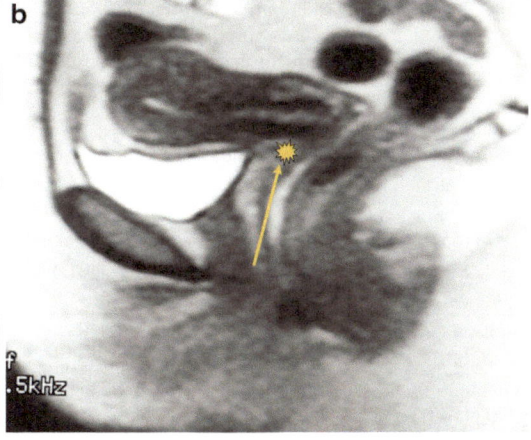

Fig. 3.2 (**a**) Magnetic resonance image (MRI) of multi-compartment ureterovaginal prolapse, sagittal view. (**b**) MRI of normal anatomic position. Star and arrow represent theoretical focal point and vector of suspension to achieve reduction of prolapse. Images provided courtesy of Dr. Shlomo Raz, Department of Urology, University of California Los Angeles, Los Angeles, CA

with a vaginal repair at the time of colposuspension [2, 14], while others suggest that adequate apical suspension will correct an anterior or posterior wall defect [15, 16].

According to DeLancey's concept of vaginal support, the sacrocolpopexy mesh aims to restore Level I support to the vaginal apex. While restoring vaginal anatomy from the level of the apex may reduce laxity in the anterior and posterior walls of the vagina, individual defects in Level II and III support are not specifically addressed by traditional sacrocolpopexy. There is no consensus in the literature as to the best approach to multi-compartment defects at the time of ASC/RASC for apical repair. Much of the evidence regarding concomitant vaginal procedures is observational and inherently biased by the practice preferences of experts. Further complicating the development of evidence for best practices are the complex outcomes reporting needs in POP surgery [8]. The objective anatomic outcomes, subjective symptom and quality of life (QOL) outcomes, related measures of voiding, sexual and defecatory function, patient preference, as well as surgical durability and risks, all must be factored into the decision for or against concomitant vaginal procedures.

There are limited short-term data demonstrating comparable outcomes between ASC and LASC/RASC in terms of anatomic outcomes, patient satisfaction, QOL, and complications [3, 10, 11, 14, 17–19]. Given this data and the conceptual similarity in anatomic restoration of the vaginal apex between ASC and RASC, the surgeon must consider how to address other compartmental defects in either case. Thus, evidence from both ASC and LASC/RASC studies can inform the decision-making process and patient counseling around concomitant vaginal surgery.

How Well Does RASC Address Anterior Compartment Defects?

A study of more than 300 physical exam findings in women with POP demonstrated a strong association and linear relationship between the pelvic organ prolapse quantification (POP-Q) points C (at the cervix or vaginal cuff) and Ba (the most prolapsed point of the anterior wall). The corresponding posterior wall point, Bp, was also associated with C, but not as strongly [20]. Thus, when advanced apical prolapse is present, anterior wall defects are very likely to be present simultaneously.

The converse may be true as well; that is, a pelvic exam on women with advanced POP (54% stage 3 POP) with simulated apical support

Table 3.1 Summary of studies reporting anterior compartment recurrence after sacrocolpopexy with and without concomitant repair demonstrates limited follow-up, variability of technique and reporting, objective anterior recurrence rates, minimal symptom recurrence, and rare subsequent anterior repair

Anterior compartment studies (n)	Mean or median follow-up (years)	Concomitant anterior repair (%)	Mesh technique	Objective anterior recurrence (%)	Symptom recurrence (%)	Subsequent anterior repair (%)
Brubaker 1995 (65)	0.25	0	Posterior mesh, distal extent NR	29	3	NR
Maher 2004 (47)	2	0[b]	Distal anterior	13	6.5[a]	0
Benson 1996 (40)	2.5	30	NR	NR	16[a]	10
Guiahi 2008 (149)	1	0	Distal posterior	15.4	NR	0.7
Snyder 1991 (116)	5	Yes, NR	Distal posterior to level of levator ani	21[a]	0–29[b]	0
Culligan 2002 (245)	2	2.4	Anterior and posterior, extent NR	9	NR	1.6[a]
Linder 2015 (70)	5	0	Y mesh, extent NR	NR	NR	2.9
Germain 2013 (52)						
Hach 2015 (101)	1.8	0	Propylene Y mesh, extent NR	NR	25[b]	0
Mueller 2016 (448)	0.25	0	Distal anterior and posterior polypropylene	NR	NR	0
Barboglio 2010 (92)	1	2.2	NR	8	NR	2.2

NR = not reported
[a]Did not report outcome by compartment
[b]see text for details

accomplishes significant reduction in point Ba. Lowder et al. reported a series of nearly 200 POP-Q exams before and after simulated support (achieved by positioning posterior blade of a standard Graves speculum over the posterior vagina to lift the apex) which revealed mean change in point Ba of 3.5 cm with apical suspension. This achieved Ba above −1 station in over half of patients [21]. By contrast, the maximum point of posterior prolapse, Bp, changed significantly less, by 1.9 cm ($p < 0.001$), with simulated apical support.

These two studies highlight DeLancey's theory of the critical role of Level I vaginal support on the anterior and posterior compartments, and particularly the former. A discussion of anterior compartment outcomes with ASC/RASC follows below and is summarized in Table 3.1.

Anterior Compartment Recurrence Without Concurrent Anterior Repair

The strong link between anterior and apical vaginal prolapse is well-demonstrated in the literature—both in their coexistence and in the ability of apical repair to improve anterior wall defects. Many surgeons feel that the reduction of cystocele accomplished with apical suspension is enough to obviate the routine need for concomitant anterior colporrhaphy when both defects are present. Modification in mesh anchoring techniques may contribute to improved cystocele reduction. Particularly during RASC, which can have longer operating room times than LASC or ASC [19], the positioning changes and maneuvering of multiple surgical access points for subsequent colporrhaphy adds to prolonged patient time in lithotomy and its associated risks. Many surgeons suggest that concurrent repair can be avoided. It may achieve more optimal anatomic outcomes, but patient relief of bothersome vaginal bulge symptoms can be achieved with reduction of prolapse proximal to the hymen [6]. Recent literature has demonstrated that, while objective anatomic outcomes are important to incorporate, definitions of surgical success should also incorporate subjective patient-based outcomes, such as relief of bothersome vaginal bulge symptoms. With such a staged approach, the number of symptomatic patients requiring a second surgery may be minimal and perhaps better selected.

Two ASC series used mesh that was broadly attached to the vagina posteriorly, as distal as the rectal reflection [22, 23]. Anatomic persistent or de novo anterior wall prolapse was noted in 25–29% of women with short-term follow-up. However, in one study prolapse symptoms were only present in 3%, and no subjective or QOL outcomes were reported in the other. Subsequent anterior repair was reported in zero patients at 3 months and one (0.7%) at 12 months in the two series. The authors concluded that cure rates for apical support were excellent with this distal posterior mesh technique, but anterior wall recurrences were common and warranted further study for optimal management. More studies are needed on patient factors and optimal surgical techniques for multi-compartment prolapse.

One randomized trial of ASC compared to vaginal vault repair with sacrospinous ligament fixation (SSLF) demonstrated similar rates of vault suspension above the hymen and relief of prolapse symptoms at 2 years [14]. One third of the 47 women in the ASC group had colposuspension for stress incontinence (SUI), which does provide some degree of anterior wall support. None of these women went on to have a subsequent repair of anterior wall defects, and three (7%) had asymptomatic grade two or higher cystocele. The cumulative risk of anterior and vault prolapse recurrence was significantly lower in the ASC group (13% vs. 45%, $p = 0.01$). An important technique point in this ASC series was

the application of a polypropylene mesh along the anterior vaginal wall to the level of the bladder trigone.

Four series of RASC without concomitant vaginal repair and with short or intermediate follow-up have recently been published [24–27]. Three of these specifically described a technique with distal anterior anchoring of mesh. Distal landmarks included the trigone or as low as the level of the urethrovesical junction. Two of these studies enrolled women with high-grade apical prolapse; the others include women with only 50–73% vault prolapse. The outcomes were heterogeneous and incompletely reported, in part due to limited follow-up. One study reported subjective outcomes using validated symptom questionnaires that met pre-defined criteria for success in 75%, and symptom scores were improved over baseline at median 2 years follow-up [25]. Another study reported symptomatic persistent or recurrent prolapse in 6% of 52 women at a median of 42 months [24]. Subsequent anterior colporrhaphy was later performed in 0–2.9% of patients at median follow-up of 13 weeks to 5 years. Higher recurrence rates coincided with longer follow-up [24, 26, 27]. These RASC-only reconstructions appear to confirm DeLancey's theory and others' observations that apical suspension is paramount, and in some cases the only repair needed, for anterior wall defects.

Anterior Compartment Recurrence After Concomitant Anterior Repair

Despite the strong link between anterior and apical vaginal prolapse, only a concomitant vaginal procedure allows the surgeon to directly address that individual compartment. Early pioneers of the ASC recommended routine concurrent anterior colporrhaphy [1, 12]. Indeed, most published series do include vaginal repairs per the surgeon's discretion. The guiding rationale and impact of this subjective expert judgment on outcomes are difficult to parse out in published trials and series. This represents an inherent systematic bias that cannot be measured without direct comparison to a series without routine colporrhaphy.

Benson et al. published a series of 40 ASC for vault and anterior wall prolapse with 30% concomitant anterior colporrhaphy [2]. At 2.5 years, 84% had resolution of symptoms, and four (11%) underwent subsequent anterior colporrhaphy. A larger series of ASC with six (2.4%) concomitant anterior repairs had only four (1.9%) subsequent prolapse repairs at 2 years [28]. This variability may be related to the inclusion criteria that favored more significant baseline anterior (as opposed to vault) prolapse, small numbers, different rates of concomitant repairs, or the mesh anchoring techniques that were not well-described in either study. Unfortunately, neither study differentiated whether any anterior wall recurrences happened in those who underwent concomitant anterior repair up front. Snyder and Krantz published one of the first series utilizing mesh anchoring distal to the apex for procidentia in 1991 by fixing polytetrafluoroethylene or dacron graft along the "full extent of the rectovaginal septum" posteriorly. Ninety-eight percent of patients were post-hysterectomy. An unspecified fraction of concomitant anterior colporrhaphies were performed per surgeon discretion, and they reported no reoperation for prolapse and 24 (21%) asymptomatic anatomic recurrences (compartment not specified) at mean 5 years follow-up [15]. Targeted investigations evaluating the effects of concomitant repair stratified by patient-specific and surgical factors have not been performed.

An RASC series by Barboglio et al. with 12 months' follow-up was published for 92 women, of whom two (2.2%) underwent concomitant anterior colporrhaphy. Ultimately, seven (8%) had anterior compartment prolapse, and two (2.2%) underwent subsequent prolapse repair (baseline performance of concomitant anterior compartment repair was not reported). The relative absence of robotic series utilizing concomitant vaginal repairs may be the result of a change in surgeon preference with time and the adoption of robotic techniques. Comparative studies, and long-term studies with uniform outcomes and follow-up, are needed to ascertain the value of anterior colporrhaphy at the time of RASC.

Regardless of whether concomitant anterior repair is used at the time of ASC, the rates of subsequent anterior repair are overall low. Whether there is a difference in the rate of reoperation for prolapse between these groups cannot be determined from these series, not only because much of the data is retrospective and not comparative, but also because the different inclusion criteria and procedure selection introduce significant bias that must be acknowledged when reviewing the outcomes. It appears that, if the anterior vaginal wall is supported by the colpopexy mesh, and the graft is attached distally, anterior repair is unlikely to be needed in many patients. An exception would be the patient desiring uterine preservation. If a posterior strip sacrocolpopexy is performed (without an attachment to the anterior vaginal wall or cervix), the anterior vaginal wall may be at higher risk of recurrence.

How Well Does RSC Address Posterior Compartment Defects?

Seventy-six percent of women with multicompartment defects have a posterior defect [6]. In response to evidence that apical suspension may address anterior compartment defects better than posterior wall defects [2], some surgeons modified the mesh attachment technique to target that anatomy [16]. While traditional posterior colporrhaphy plicates the posterolateral rectovaginal fascia into the midline in a compensatory reconstruction that imposes a barrier between rectum and vagina, distal mesh anchoring on the vagina during sacrocolpopexy can restore the normal fascial continuity between level III and level II supports, as described by DeLancey [29]. Pulling the perineal body superiorly toward the apex will repair some types of rectocele and perineal descent. However, if the defect is a disruption of the lateral attachments of the perineal membrane (urogenital diaphragm), this cannot be addressed from an abdominal approach and may need to be approached vaginally.

Some surgeons advocate for traditional posterior repair with perineorrhaphy or defect-directed repair by the vaginal approach at the time of ASC [30, 31]. Others have proposed that posterior support can be adequately achieved from the abdominal approach alone with distal mesh anchoring [15, 16]. Unfortunately, discrete comparative data to clarify outcomes by a particular approach are muddled by the surgeon practice preferences utilized in retrospective sacrocolpopexy series. The available evidence outcomes for ASC/RASC on the posterior compartment are reviewed below (summarized in Table 3.2).

Posterior Compartment Recurrence Without Concomitant Posterior Repair

Two series reported outcomes for ASC-only repairs performed using distal anchoring of synthetic mesh to the rectovaginal junction in 116 women and to the rectal reflection in 149 women [15, 23]. The former series stated 93% of patients had "restoration of a functional vagina ... and nonrecurrence of presenting symptoms" at

Table 3.2 Summary of studies reporting posterior compartment recurrence after sacrocolpopexy demonstrates limited follow-up, variability of technique and reporting, higher rates of concomitant posterior repair, low need for subsequent posterior repair

Posterior compartment studies (n)	Mean or median follow-up (years)	Concomitant posterior repair (%)	Mesh technique	Objective posterior recurrence (%)	Symptom recurrence (%)	Subsequent posterior repair (%)
Maher 2004 (47)	2	23	7–8 cm along posterior wall	33	6.5[a]	2.1
Condiff 1997 (19)	0.2	10.5	Distal to posterior vaginal fascia or perineal body	0	0[b]	0
Snyder 1991 (116)	5	0	Distal posterior to level of levator ani	21[a]	0–29[b]	0
Benson 1996 (40)	2.5	45	NR	NR	16[a]	5
Guiahi 2008 (149)	1	0	Distal posterior	8.1	NR	0.7
Culligan 2002 (245)	2	25	Anterior and posterior, extent NR	5.7	NR	1.6[a]
Linder 2015 (70)	5	0	Y mesh, extent NR	NR	NR	1.4
Germain 2013 (52)	3.5	0	Two prolene strips, distal posterior	1.9	1.9	1.9[a]
Hach 2015 (101)	1.8	0	Polypropylene Y mesh, extent NR		25[b]	0
Mueller 2016 (448)	0.25	0	Distal anterior and posterior polypropylene	NR	NR	0.9
Crane 2013 (70)	1	27	Distal anterior to perineal body	NR	18.2	11.7
Aslam 2015 (125)	1	37	Distal anterior and posterior	12.8	NR	0
Matthews 2012 (85)	0.5	39	Distal posterior	5.9	NR	1.2

NR = not reported
[a]Did not report outcome by compartment
[b]See text for details

5 years follow-up. There were 24 (21%) single compartment anatomic recurrences without symptoms and no patients underwent subsequent reoperation. The latter series reported that 12 (8%) had persistent posterior compartment prolapse and one (0.7%) had a subsequent vaginal repair at 1 year. The authors concluded that apical suspension, as achieved using distal mesh anchoring, could restore the posterior compartment anatomy.

Four robotic series reported outcomes without concurrent posterior colporrhaphy. Median satisfaction on a 10-point Likert scale was 10 at 7 years follow-up in one series of 70 patients with stage III–IV POP [26]. Subsequent posterior colporrhaphy rates for RASC when the distal extent of mesh attachment was not described were 0–1.4% at a median of 2–5 years [25, 26]. Reoperation rates for the posterior compartment with mesh attached 2–3 cm proximal to the perineal body were 0% at 3 months [27]. Symptomatic posterior wall recurrence was reported in 1/52 (1.9%) at a median 3.5 years follow-up after RASC by a similar technique [24], but it was seen in up to 25% at 22 months in a heterogeneous group (only 73% vault POP at baseline) without a clear description of the distal mesh anchoring point [25]. The authors concluded that concomitant vaginal repairs do not improve outcomes and could feasibly be performed in a staged manner, if necessary, after RASC or LASC.

Posterior Compartment Recurrence After Concomitant Posterior Repair

Rates of concomitant posterior colporrhaphy at the time of ASC range in the literature from 10.5 to 45% [2, 14, 16, 28]. This variability reflects the differences in study populations and subjective surgeon preferences. The inclusion criteria for the studies vary markedly; one study included vault prolapse patients with 74% having at least grade two rectocele [14], another had predominantly high-grade POP, but all patients exhibited perineal descent on defecography [16]; and another included predominant anterior wall or

vault prolapse but half of the patients also exhibited perineal descent [2]. The distalmost mesh anchoring point ranged from 7 to 8 cm distal to the vaginal apex on the posterior vaginal [14] to anchoring on the perineal body [16], or was not described [2, 28, 32]. Anatomic recurrences in the posterior compartment were reported in 5.7–33% [14, 28] at a mean of 2 years depending on the definition used. The distal point of posterior wall prolapse (Bp) was reported to improve from 0 to −3 cm ($p = 0.009$) after surgery in one series [16] and was not significantly different between ASC with or without concomitant repair in another (−2.0 vs. −3.0, $p = 0.18$) [32]. Selection bias may contribute to the latter finding. Symptomatic prolapse was present in 6–16% at a mean of 2–2.5 years [2, 14], and subsequent posterior colporrhaphy was performed in 1.6–5% at a mean of 2–2.5 years [2, 14, 28].

Several robotic series have been published with concomitant posterior colporrhaphy or perineorrhaphy per surgeon discretion. Again, the impact of the surgeon-selected treatment algorithm on the outcome is difficult to ascertain from retrospective studies. Furthermore, the study populations and outcomes measures are heterogeneous not only in the entire body of sacrocolpopexy and concomitant repair literature, but within the robotic series specifically.

Concomitant posterior colporrhaphy was performed in 27–39% of RASC cases [33–35]. The distal attachments of sacrocolpopexy mesh were described as far as the perineal body [33, 35] and as a "deep dissection" of both anterior and posterior vaginal walls to address all three compartments [34]. One RASC series compared anatomic outcomes of RASC with concomitant vaginal repair for the posterior compartment to vaginal POP repair alone and demonstrated slightly less support in the former group (Bp −2.5 vs. −3.0, $p = 0.01$), though the clinical significance of that difference is unclear [33]. Anatomic recurrence was 5.9–23% at 6–12 months [34, 35], with one series reporting no difference between RASC alone or concomitant repair (with prolapse beyond the hymen as the endpoint, $p = 0.88$) [34]. Baseline POP stage IV did predict anatomic failure ($p < 0.001$). Symptomatic recurrence was reported in 18% at 1 year and there was again no difference between RASC alone and the concomitant repair cohort [33]. Zero to 11.7% of patients in these series ultimately had reoperation for posterior colporrhaphy at 6 months to 1 year [33–35].

Finally, a meta-analysis of RSC series with a total of 577 patients and mean follow-up of 27 months found the reoperation rate for prolapse was 3.3%, with 2.5% being nonapical [36]. The majority of those reoperations were for posterior repair, despite an overall rate of 18.5% concomitant posterior repairs in the combined analysis. The authors suggested that a posterior colporrhaphy at the time of RSC may be indicated for patients with significant posterior compartment defects to avoid subsequent surgery. However, it was not clear from the available evidence whether these posterior compartment defects were present at baseline or developed de novo. The decision to perform a concomitant posterior repair should be a shared one with the patient, specifically discussing the risk of dyspareunia that may develop with a posterior repair.

Impact on Genital Hiatus

Enlarged genital hiatus is thought to reflect levator injury or dysfunction and may be both a risk factor for POP and the result of longstanding POP [37, 38]. DeLancey described how the levator ani muscles relieve connective tissue stress on the perineal body and membrane [29], but a large gap in the levator ani permits further connective tissue trauma and thereby POP progression.

The genital hiatus size is specifically believed to contribute to posterior compartment symptoms and reflect the degree of perineal descent [16, 39]. Fialkow et al. measured perineal descent by comparing the position of the perineal body during strain with an imaginary line connecting the ischial tuberosities. They found that posterior compartment symptoms in prolapse were associated with an enlarged genital hiatus >3 cm, resulting in perineal descent >2 cm. Thus, some surgeons have proposed that pelvic floor reconstruction that decreases the hiatus reflects resto-

ration of Level III perineal support, and this may be associated with improvement in posterior compartment symptoms [16].

Several investigators have demonstrated a decrease in genital hiatus size after ASC and selective posterior colporrhaphy or perineorrhaphy [16, 28]. Interestingly, Guiahi et al. found that posterior wall topography was restored from ASC with distal mesh anchoring and no concomitant posterior colporrhaphy or perineorrhaphy. Specifically, there was a decrease in genital hiatus size from 4.0 to 3.0 cm ($p = 0.001$) and no significant change in perineal body measurement ($p = 0.395$) after surgery [23]. They suggested that ASC restored posterior wall and perineal topography without a concomitant vaginal procedure and questioned the necessity of a separate vaginal repair which is associated with unique risks.

In contrast, Crane et al. published a series of RASC with posterior colporrhaphy as indicated and compared the outcomes of women with and without concomitant posterior repairs [33]. Both groups had a decrease in genital hiatus size after surgery, though the concomitant repair group had a significantly smaller hiatus size (3.0 vs. 3.5 cm, $p = 0.01$). Perineal body measurements were similar. It is difficult to ascertain the impact of posterior repair since some difference in baseline factors prompted the surgeon to select colporrhaphy; enlarged hiatus itself was one cited indication for concomitant vaginal repair. Yet even the RASC-only group of 56 patients had a decrease in genital hiatus from mean 5.0 to 3.5 cm (no statistics reported).

Furthermore, Aslam et al. reported a series of 125 RASC with a distal mesh anchoring technique and posterior colporrhaphy in 37% of patients [34]. Prolapse beyond the hymen defined anatomic failure in this cohort and occurred in 23% at 1 year. The authors noted that genital hiatus size was larger in the failure group compared to the success group (5.1 vs. 4.6 cm, $p = 0.05$). Altering the genital hiatus is an option. Many women will do well with robotic apical suspension alone. Alternatively, an enlarged genital hiatus can be addressed and options discussed. When offered, some women, especially those who are sexually active, may choose to narrow an enlarged genital hiatus and provide support to an area weakened by childbirth injury. Therefore, perineorrhaphy with or without distal rectocele repair to narrow genital hiatus and restore support can be discussed when discussing the risks and benefits of surgery.

Bowel Symptom Impact

Functional disorders of the gastrointestinal tract are common in advanced POP and pelvic floor disorders [40]. Constipation, straining to defecate, need for splinting, and prolonged pudendal nerve terminal motor latency (an objective sign of pudendal neuropathy related to incontinence) are all more commonly found in women with POP or pelvic floor disorders than in women without POP or pelvic floor disorders. It is not clear, however, whether prolonged defecatory dysfunction might contribute to prolapse development, or whether POP may lead to defecatory dysfunction by an obstructive mechanism. Likewise, surgeons have postulated that ASC might benefit or compromise defecation. If the etiology of dysfunction is obstructive, a vault suspension might alleviate blockage and eliminate the need for straining. The contrary argument states that extensive dissection between the vagina and rectum might exacerbate or even cause defecatory dysfunction. A 2004 review of ASC literature described that the data on defecatory dysfunction are limited due to the paucity of prospective studies, poorly described baseline bowel function, variability in surgical technique and follow-up duration, as well as the confounding effects of age, estrogen status, and comorbidities [12]. Data on constipation and ASC are conflicting, with some studies reporting improvement and others reporting de novo or worsening constipation after surgery [12, 14].

An analysis of baseline symptoms of the CARE trial participants, a landmark multicenter randomized trial of ASC with or without Burch colposuspension (an anti-incontinence procedure), found that prolapse stage does not directly correlate with bowel symptoms [41]. Women with advanced POP reported bowel symptoms that included constipation, straining to defecate, splinting, and anal incontinence. However, validated bowel symptom questionnaires, POP stage, and POP-Q exam measurements were not associated across multiple analyses except that the Colorectal-Anal Distress Inventory (CRADI) obstructive subscale scores were actually higher (indicating more bother) in stage II compared to stage III and IV ($p = 0.01$).

One year after ASC with or without posterior colporrhaphy, >80% of CARE trial participants reported resolution of their bowel symptoms including: need for splinting, incomplete defecation, fecal incontinence, and pain prior to defecation [32]. These symptoms may result not only from posterior vaginal prolapse, but associated enterocele or perineal body descent, which may or may not be addressed with isolated posterior colporrhaphy. And remarkably, vault suspension with ASC resolved the majority of bowel symptoms whether or not this concomitant repair was performed. Thus, even though symptoms and prolapse stage could not be directly linked in a cross-sectional analysis, the outcome that vault suspension resolves most of the bowel symptoms does imply an association with moderate to severe POP. Similar findings were reported in smaller series [16, 42], while others have reported minimal impact of ASC on defecatory dysfunction [14, 43].

Crane et al. reported bowel symptoms in a series of RASC with posterior colporrhaphy per surgeon discretion [33]. Over half of the women reported baseline outlet constipation (sensation of incomplete bowel emptying with need to strain or splint). One year after surgery, 56% of outlet constipation resolved and 44% was persistent and there was no difference between RASC with or without colporrhaphy. De novo outlet constipation was reported in 14%. The authors concluded that there was a high rate of persistent outlet constipation and moderate de novo outlet constipation. Over half of baseline defecatory symptoms resolved, and concomitant posterior colporrhaphy did not appear to significantly impact these outcomes. Another RASC series by Lewis et al. had similar findings in a series of 423 patients, though the authors noted a significant difference in baseline symptoms between RASC patients with and without colporrhaphy (CRADI 25.0 vs. 20.1, $p = 0.049$) [44]. This suggests selection bias may be an important factor present in this study and others. Further prospective analysis and rigorous reporting are needed to illuminate whether posterior colporrhaphy with RASC is beneficial for bowel symptoms.

Sexual Function Impact

One classically cited risk of vaginal surgery is the development of scar, pain, and subsequent dyspareunia or other negative effects on sexual function. Posterior colporrhaphy is associated with a 17–19% risk of postoperative dyspareunia [45, 46]. The impact of combined abdominal and vaginal procedures on sexual function is difficult to assess because of the interaction of multiple possibly confounding factors such as vault tension and axis, mesh anchoring, vaginal scar, prior surgery, etc. Adding this separate risk to any changes occurring with abdominal vault suspension is a theoretical concern when considering concomitant vaginal surgery. Most women who are sexually active before ASC remain so afterwards (including ASC with concomitant posterior colpoperineorrhaphy) [12, 14]. Common study design flaws in sexual function outcomes are failure to capture dyspareunia when it causes a woman to cease sexual activity, underestimating the problem, non-utilization of validated sexual function instruments, and discrepancies in using the entire cohort as a denominator versus only sexually active women at the relevant time point. Besides the presence of all of these confounders, few researchers have looked at sexual function as a primary outcome. The evidence for impact of ASC/RASC with or without concomitant vaginal repair is limited and contradictory.

A systematic review of vaginal and abdominal apical suspension complications cited a low rate of dyspareunia with either approach (1.5%) [10]. It was not specified if this represented de novo occurrence. Other retrospective studies support the finding of no significant difference between dyspareunia rates in ASC and vaginal approach

sacrospinous ligament fixation [2, 14], or between RASC and vaginal approach uterosacral ligament suspension, including concomitant repairs in both groups [47]. There were significantly more sexually active women in the RASC group (83% vs. 42%, $p = 0.001$), which reflects a commonly encountered selection bias in these studies.

In contrast, a Cochrane review of ASC and vaginal vault suspensions (the analysis combined both sacrospinous and uterosacral ligament suspensions) reported a lower rate of dyspareunia after ASC (RR, 0.39, $p = 0.019$) [3]. This review included trials utilizing concomitant compartment repairs in both groups.

Retrospective studies of pain with intercourse found a 13–32% prevalence of postoperative dyspareunia after ASC (8.7–10.5% de novo), but resolution of 56–89% of preoperative dyspareunia [14, 48]. Comparably high rates of resolution of dyspareunia and moderate rates of de novo occurrence have been reported after isolated colporrhaphy [46]. It is difficult to draw any linear conclusions for expected sexual function outcomes with the current literature addressing dyspareunia in RASC with or without vaginal repairs. The relationship is complex. Regardless of surgical approach, it appears possible to improve, worsen, or not change dyspareunia and sexual function. All of these possible outcomes should be discussed with the patient during surgical counseling.

Mesh Anchoring Techniques

Many pelvic floor surgeons have adapted the principles of ASC with a distal mesh anchoring technique in an attempt to address Level II or III support at the time of apical suspension [12]. Mesh anchoring with no anterior fixation may be associated with anatomic recurrence in as many as one third of patients [22]. No direct or prospective comparisons of these techniques have been published.

Different opinions exist on whether the support achieved obviates the need for concomitant vaginal repair. Distal dissection and synthetic mesh graft placement between the rectum or bladder and vagina may be of concern to the pelvic floor surgeon given the controversy surrounding transvaginal mesh. Rapid adoption of synthetic mesh-augmented prolapse repairs in a short period of time led to relatively high rates of complications requiring surgical intervention [49]. Although current evidence suggests transabdominal placement of synthetic mesh grafts is relatively safe, the distal mesh anchoring technique warrants close attention with regard to intraoperative injuries or postoperative pain. The risk of sacrocolpopexy mesh erosion into the bladder is a concern that should be considered, as there is a small but known risk of erosion into adjacent organs. These types of erosions may require major reconstruction to manage the serious nature of a sacrocolpopexy mesh erosion into the bladder; particularly if located near the trigone. The location and extent of the mesh placement may require significant reconstruction including cystorrhaphy, ureteral reimplantation, and even possibly urinary diversion. Long-term follow-up is warranted to monitor for erosion rates and other complications.

A few RASC/ASC series with distal mesh anchoring reported visceral complications and open conversion rates. Cystotomies were repaired intraoperatively in 1.3–5.3% of cases where anterior dissection was performed to the level of the trigone [14, 16, 27, 35, 50]. Intraoperative bowel injuries occurred in 0–2.3% and were also managed intraoperatively in cases where the posterior dissection extended just proximal to the perineal body [27, 35]. About 0–5% of cases were converted to open laparotomy [27, 35, 50] and 1.2% had a ureteral injury [50]. Postoperatively, 1.2–4.3% suffered bowel complications (small bowel obstruction, ileus, or port site hernia), and up to half of these required reoperation [14, 27, 50]. Matthews et al. [35] found that prior reconstructive pelvic surgery was a risk factor for intraoperative injury in their series and suggested that less extensive distal dissection would be reasonable in patients with significant scar tissue from prior pelvic surgery. Not all RASC/ASC series described the distal extent of their vaginal dissection and mesh anchoring.

There are no comparative or long-term trials that describe the impact of mesh anchoring technique on reoperation rates or symptoms. Distal attachment appears to be safe based on observational data and has conceptual plausibility as an alternative approach to other compartmental defects during vault suspension compared to concomitant vaginal surgery. Anchoring techniques allow options for individualizing the apical suspension to support a particular patient's pelvic floor defects—more distal dissection and anchoring may target Level II or III weaknesses when present. However, rigorous comparative study would be required to confirm any practical benefit of distal mesh anchoring techniques. The effect of tensioning on prolapse outcomes, complications, and recurrence is also difficult to measure. Surgeons vary their tensioning of sacrocolpopexy mesh from loosely placed to neutral to somewhat taut. Adjusting the placement of the apex of the mesh can also vary the resulting support. Patient factors also vary, including multi-compartment defects versus loss of primarily apical support, symptoms and goals of treatment, the elasticity of the tissues, vaginal length, and pelvic and sacral dimensions. Some surgeons feel that an adequately tensioned sacrocolpopexy results in elimination of cystocele defects, provides relief of symptoms and support, and prevents prolapse recurrence. Sacrocolpopexy mesh tensioning is an art which is achieved with experience and with a deep understanding of the anatomy, consideration for patient symptoms, and possible complications associated with the procedure including pain, dyspareunia, vaginal exposures, and erosions of mesh into the bladder.

Conclusions

Long-term (greater than 4-year) comparative data on RSC outcomes is lacking in the literature. The populations included in published series are heterogeneous, as are the surgical approaches used to treat them. Although outcomes are grossly similar and demonstrate positive surgical outcomes, prospective comparative trials would be needed to clearly establish whether an algorithm including selective concomitant vaginal surgery is beneficial or not. Furthermore, many studies do not differentiate between persistent and recurrent prolapse, or between symptomatic or asymptomatic recurrence. These points must be clearly distinguished to establish best practice patterns for complex pelvic floor disorders. Inconsistent reporting of anatomic versus functional outcomes measures limits the comparability of published series. The relevance of objective outcomes to patient satisfaction has also been called into question [6]. Recent guidelines [8] and consensus statements by pelvic floor researchers advocating improved quality of POP outcomes studies [51] should lead to improved uniformity and applicability of outcomes measures in the future.

The impact of RSC with or without concomitant vaginal repair on voiding, defecatory, and sexual function is unclear. Multiple confounding variables and the limitations of retrospective studies using different study inclusion criteria and primary outcomes measures limit the quality of the literature on these important outcomes.

The best advice for surgical decision-making with the available options and literature is to individualize the choice to the patient's needs and goals. Relevant clinical factors including age, health, fertility status, sexual activity, presence of dyspareunia, and vaginal length should be considered [52]. In the pelvic floor outcomes literature, the paramount importance of patient goals and expectations for surgery is being recognized and utilized as a benchmark to define surgical success [6, 9, 53]. There is a great deal of data on anatomic single compartment recurrence rates, but this measure has gradually become less relevant to patients and surgeons as an outcome because it may not correlate with patient's bother and satisfaction [54]. The evidence for and against concomitant vaginal procedures at the time of RSC is heterogeneous and poses additional research questions. The ultimate choice of whether or not to pursue concomitant vaginal repairs should be based on a discussion of patient goals and expectations for surgery, the known risks and benefits of available surgical approaches, and should ultimately rest on the shared decision-making of patient and surgeon.

References

1. Lane FE. Repair of posthysterectomy vaginal-vault prolapse. Obstet Gynecol. 1962;20:72.
2. Benson JT, Lucente V, McClellan E. Vaginal versus abdominal reconstructive surgery for the treatment of pelvic support defects: a prospective randomized study with long-term outcome evaluation. Am J Obstet Gynecol. 1996;175:1418–21.
3. Maher C, Feiner B, Baessler K, Schmid C. Surgical management of pelvic organ prolapse in women. Cochrane Database Syst Rev. 2013;(4):CD004014. doi:10.1002/14651858.CD004014.pub5. Review. Update in: Cochrane Database Syst Rev. 2016 Nov 30;11:CD004014.
4. Chesson R, Hallner B. Why complex pelvic organ prolapse should be repaired vaginally. Curr Opin Urol. 2013;23:312–6.
5. Fialkow MF, Newton KM, Lentz GM, Weiss NS. Lifetime risk of surgical management for pelvic organ prolapse or urinary incontinence. Int Urogynecol J Pelvic Floor Dysfunct. 2008;19:437–40.
6. Olsen AL, Smith VJ, Bergstrom JO, Colling JC, Clark AL. Epidemiology of surgically managed pelvic organ prolapse and urinary incontinence. Obstet Gynecol. 1997;89:501–6.
7. Barber MD, Brubaker L, Nygaard I, Wheeler TL, Schaffer J, Chen Z, et al. Defining success after surgery for pelvic organ prolapse. Obstet Gynecol. 2009;114:600–9.
8. Toozs-Hobson P, Freeman R, Barber M, Maher C, Haylen B, Athanasiou S, et al. An International Urogynecological Association (IUGA)/International Continence Society (ICS) joint report on the terminology for reporting outcomes of surgical procedures for pelvic organ prolapse. Int Urogynecol J. 2012;23(5):527–35.
9. Elkadry EA, Kenton KS, FitzGerald MP, Shott S, Brubaker L. Patient-selected goals: a new perspective on surgical outcome. Am J Obstet Gynecol. 2003;189:1551–8.
10. Diwadkar GB, Barber MD, Feiner B, Maher C, Jelovsek JE. Complication and reoperation rates after apical vaginal prolapse surgical repair: a systematic review. Obstet Gynecol. 2009;113:367–73.
11. Jia X, Glazener C, Mowatt G, Jenkinson D, Fraser C, Bain C, et al. Systematic review of the efficacy and safety of using mesh in surgery for uterine or vaginal vault prolapse. Int Urogynecol J. 2010;21(11):1413–31.
12. Nygaard IE, McCreery R, Brubaker L, Connolly A, Cundiff G, Weber AM, et al. Abdominal sacrocolpopexy: a comprehensive review. Obstet Gynecol. 2004;104:805–23.
13. DeLancey JO. Anatomic aspects of vaginal eversion after hysterectomy. Am J Obstet Gynecol. 1992;166:1717–24.
14. Maher CF, Qatawneh AM, Dwyer PL, Carey MP, Cornish A, Schluter PJ. Abdominal sacral colpopexy or vaginal sacrospinous colpopexy for vaginal

vault prolapse: a prospective randomized study. Am J Obstet Gynecol. 2004;190:20–6.

15. Snyder TE, Krantz KE. Abdominal-retroperitoneal sacral colpopexy for the correction of vaginal prolapse. Obstet Gynecol. 1991;77:944–9.

16. Cundiff GW, Harris RL, Coates K, Low VHS, Bump RC, Addison WA. Abdominal sacral colpoperineopexy: a new approach for correction of posterior compartment defects and perineal descent associated with vaginal vault prolapse. Am J Obstet Gynecol. 1997;177:1345–55.

17. Freeman RM, Pantazis K, Thomson A, Frappell J, Bombieri L, Moran P, et al. A randomised controlled trial of abdominal versus laparoscopic sacrocolpopexy for the treatment of post-hysterectomy vaginal vault prolapse: LAS study. Int Urogynecol J. 2013;24:377–84.

18. Paraiso MFR, Jelovsek JE, Frick A, Chen CCG, Barber MD. Laparoscopic compared with robotic sacrocolpopexy for vaginal prolapse: a randomized controlled trial. Obstet Gynecol. 2011;118:1005–13.

19. Anger JT, Mueller ER, Tarnay C, Smith B, Stroupe K, Rosenman A, et al. Robotic compared with laparoscopic sacrocolpopexy: a randomized controlled trial. Obstet Gynecol. 2014;123:5–12.

20. Rooney K, Kenton K, Mueller ER, FitzGerald MP, Brubaker L. Advanced anterior vaginal wall prolapse is highly correlated with apical prolapse. Am J Obstet Gynecol. 2006;195:1837–40.

21. Lowder JL, Park AJ, Ellison R, Ghetti C, Moalli P, Zyczynski H, et al. The role of apical vaginal support in the appearance of anterior and posterior vaginal prolapse. Obstet Gynecol. 2008;111:152–7.

22. Brubaker L. Sacrocolpopexy and the anterior compartment: support and function. Am J Obstet Gynecol. 1995;173:1690–5.

23. Guiahi M, Kenton K, Brubaker L. Sacrocolpopexy without concomitant posterior repair improves posterior compartment defects. Int Urogynecol J Pelvic Floor Dysfunct. 2008;19:1267–70.

24. Germain A, Thibault F, Galifet M, Scherrer M-L, Ayav A, Hubert J, et al. Long-term outcomes after totally robotic sacrocolpopexy for treatment of pelvic organ prolapse. Surg Endosc. 2013;27:525–9.

25. Hach CE, Krude J, Reitz A, Reiter M, Haferkamp A, Buse S. Midterm results of robot-assisted sacrocolpopexy. Int Urogynecol J. 2015;26:1321–6.

26. Linder BJ, Chow GK, Elliott DS. Long-term quality of life outcomes and retreatment rates after robotic sacrocolpopexy. Int J Urol. 2015;22:1155–8.

27. Mueller MG, Jacobs KM, Mueller ER, Abernethy MG, Kenton KS. Outcomes in 450 women after minimally invasive abdominal sacrocolpopexy for pelvic organ prolapse. Female Pelvic Med Reconstr Surg. 2016;22:267–71.

28. Culligan PJ, Murphy M, Blackwell L, Hammons G, Graham C, Heit MH. Long-term success of abdominal sacral colpopexy using synthetic mesh. Am J Obstet Gynecol. 2002;187:1473–80.

29. DeLancey JOL. Structural anatomy of the posterior pelvic compartment as it relates to rectocele. Am J Obstet Gynecol. 1999;180:815–23.

30. Addison WA, Livengood CH, Sutton GP, Parker RT. Abdominal sacral colpopexy with Mersilene mesh in the retroperitoneal position in the management of posthysterectomy vaginal vault prolapse and enterocele. Am J Obstet Gynecol. 1985;153:140–6.

31. Addison WA, Cundiff GW, Bump RC, Harris RL. Sacral colpopexy is the preferred treatment for vaginal vault prolapse. J Gynecol Tech. 1996;2:69–74.

32. Bradley CS, Nygaard IE, Brown MB, Gutman RE, Kenton KS, Whitehead WE, et al. Bowel symptoms in women 1 year after sacrocolpopexy. Am J Obstet Gynecol. 2007;197:642. e1–8

33. Crane AK, Geller EJ, Matthews CA. Outlet constipation 1 year after robotic sacrocolpopexy with and without concomitant posterior repair. South Med J. 2013;106:409–14.

34. Aslam MF, Osmundsen B, Edwards SR, Matthews C, Gregory WT. Preoperative prolapse stage as predictor of failure of sacrocolpopexy. Female Pelvic Med Reconstr Surg. 2016;22(3):156–60.

35. Matthews CA, Carroll A, Hill A, Ramakrishnan V, Gill EJ. Prospective evaluation of surgical outcomes of robot-assisted sacrocolpopexy and sacrocervicopexy for the management of apical pelvic support defects. South Med J. 2012;105:274–8.

36. Hudson CO, Northington GM, Lyles RH, Karp DR. Outcomes of robotic sacrocolpopexy: a systematic review and meta-analysis. Female Pelvic Med Reconstr Surg. 2014;20:252–60.

37. Pierce CB, Hallock JL, Blomquist JL, Handa VL. Longitudinal changes in pelvic organ support among parous women. Female Pelvic Med Reconstr Surg. 2012;18:227–32.

38. Khunda A, Shek KL, Dietz HP. Can ballooning of the levator hiatus be determined clinically? Am J Obstet Gynecol. 2012;206:246. e1–4

39. Fialkow MF, Gardella C, Melville J, Lentz GM, Fenner DE. Posterior vaginal wall defects and their relation to measures of pelvic floor neuromuscular function and posterior compartment symptoms. Am J Obstet Gynecol. 2002;187:1443–8.

40. Spence-Jones C, Kamm MA, Henry MM, Hudson CN. Bowel dysfunction: a pathogenic factor in uterovaginal prolapse and urinary stress incontinence. Br J Obstet Gynaecol. 1994;101:147–52.

41. Bradley CS, Brown MB, Cundiff GW, Goode PS, Kenton KS, Nygaard IE, et al. Bowel symptoms in women planning surgery for pelvic organ prolapse. Am J Obstet Gynecol. 2006;195:1814–9.

42. Marinkovic SP, Stanton SL. Triple compartment prolapse: sacrocolpopexy with anterior and posterior mesh extensions. BJOG. 2003;110:323–6.

43. Pilsgaard K, Mouritsen L. Follow-up after repair of vaginal vault prolapse with abdominal colposacropexy. Acta Obstet Gynecol Scand. 1999;78:66–70.

44. Lewis C, Salamon C, Priestley JL, Gurshumov E, Culligan P. Prospective cohort study of bowel function after robotic sacrocolpopexy. Female Pelvic Med Reconstr Surg. 2014;20:87–9.
45. Abramov Y, Gandhi S, Goldberg RP, Botros SM, Kwon C, Sand PK. Site-specific rectocele repair compared with standard posterior colporrhaphy. Obstet Gynecol. 2005;105:314–8.
46. Weber AM, Walters MD, Piedmonte MR. Sexual function and vaginal anatomy in women before and after surgery for pelvic organ prolapse and urinary incontinence. Am J Obstet Gynecol. 2000;182:1610–5.
47. De La Cruz JF, Myers EM, Geller EJ. Vaginal versus robotic hysterectomy and concomitant pelvic support surgery: a comparison of postoperative vaginal length and sexual function. J Minim Invasive Gynecol. 2014;21:1010–4.
48. Baessler K, Schuessler B. Abdominal sacrocolpopexy and anatomy and function of the posterior compartment. Obstet Gynecol. 2001;97:678–84.
49. Sullivan ES, Longaker CJ, Lee DPYH. Total pelvic mesh repair. Dis Colon Rectum. 2001;44:857–63.
50. Akl MN, Long JB, Giles DL, Cornella JL, Pettit PD, Chen AH, et al. Robotic-assisted sacrocolpopexy: technique and learning curve. Surg Endosc. 2009;23:2390–4.
51. Nygaard I, Chai TC, Cundiff GW, DeLancey JOL, FitzGerald MP, Heit M, et al. Summary of research recommendations from the inaugural American Urogynecologic Society Research Summit. Female Pelvic Med Reconstr Surg. 2011;17:4–7.
52. Dwyer PL. Choice of pelvic organ prolapse surgery: vaginal or abdominal, native tissue or synthetic grafts, open abdominal versus laparoscopic or robotic. Int Urogynecol J. 2014;25:1151–2.
53. Brubaker L, Shull B. EGGS for patient-centered outcomes. Int Urogynecol J Pelvic Floor Dysfunct. 2005;16(3):171.
54. Pham T, Kenton K, Mueller E, Brubaker L. New pelvic symptoms are common after reconstructive pelvic surgery. Am J Obstet Gynecol. 2009;200:88–e1–5.

Concomitant Management of Occult and Symptomatic Stress Urinary Incontinence

Steven J. Weissbart and Ariana L. Smith

Introduction

Millions of women worldwide have stress urinary incontinence (SUI) and experience significant bother from the inability to adequately store urine during laughing, sneezing, or exertion [1]. Women suffering from SUI may feel socially embarrassed, experience perineal skin irritation, and avoid exercise [1–3]. Additionally, many women with SUI incur significant financial costs from managing their incontinence [4]. Unfortunately, despite the morbidity associated with SUI, many women with SUI do not seek medical care and may consider SUI to be a normal aspect of aging [5]. Therefore, health care providers should consistently ask women about the presence of urinary incontinence and provide appropriate management when indicated.

Women with pelvic organ prolapse (POP) are at elevated risk of having SUI [6], and SUI management in women undergoing prolapse repair can be challenging. While many women with POP experience SUI preoperatively, a considerable proportion of women develop new SUI after reconstructive surgery and in essence have SUI "unmasked" by prolapse repair. Therefore, pelvic surgeons must address the presence of preexisting SUI during prolapse repair and additionally consider the possibility of SUI occurring postoperatively.

In this chapter, we discuss the concomitant management of SUI during robotic female pelvic floor reconstruction. Although information in this chapter is intended to aid surgeons performing robotic surgery, the majority of data on this topic has been accumulated from studies that predate the widespread use of robotic technology in the field of female pelvic medicine and reconstructive surgery. Nonetheless, the principles of managing SUI during prolapse repair that were gleaned from the open and straight-laparoscopic surgical experience are extremely applicable to managing SUI during robotic pelvic floor reconstruction.

S.J. Weissbart, M.D. (✉)
Department of Urology, Stony Brook University,
Health Science Tower, Level 9, Room 040,
Stony Brook, NY 11794, USA
e-mail: steven.weissbart@stonybrookmedicine.edu

A.L. Smith, M.D.
Department of Surgery, Perelman School of
Medicine, University of Pennsylvania Health System,
800 Walnut Street, Philadelphia, PA 19107, USA
e-mail: ariana.smith@uphs.upenn.edu

© Springer International Publishing AG 2018
J.T. Anger, K.S. Eilber (eds.), *The Use of Robotic Technology in Female Pelvic Floor Reconstruction*, DOI 10.1007/978-3-319-59611-2_4

Background

Definitions

Women with POP may report the symptom of SUI and/or demonstrate the sign of SUI during consultation. The International Continence Society (ICS) defines the symptom of SUI as the "complaint of involuntary leakage on effort or exertion, or on sneezing or coughing" and the sign of SUI as the "observation of involuntary leakage from the urethra, synchronous with exertion/effort, or sneezing or coughing" [7]. SUI on prolapse reduction, or "occult" SUI, is defined by the ICS as "stress incontinence only observed after reduction of coexistent prolapse" [8]. Although not defined by the ICS, de novo SUI is commonly referred to as new SUI that occurs, or is "unmasked," after prolapse repair.

These definitions have been fundamental to categorizing three different subgroups of women with POP that may be seen during preoperative consultation: (1) women with POP and the symptom and/or sign of SUI (i.e., complain of SUI or demonstrate SUI on nonreduced testing), (2) women with POP who only have the sign of SUI on prolapse reduction (i.e., women with occult SUI), and (3) women with POP without any symptom or sign of SUI.

As will be discussed in this chapter, classifying women with POP according to these subgroups is clinically meaningful as women in each subgroup have different probabilities of experiencing SUI after prolapse repair.

Pathophysiology

The pathophysiology of SUI in women with POP is not without controversy. While on an elementary level, SUI ensues when increased intra-abdominal pressure on the bladder overcomes outlet resistance, the precise anatomical and physiological deficiencies leading to SUI are debatable, and there are likely differing etiologies of SUI in women with POP. SUI has traditionally been classified as occurring as a result of urethral hypermobility, intrinsic sphincter deficiency (ISD), or both.

The two widely held theories describing the pathophysiology of urethral hypermobility and

SUI are *the hammock theory* (Fig. 4.1) and *the integral theory* (Fig. 4.2). According to DeLancey's hammock theory, SUI ensues due to a deficiency of a so-called "hammock" to support and compress the bladder neck/urethra during states of increased abdominal pressure [9]. Using cadaveric dissection, he described that the bladder neck/urethra rests on a hammock formed by the pubocervical fascia, which is attached to the levator ani muscle at the arcus tendineus fascia pelvis. During states of increased intra-abdominal pressure, this hammock acts as a backboard, which compresses the bladder neck/urethra and prevents incontinence. Anatomic deficiencies of the pubocervical fascia and/or neuromuscular injury to the levator ani muscle can therefore compromise the hammock and cause SUI. The hammock theory also substantiates the common co-occurrence of SUI and POP. Deficiencies of the pubocervical fascia are also considered to be an etiology for anterior vaginal wall prolapse [11].

Petros and Ulstem's integral theory suggests that pelvic floor disorders such as SUI, POP, urinary urgency, impaired bowel and bladder emptying, and some forms of pelvic pain are all related to laxity in the vagina or its supporting structures, such as its ligaments [12]. Pertaining to SUI, their theory suggests that urethral closing is under muscle control via ligamentous/connective tissue

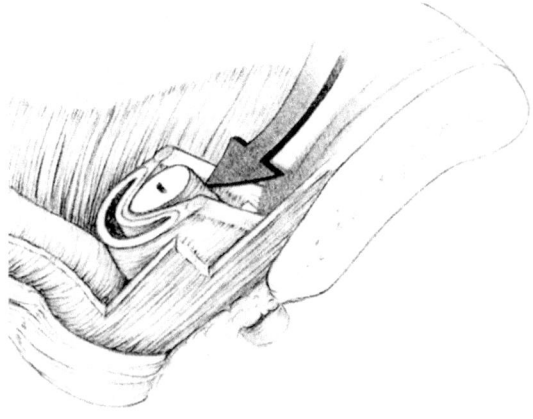

Fig. 4.1 As suggested by the *hammock theory*, the urethra is compressed against the pubocervical fascia of the anterior vaginal wall to provide continence. From DeLancey [9]; with permission

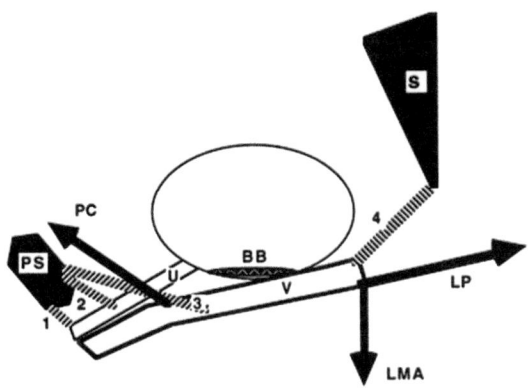

Fig. 4.2 As suggested by the *integral theory*, the urethra (U) is closed via muscle contraction/forces (*arrows*). Other structures represented in this figure include the vagina (V), bladder base (BB), anterior pubourethral ligament (1), midurethral part of pubourethral ligament (2), vaginal part of pubourethral ligament (3), uterosacral ligament (4), Hammock closure muscle (PC), Levator plate (LP), longitudinal muscle of the anus (LMA), sacrum (S), and pubic symphysis (PS). From Petros [10]; with permission

attachments to the urethra. Therefore, injury to the urethral ligaments/connective tissue can prevent appropriate transmission of the muscle activity required to close the urethra. Similar ligamentous/connective tissue injury may additionally contribute to the development of POP.

The hammock and integral theories have been pivotal to explaining the pathophysiology of SUI and its relationship to POP, although they do not describe the pathophysiology of ISD, which was introduced by McGuire [13]. SUI may be caused by inherent failure of the urethral sphincter to close, and this may occur in the presence or absence of urethral hypermobility. Among other factors, urethral sphincter competence is dependent upon intact neurologic control and appropriate watertight apposition of the urethral mucosa. Therefore, neural injury, as well as urethral mucosal deficiency (e.g., due to radiation, trauma, or ischemia), may lead to ISD and SUI. Clinically, ISD may be a potential reason for diminished SUI treatment efficacy [14]. In fact, it can be argued that, since most women develop urethral hypermobility after vaginal delivery yet have no SUI, some degree of ISD must be present for SUI to develop, regardless of the presence of urethral hypermobility.

While the underlying mechanism for SUI in women with POP may be urethral hypermobility, ISD, or both, advanced POP is well-known to potentially "mask" underlying SUI by displacing the bladder neck and "kinking" the urethra. In a study of 237 women with symptomatic POP, prolapse stage was inversely related to reported SUI [15], and in a urodynamic study of women with advanced prolapse, maximum urethral closure pressure decreased by 31% upon prolapse reduction [16]. Thus, underlying anatomic and physiologic deficiencies responsible for causing SUI may be obscured by POP and first become apparent postoperatively.

Incidence

Women with POP have a markedly elevated overall incidence of concomitant SUI versus women without POP, and studies have reported SUI occurring in as many as 80% of women with POP [17–19]. However, the exact overall rate of SUI in women with POP is unclear, owing to varying SUI definitions used in the literature and the dynamic nature of SUI in women with POP. While the natural history of POP progression (from low stages to high stages) is debatable [20], women with low-stage POP and SUI may potentially have continence restored by advancement of prolapse to a higher stage. Not uncommonly, women with POP who are presently continent can report a history of SUI that resolved without treatment. Therefore, the exact overall incidence of SUI in women with POP is difficult to determine. Nonetheless, it is clearly important for surgeons to appreciate the strong epidemiological relationship between POP and SUI.

Likewise, it is imperative for robotic pelvic surgeons to understand the general rates of SUI that can occur after pelvic floor reconstruction. Over the past decade, considerable research has been conducted to ascertain these rates and has provided a basis for performing an anti-incontinence procedure at the time of prolapse repair in some women (Table 4.1). While reported rates of postoperative SUI vary across studies, the data have generally suggested that the occurrence of postoperative SUI is dependent upon two factors: (1) the

Table 4.1 Randomized clinical trials reporting rates of subjective and objective postoperative SUI

Study	Randomization arms	Rate of postoperative subjective SUI	Rate of postoperative objective SUI
Brubaker et al. [21] (CARE) [n = 322](women in the trial did not report preoperative SUI)	1. Open sacrocolpopexy and Burch colposuspension	1. 19% (at postoperative month-3)	1. 4.7% (at postoperative month-3)
	2. Open sacrocolpopexy only	2. 39.7% (at postoperative month-3)	2. 8.6% (at postoperative month-3)
Liapis et al. [22] [n = 82] (women in the trial had occult SUI)	1. Vaginal POP repair and TVT-O	1. 18.6% (at postoperative month-3)	1. 9.3% (at postoperative month-3)
	2. Vaginal POP repair only	2. 23% (at postoperative month-3)	2. 28.1% (at postoperative month-3)
Schierlitz et al. [23] [n = 80] (women in the trial had preoperative occult SUI or asymptomatic urodynamic SUI and the study included vaginal and abdominal POP repairs)	1. POP repair and TVT	Rates not reported	1. 15% (at postoperative month-6)
	2. POP repair only	No change in Median UDI-6 question 3 score in either group (at postoperative months- 6 and 24)	2. 66% (at postoperative month-6)
van der Ploeg et al. [24] (CUPIDO-1) [n = 138](women in the trial had subjective SUI or objective SUI on non-reduced test)	1. Vaginal POP repair and midurethral sling	1. 22% (at postoperative month-12)	1. 16% (at postoperative month-12)
	2. Vaginal POP repair only	2. 61% (at postoperative month-12)	2. 44% (at postoperative month-12)
van der Ploeg et al. [25] (CUPIDO-2) [n = 91](women in the trial had occult SUI)	1. Vaginal POP repair and midurethral sling	1. 14% (at postoperative month-12)	1. 0% (at postoperative month-12)
	2. Vaginal POP repair only	2. 52% (at postoperative month-12)	2. 35% (at postoperative month-12)
Wei et al. [26] (OPUS) [n = 337](women in the trial did not report preoperative SUI and the postoperative incontinence outcome was not restricted to SUI, i.e., incuded stress, urgency, or mixed incontinence)	1. Vaginal POP repair and midurethral sling	1. 9.4% (at postoperative month-3)	1. 6.3% (at postoperative month-3)
	2. Vaginal POP repair only	2. 24.8% (at postoperative month-3)	2. 34.4% (at postoperative month-3)

Abbreviation: *TVT* tension-free vaginal tape

presence of preoperative SUI and (2) the performance of an anti-incontinence procedure at the time of surgery [21, 26–28].

Women with preoperative SUI (i.e., complain of SUI or demonstrate SUI on a non-reduced test) who do not undergo a concomitant anti-incontinence procedure appear to have the highest rate of postoperative SUI. The CUPIDO-1 study was a European multicenter randomized trial comparing vaginal prolapse repair with and without concomitant midurethral sling in women with POP and symptomatic or objective SUI (on non-reduced testing). Fifty-seven percent of women undergoing isolated prolapse repair reported bothersome SUI, had objective evidence of SUI, or were treated for SUI at 1 year postoperatively [24]. Another randomized trial, which compared prolapse repair with and without concomitant midurethral sling in women with POP and preoperative SUI (women with SUI upon prolapse reduction with a pessary were included), found that 71% of women undergoing isolated prolapse repair experienced SUI at postoperative month three [29].

Women with preoperative SUI who undergo a concomitant anti-incontinence procedure have a lower rate of postoperative SUI. In the CUPIDO-1 study, 78% of women undergoing concomitant midurethral sling placement experienced absence of SUI in comparison to 39% of women undergoing isolated prolapse repair [24]. Additionally, while 16% of women receiving a concomitant midurethral sling demonstrated SUI postoperatively, 44% of women who underwent an isolated prolapse repair had demonstrable SUI. The 16% objective failure rate of concomitant midurethral sling placement in this trial appears similar to the objective failure rate of midurethral slings in the Trial Of Mid-Urethral Slings (TOMUS), a multicenter randomized trial comparing retropubic to transobturator midurethral slings [30]. Failure rates could be due to surgical technique, as prophylactic slings at the time of POP repair may potentially be tensioned to loosely and result in postoperative SUI.

Women with occult SUI prior to prolapse repair appear to be at elevated risk of postoperative SUI (i.e., de novo SUI) compared to stress continent women, and performing a concomitant anti-incontinence procedure decreases their risk of postoperative incontinence [27, 28, 31]. The

Colpopexy and Urinary Reduction Efforts (CARE) study was a large multicenter trial investigating the effects of performing a concomitant Burch colposuspension at the time of sacrocolpopexy in women without SUI symptoms [21]. Participants in the study were randomized to sacrocolpopexy versus sacrocolpopexy with concomitant Burch colposuspension, and participants underwent urodynamic testing preoperatively (with and without prolapse reduction). The rate of occult SUI in the study was 27%, and women with preoperative occult incontinence more frequently reported SUI postoperatively whether or not they underwent concomitant Burch colposuspension [31]. Among women who did not undergo a Burch colposuspension, 58% with preoperative occult SUI reported SUI postoperatively compared to 38% who did not demonstrate occult SUI preoperatively. Among women undergoing concomitant Burch colposuspension, 32% with preoperative occult SUI reported SUI postoperatively, compared to 21% who did not demonstrate occult SUI preoperatively.

Another multicenter randomized trial (Outcomes Following Vaginal Prolapse Repair and Midurethral Sling, OPUS), which investigated the effects of concomitantly placing a midurethral sling at the time of vaginal prolapse repair, confirmed an elevated rate of postoperative SUI in women with preoperative occult SUI [26]. This trial also substantiated a role for concomitant SUI treatment. In the OPUS trial, 34% of women demonstrated SUI on preoperative prolapse reduction testing, and there was a clear reduction in postoperative urinary incontinence in these women by placement of a concomitant midurethral sling (at postoperative month three, 30% of women receiving a concomitant midurethral sling experienced urinary incontinence compared to 72% of women who did not).

Women who are stress continent before surgery (i.e., no subjective/objective SUI, including no occult SUI) appear to have the lowest risk of postoperative SUI [26, 31]. However, the rate of postoperative SUI is also decreased in these women by performing an anti-incontinence procedure at the time of POP repair [26, 31]. As previously mentioned, the rates of postoperative SUI in women who did not have occult incontinence in the CARE trial were 38% (no Burch group) and 21% (Burch group) [21, 31]. In the OPUS trial, the rates of postoperative urinary incontinence in women who did not have occult SUI were 38% (no midurethral sling group) and 21% (midurethral sling group) [26]. These results were similar to the findings in the CUPIDO-2 study, which also compared postoperative SUI rates among women with and without occult SUI [25]. Thus, although stress continent women may have a lower rate of postoperative SUI, they still remain at risk.

Other factors, such as type of prolapse repair, may potentially influence the incidence of postoperative SUI. While large randomized trials have established the safety and efficacy of robotic pelvic floor repair, there is no high-quality evidence at this time that assesses if using robotic technology in pelvic floor reconstruction affects postoperative SUI rates [32]. However, findings from a meta-analysis suggested that between 10 and 25% of women undergoing isolated robotic sacrocolpopexy need subsequent anti-incontinence surgery [32]. The excellent support of the anterior vaginal wall with sacrocolpopexy (either open, laparoscopic, or robotic) is likely to result in higher rates of postoperative SUI than other POP procedures that have less of a "straightening" effect on the bladder neck.

Preoperative Decision Making

Deciding whether or not to perform an anti-incontinence procedure at the time of robotic pelvic floor reconstruction can be challenging. As discussed in the previous section (*Incidence*), women with POP have a high rate of SUI preoperatively and a considerable risk of experiencing persistent SUI or developing de novo SUI after prolapse repair. On the other hand, concomitantly treating SUI during prolapse repair poses additional surgical risks and not all women undergoing isolated prolapse repair experience SUI postoperatively. Therefore, pelvic surgeons are faced with a clear dilemma during reconstructive surgical planning. Adding another layer of complexity to this dilemma is the fact that opposing conclusions can be drawn from examining the same data on the topic [33, 34]. For

example, data from the CARE trial can be used to support one of three strategies: (1) always perform an anti-incontinence procedure during POP repair, (2) never perform an anti-incontinence procedure during POP repair, and (3) selectively perform an anti-incontinence procedure during POP repair.

Multiple strategies for managing SUI at the time of pelvic floor reconstruction have been adapted, and there is no gold standard method of management [35]. While SUI can be markedly bothersome to women, it is rarely life-threatening, and treatment is considered elective. Therefore, the decision to perform an anti-incontinence procedure at the time of robotic pelvic floor reconstruction should be handled on an individual basis and reflect the patient's risk of postoperative SUI and treatment goals [36, 37]. The risks and benefits of performing a concomitant anti-incontinence procedure should always be discussed with the patient during counseling and the informed consent process. Understanding the advantages and disadvantages of concomitantly performing an anti-incontinence procedure provides the foundation for counseling.

Advantages of Performing a Concomitant Anti-incontinence Procedure

There are multiple benefits of performing a concomitant anti-incontinence procedure at the time of prolapse repair. In many clinical trials, concomitant anti-incontinence procedures led to a reduction in the rate of postoperative SUI [27, 28]. Thus, for many women, performing an anti-incontinence procedure at the time of prolapse repair can obviate the need for further SUI therapy. As many as 56% of women with preoperative SUI undergoing isolated prolapse repair may proceed to subsequent anti-incontinence surgery [29]. Needless to say, those women undergoing subsequent anti-incontinence surgery are then exposed to the risks of an initial anti-incontinence operation (e.g., voiding dysfunction, mesh exposure, pain), plus the additional risks of undergoing a second operative intervention, including anesthetic risks. Therefore, performing a concomitant anti-incontinence procedure during prolapse repair may potentially prevent the need for a future operative intervention.

After an isolated prolapse repair, some women with postoperative SUI may elect to not undergo subsequent incontinence surgery and may experience continued bother from SUI. While as many as 56% of women undergoing isolated prolapse repair proceeded to subsequent anti-incontinence surgery, 21% of women with postoperative SUI elected not to return to the operating room for treatment [29]. Furthermore, in a retrospective study of 100 women who underwent isolated POP repair, 32% of women with postoperative SUI reported their incontinence to be bothersome [38]. Therefore, these women may have potentially benefitted from the performance of a concomitant anti-incontinence procedure; granted, the relationship between SUI bother and the decision to undergo anti-incontinence surgery is unclear. However, aside from operative intervention, women undergoing isolated prolapse repair more frequently undergo additional non-operative SUI treatment, such as physiotherapy, compared to women undergoing concomitant anti-incontinence surgery [24].

Thus, the overall advantages of performing anti-incontinence surgery at the time of prolapse repair are: (1) decreased occurrence of postoperative SUI, (2) decreased need for future SUI surgical therapy, (3) decreased need for further non-operative SUI therapy, and (4) empiric treatment of women who may experience bothersome postoperative SUI, yet wish to avoid a second operative intervention.

Disadvantages of Performing a Concomitant Anti-incontinence Procedure

There are also disadvantages of performing concomitant anti-incontinence surgery at the time of prolapse repair. While anti-incontinence surgery decreases the rate of postoperative SUI, many women undergoing isolated prolapse repair do not experience bothersome SUI postoperatively. In women without preexisting SUI, data from the CARE trial demonstrated that only 25% reported bothersome SUI after isolated prolapse repair [21]. Thus, performing an anti-incontinence procedure in women without preexisting SUI may be unnecessary. Furthermore, approximately 39% of women with preexisting SUI reported resolution of SUI after isolated prolapse repair [39]. Thus, prolapse repair alone may, perhaps, lead to SUI resolution in some women [40].

Women who experience postoperative SUI may not be significantly bothered by their incontinence, and women with postoperative SUI still frequently report surgical satisfaction [41, 42]. In the CUPIDO-1 study, although 61% of women undergoing isolated prolapse repair reported SUI, only 17% underwent subsequent anti-incontinence surgery [24]. Additionally, 7 year CARE data found that only 13 women who underwent isolated prolapse repair underwent subsequent SUI surgery (including injection therapy) [43]. Therefore, it may be unnecessary to perform an anti-incontinence procedure in women at the time of prolapse repair, as postoperative SUI may not always be bothersome or result in further treatment.

Undergoing concomitant anti-incontinence surgery at the time of prolapse repair exposes women to additional adverse events. Women undergoing concomitant midurethral sling placement in the OPUS trial had more urinary tract infections (31% vs. 18%; $p = 0.008$), more episodes of major bleeding or vascular complications (3% vs. 0%; $p = 0.03$), incomplete bladder emptying (at multiple time points), and the need for urethrolysis (2.4% vs. 0%; $p = 0.06$) [26]. Furthermore, women undergoing concomitant midurethral sling had longer operative times and larger operative blood loss, albeit only by 11 min ($p = 0.05$) and 24 mL ($p = 0.03$), respectively. Notably, in a different study of women undergoing transvaginal POP repair, the rate of surgical intervention to correct obstruction after concomitant midurethral sling placement was equal to the rate of subsequent surgical intervention for SUI (8.5% vs. 8.3%) [44].

Thus, the overall disadvantages of performing anti-incontinence surgery at the time of prolapse repair are: (1) unnecessarily treating women for SUI (i.e., overtreatment) and (2) potentially exposing women to adverse events.

De Novo Storage Symptoms

Developing new urinary urgency and/or urge incontinence is a well-known phenomenon that can occur after isolated anti-incontinence surgery [45]. While women who undergo concomitant anti-incontinence surgery at the time of prolapse repair may theoretically be at increased risk of experiencing de novo storage symptoms, the data suggests otherwise. In the CARE and OPUS trials, women who underwent concomitant anti-incontinence procedures did not have worse storage symptoms, and a meta-analysis found that the development of postoperative urge urinary incontinence was unrelated to whether an anti-incontinence procedure at the time of prolapse repair [21, 26, 28, 46]. Notably, storage symptoms can often improve after isolated prolapse repair [47], and whether anti-incontinence surgery diminishes or augments this improvement is unclear. Therefore, in regard to storage symptoms, there is no clear advantage or disadvantage to performing concomitant anti-incontinence surgery at the time of prolapse repair.

Approach to Treatment

Ideally, an anti-incontinence procedure would only be performed in women who would experience postoperative SUI, be bothered by SUI, and be at low risk of having complications. Unfortunately, accurately identifying women with these exact characteristics is challenging. Therefore, three common strategies to manage SUI at the time of prolapse repair have been adopted: the universal approach, the staged approach, and the selective approach (Fig. 4.3).

In the universal approach, surgeons perform an anti-incontinence procedure in all women undergoing prolapse repair, irrespective of preoperative testing and SUI risk factors (women who have already undergone midurethral sling placement may be excluded from this approach). While this approach minimizes undertreatment, it exposes women to overtreatment and additional surgical complications. In the staged approach, surgeons never perform a concomitant anti-incontinence procedure, irrespective of preoperative testing and SUI risk factors, and subsequently offer anti-incontinence surgery to only those women with bothersome SUI postoperatively. While this approach minimizes overtreatment, it exposes women to undertreatment, as some women will have to undergo a subsequent anti-incontinence intervention. Additionally, with this approach, women with postoperative SUI who elect to not undergo a second operative intervention may experience persistent bother from their incontinence. In the selective approach, surgeons incorporate preoperative testing and SUI risk factors in their decision to perform a concomitant SUI procedure. This approach has the benefits of balancing overtreatment and undertreatment and is predicated on identifying those women who will be at the highest risk of postoperative SUI [35].

Understanding the number of women who need to be treated (i.e., number needed to treat [NNT]) with anti-incontinence surgery to prevent a case of postoperative SUI highlights the benefit of using a selective approach. In women with preoperative coexisting SUI (i.e., not occult SUI), data from a meta-analysis suggested that two women would need to be treated with anti-incontinence surgery to prevent a case of postoperative SUI [28]. Therefore, pelvic surgeons may elect to perform concomitant anti-incontinence surgery in women with preexisting symptomatic SUI. On the other hand, in women without symptomatic SUI preoperatively, the number of anti-incontinence procedures that would need to be performed to reduce a case of postoperative SUI is considerably higher and is markedly dependent upon the presence of occult SUI preoperatively. According to the CARE data, 5.4 Burch colposuspensions would have to be performed to prevent one case of postoperative SUI, and according to the OPUS data, 3.9 midurethral slings would have to be placed to reduce one case of postoperative SUI [21, 26, 48]. However, results of preoperative occult stress testing significantly alter the NNT. In the CARE trial, the NNT among women with occult incontinence was 3.8 as opposed to 5.7 in women without occult SUI, and the NNT among women with occult incontinence in the OPUS trial was 2.4 versus 5.7 in women without occult SUI. Therefore, preoperatively testing for occult SUI provides a key data point for surgeons using the selective approach.

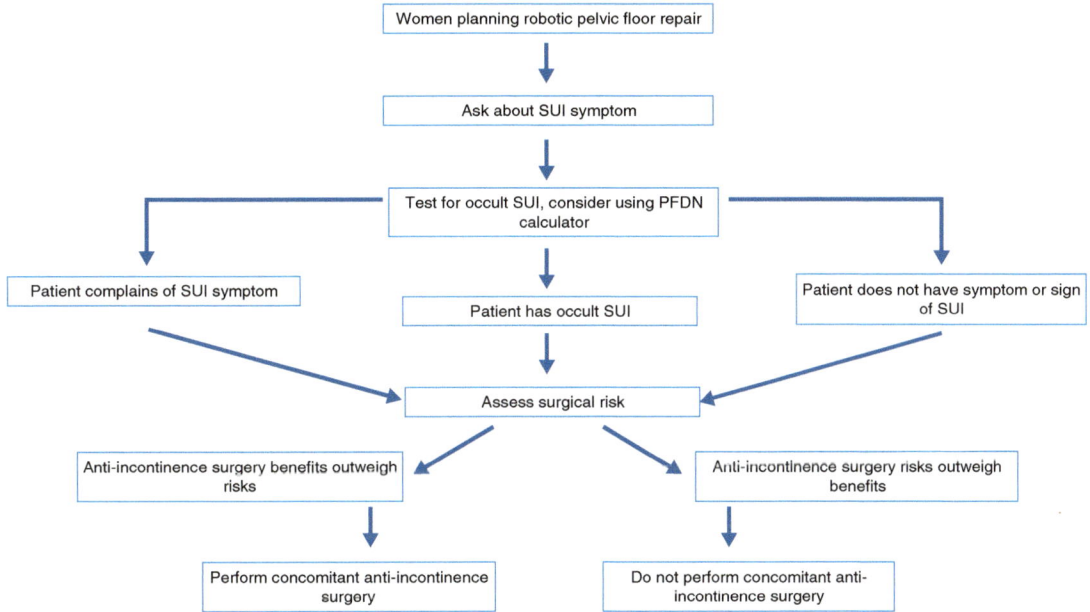

Fig. 4.3 Example of a selective approach to managing SUI at the time of POP repair. *PFDN* pelvic floor disorders network

Testing for Occult Incontinence

While it may be important to test for occult SUI for surgical planning purposes, unfortunately, there is no superior method for testing. On a basic level, testing is performed by reducing prolapse and asking women to cough or Valsalva with a filled bladder. However, the prolapse reduction technique and bladder volume during testing clearly affect test results [49]. Visco et al. investigated the test characteristics of commonly utilized methods of detecting occult SUI, including using a pessary, forceps, swab, speculum, and manual reduction [31]. They found an overall occult SUI detection rate of 19%, and that using a pessary was associated with the lowest rate of detecting occult SUI (6%), while using a speculum was associated with the highest rate of detecting occult SUI (30%). In addition to simple office testing, urodynamics may also be used to detect occult SUI (as well as measure the maximum urethral closure pressure, MUCP). While urodynamics, with or without POP reduction, may be useful for multiple reasons in women with POP [50], data have not suggested a particular benefit in detecting occult SUI compared to other office testing

[48]. Furthermore, measuring the MUCP (which changes with prolapse reduction [16]) may be unnecessary as it has not been reliably shown to predict risk of occult incontinence or surgical outcomes. Although the optimal method for occult SUI testing is unclear, surgeons may find some form of testing to be useful in their practice. On the other hand, leading experts in the field are not in agreement about considering occult SUI testing as a quality of care indictor [51].

In addition to urodynamics, an online calculator (created by the Pelvic Floor Disorders Network, [PFDN], available at http://www.r-calc.com/ExistingFormulas.aspx?filter=CCQHS) can be used to predict a patient's risk of developing de novo postoperative SUI [52]. In examining the OPUS data, the PFDN found seven factors that were predictive of developing postoperative SUI and are integrated into their calculator: age at surgery, number of vaginal births, body mass index (BMI), preoperative stress test result, performance of an anti-incontinence procedure, incontinence associated with urgency, and diagnosis of diabetes [52]. Notably, their prediction model actually outperformed a panel of 22 experts as well as a preoperative prolapse reduction stress test alone.

Economic Considerations

The three different strategies of managing SUI at the time of pelvic floor reconstruction (i.e., universal, staged, selective) are not likely equivalent in cost. However, studies comparing the cost-effectiveness between strategies demonstrate conflicting results. In a cost-effectiveness analysis based upon CARE data and Medicare reimbursement rates, the universal approach was found to be the most cost-effective strategy and had an incremental cost-effectiveness ratio of $2867 per quality-adjusted life year compared to the strategy of only performing sacrocolpopexy [53]. However, a different study comparing prolapse repair with midurethral sling ($n = 16$) to prolapse repair alone ($n = 14$) reported differential cost savings when using a selective strategy to manage SUI at the time of prolapse repair [41]. Women in this study underwent different types of prolapse repair (abdominal sacrocolpopexy, sacrospinous ligament suspension, etc.).

Surgical Technique

Synthetic midurethral sling placement and Burch colposuspension are two commonly utilized procedures to treat SUI at the time of POP repair [54]. Historically, other procedures, such as anterior colporraphy, paravaginal repair, transvaginal needle suspension, and Marshall-Marchetti-Krantz urethropexy, were used to surgically treat SUI, but they have been associated with poor efficacy and/or high complication rates [55–58]. Autologous facial sling placement can be used to treat SUI during a concomitant prolapse repair [59], but the incision needed for harvesting rectus fascia or fascia lata may defeat the purpose of performing a minimally invasive robotic repair. While urethral bulking agents can be injected during prolapse repair, surgeons may elect to use bulking agents in the office setting for women who experience postoperative SUI. Artificial urinary sphincter placement is no longer routinely performed for women [60].

There are no direct comparative data examining the safety and efficacy of synthetic midurethral sling placement versus robotic Burch colposuspension at the time of robotic pelvic floor reconstruction. However, a meta-analysis (not limited to women undergoing prolapse repair) found that midurethral sling placement and laparoscopic Burch colposuspension appear to have equivalent efficacy [61]. Notably, bladder perforations were more frequent in women undergoing midurethral sling placement, while de novo storage symptoms were more common in women undergoing laparoscopic Burch colposuspension [61].

Midurethral Sling

Synthetic midurethral slings are macroporous monofilament polypropylene meshes that are placed underneath the midurethra via a retropubic or transobturator approach. Retropubic midurethral slings can be inserted in either a bottom-to-top or top-to-bottom fashion, and transobturator slings can be inserted in either an out-to-in or in-to-out fashion. While data specifically comparing midurethral sling approaches in women with prolapse are lacking, overall data from women with SUI suggests that retropubic and transobturator slings are equally effective [30, 62]. One exception may be women with ISD, for whom retropubic slings may be superior [63]. Retropubic slings and transobturator slings are associated with different complication profiles [30, 61]. Retropubic slings are associated with increased rates of bladder perforation and voiding dysfunction, while transobturator slings are associated with increased rates of groin pain [30, 61] and possibly mesh extrusion [64]. Although uncommon, retropubic slings are also associated with an increased risk of bowel injury, which may be heightened in the women with previous abdominal/inguinal surgery [45]. Studies are conflicting as to whether operative time, blood loss, and sexual function are equivalent between the two sling types.

Mini-slings are also macroporous monofilament polypropylene meshes, but they are shorter than full-length slings. These slings are placed via a single vaginal incision and are thought to pose less risk than full-length slings. However, a meta-analysis found mini-slings to be less efficacious than full-length slings in terms of subjective and objective cure rates [65]. Regardless, they may have a role in women who are undergoing robotic pelvic floor repair, as they may improve incontinence while posing less surgical risk [66].

The surgical technique for placing a full-length midurethral sling during prolapse repair is similar to placement in women without prolapse and has been previously described [67]. In brief, after robotic pelvic floor repair is completed, the robot is undocked, and attention is turned to the vagina. Cystoscopy (with a 70° lens) may be performed at this point (to visualize ureteral jets and assess bladder wall integrity), or it may be deferred until after the midurethral sling trocars have been passed. The robot should be kept sterile until after cystoscopy is completed so that it may be quickly redocked in the event of suspected ureteral or bladder injury. Midurethral sling placement is carried forth by identifying the midurethra with the aid of a Foley catheter, dissecting bilateral vaginal flaps with Metzenbaum scissors (with or without the aid of prior hydrodissection) and passing the sling trocars in a retropubic or transobturator fashion. Cystoscopy is conducted to rule out bladder perforation and a Foley catheter is reinserted. The vaginal mucosa is inspected to rule out vaginal perforation, the sling is tensioned, and the vaginal incision is closed with a delayed absorbable suture. The trocar exit sites may be closed with skin adhesive, and vaginal packing with or without estrogen cream may be used.

Burch Colposuspension

Burch colposuspension was a frequently used procedure to correct SUI in women prior to the advent of synthetic midurethral slings. However, midurethral slings are more commonly used to treat SUI given their advantage of avoiding abdominal entry [68]. Yet, for surgeons who are already operating within the abdomen, Burch colposuspension has a valuable role in treating SUI and a robotic Burch colposuspension can be performed after robotic pelvic floor repair is completed.

The surgical technique for performing a robotic Burch colposuspension has been adapted from the open and straight-laparoscopic surgical experience and has been previously described (Fig. 4.4) [69]. In brief, after robotic prolapse repair is completed, the robot is kept docked and the Burch colposuspension proceeds through the previously placed robotic ports. A Foley catheter is inserted if not already in place. Using a monopolar scissor, the space of Retzius is entered by incising the peritoneum of the anterior abdominal wall (the bladder may be temporarily backfilled to aid in dissection) and dissection is carried to the pubic symphysis. Cooper's ligament is identified as well as an area of anterior vaginal wall that is adjacent to the midurethra to bladder neck. Bilaterally, sutures are then passed 2 cm lateral to the urethra at this anterior vaginal wall location and are gently approximated to Cooper's ligament. Special care is taken during knot-tying to avoid placing undue tension on the vagina/urethra. The robot may be undocked, but should be kept sterile until after cystoscopy is completed. Cystoscopy (with a 70° lens) is conducted to visualize ureteral jets, assess bladder wall integrity, and ensure absence of suture intravesically and intraurethrally, and a Foley catheter is reinserted. The vagina is examined to ensure absence of suture penetrating the vaginal lumen. The Burch colposuspension concludes by closure of the peritoneum with an absorbable suture and the robotic port sites are closed in the standard fashion.

Postoperative Care and Complications

The postoperative care of women who undergo concomitant anti-incontinence surgery during robotic pelvic floor repair includes providing a trial of void and ensuring adequate bladder emptying. While Foley catheters in general are ideally removed as soon as possible after surgery, the optimal timing of providing a postoperative trial of void after robotic pelvic floor repair is unclear. Needless to say, a longer period of bladder catheterization may be required in cases of

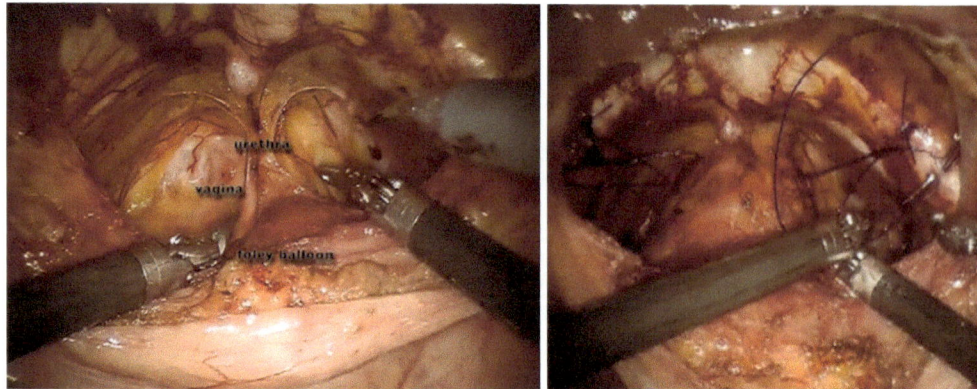

Fig. 4.4 Robotic Burch colposuspension showing sutures placed into Cooper's ligament bilaterally. From Francis et al. [69]; with permission

cystotomy, ureteral injury, or urethrotomy. The risks and benefits of administering prophylactic antibiotics to prevent urinary tract infection should be considered. If used, antibiotics may be administered while the Foley catheter is in place or at the time of Foley catheter removal [70].

Surgical trials comparing different anti-incontinence procedures have provided high-quality evidence of the complication rates associated with anti-incontinence surgery [30, 71]. Unfortunately, these complication rates may not be perfectly applicable to women undergoing concomitant anti-incontinence surgery at the time of robotic pelvic floor repair. In a study examining Medicare claims, women who underwent concomitant anti-incontinence and prolapse surgery had a higher rate of outlet obstruction compared to women who underwent isolated anti-incontinence surgery (9.4 vs. 5.5%) [72]. A different study reported a 20% midurethral sling failure rate in women undergoing concomitant tension-free vaginal tape (TVT) at the time of robotic sacrocolpopexy [73]. The authors of this study speculated that this high failure rate may be attributable to "overcorrection" of the anterior vaginal wall that may occur during robotic prolapse repair. This indicates that sling tensioning should be tailored to the degree of urethral hypermobility that results after the sacrocolpopexy. Further study is needed to clarify the effect of robotic prolapse repair on anti-incontinence outcomes.

Conclusions

Women with POP have a high rate of preexisting SUI as well as have a high rate of postoperative SUI. Performing a concomitant anti-incontinence procedure at the time of robotic pelvic floor repair can decrease postoperative SUI risk, although anti-incontinence procedures are associated with additional risks. Further, not all women undergoing isolated prolapse repair experience postoperative SUI. As there is no gold standard method of managing SUI at the time of robotic pelvic floor repair, surgeons should individually consider the advantages and disadvantages of performing a concomitant anti-incontinence procedure in each patient. Discussing and defining surgical goals with women may lead to increased patient satisfaction postoperatively.

References

1. Fultz NH, Burgio K, Diokno AC, Kinchen KS, Obenchain R, Bump RC. Burden of stress urinary incontinence for community-dwelling women. Am J Obstet Gynecol. 2003;189(5):1275–82.
2. Lagro-Janssen T, Smits A, Van Weel C. Urinary incontinence in women and the effects on their lives. Scand J Prim Health Care. 1992;10(3):211–6.
3. Gray M, Ratliff C, Donovan A. Perineal skin care for the incontinent patient. Adv Skin Wound Care. 2002;15(4):170–5.

4. Chong EC, Khan AA, Anger JT. The financial burden of stress urinary incontinence among women in the United States. Curr Urol Rep. 2011;12(5):358–62.
5. Mitteness LS. Knowledge and beliefs about urinary incontinence in adulthood and old age. J Am Geriatr Soc. 1990;38(3):374–8.
6. Bai S, Jeon M, Kim J, Chung K, Kim S, Park K. Relationship between stress urinary incontinence and pelvic organ prolapse. Int Urogynecol J. 2002;13(4):256–60.
7. Abrams P, Cardozo L, Fall M, Griffiths D, Rosier P, Ulmsten U, et al. Standardisation Subcommittee of the International Continence Society. The standardisation of terminology of lower urinary tract function: report from the Standardisation Sub-committee of the International Continence Society. Neurourol Urodyn. 2002;21(2):167–78.
8. Haylen BT, De Ridder D, Freeman RM, Swift SE, Berghmans B, Lee J, et al. An International Urogynecological Association (IUGA)/International Continence Society (ICS) joint report on the terminology for female pelvic floor dysfunction. Int Urogynecol J. 2010;21(1):5–26.
9. DeLancey JO. Structural support of the urethra as it relates to stress urinary incontinence: the hammock hypothesis. Am J Obstet Gynecol. 1994;170(6):1713–23.
10. Petros PP, Skilling P. Pelvic floor rehabilitation in the female according to the integral theory of female urinary incontinence: first report. Eur J Obstet Gynecol Reprod Biol. 2001;94(2):264–9.
11. DeLancey JO. Anatomic aspects of vaginal eversion after hysterectomy. Am J Obstet Gynecol. 1992;166(6):1717–28.
12. Petros PEP, Ulmsten UI. An integral theory of female urinary incontinence. Acta Obstet Gynecol Scand Suppl. 1990;69(S153):7–31.
13. McGuire EJ, Lytton B. Pubovaginal sling procedure for stress incontinence. J Urol. 1978;119(1):82–4.
14. Paick J-S, Ku JH, Shin JW, Son H, Oh S-J, Kim SW. Tension-free vaginal tape procedure for urinary incontinence with low Valsalva leak point pressure. J Urol. 2004;172(4):1370–3.
15. Ellerkmann RM, Cundiff GW, Melick CF, Nihira MA, Leffler K, Bent AE. Correlation of symptoms with location and severity of pelvic organ prolapse. Am J Obstet Gynecol. 2001;185(6):1332–8.
16. Mueller E, Kenton K, Mahajan S, FitzGerald M, Brubaker L. Urodynamic prolapse reduction alters urethral pressure but not filling or pressure flow parameters. J Urol. 2007;177(2):600–3.
17. Richardson DA, Bent AE, Ostergard DR. The effect of uterovaginal prolapse on urethrovesical pressure dynamics. Am J Obstet Gynecol. 1983;146(8):901–5.
18. Bergman A, Koonings PP, Ballard CA. Predicting postoperative urinary incontinence development in women undergoing operation for genitourinary prolapse. Am J Obstet Gynecol. 1988;158(5):1171–5.
19. Chaikin DC, Groutz A, Blaivas JG. Predicting the need for anti-incontinence surgery in continent women undergoing repair of severe urogenital prolapse. J Urol. 2000;163(2):531–4.
20. Dietz HP. Prolapse worsens with age, doesn't it? Aust N Z J Obstet Gynaecol. 2008;48(6):587–91.
21. Brubaker L, Cundiff GW, Fine P, Nygaard I, Richter HE, Visco AG, et al. Abdominal sacrocolpopexy with Burch colposuspension to reduce urinary stress incontinence. N Engl J Med. 2006;354(15):1557–66.
22. Liapis A, Bakas P, Georgantopoulou C, Creatsas G. The use of the pessary test in preoperative assessment of women with severe genital prolapse. Eur J Obstet Gynecol Reprod Biol. 2011;155(1):110–3.
23. Schierlitz L, Dwyer P, Rosamilia A, Murray C, Thomas E, Taylor N, et al. A prospective randomised controlled study comparing vaginal prolapse repair with and without tension free vaginal tape (TVT) in women with severe pelvic organ prolapse and occult stress incontinence. Neurourol Urodyn. 2007;26(5):743–4.
24. Ploeg J, Oude Rengerink K, Steen A, Leeuwen J, Stekelenburg J, Bongers M, et al. Transvaginal prolapse repair with or without the addition of a midurethral sling in women with genital prolapse and stress urinary incontinence: a randomised trial. BJOG. 2015;122(7):1022–30.
25. van der Ploeg JM, Rengerink KO, van der Steen A, van Leeuwen JHS, van der Vaart CH, Roovers J-PW, et al. Vaginal prolapse repair with or without a midurethral sling in women with genital prolapse and occult stress urinary incontinence: a randomized trial. Int Urogynecol J. 2016;27(7):1029–1038.
26. Wei JT, Nygaard I, Richter HE, Nager CW, Barber MD, Kenton K, et al. A midurethral sling to reduce incontinence after vaginal prolapse repair. N Engl J Med. 2012;366(25):2358–67.
27. Matsuoka PK, Pacetta AM, Baracat EC, Haddad JM. Should prophylactic anti-incontinence procedures be performed at the time of prolapse repair? Systematic review. Int Urogynecol J. 2015;26(2):187–93.
28. Ploeg J, Steen A, Oude Rengerink K, Vaart C, Roovers J. Prolapse surgery with or without stress incontinence surgery for pelvic organ prolapse: a systematic review and meta-analysis of randomised trials. BJOG. 2014;121(5):537–47.
29. Borstad E, Abdelnoor M, Staff AC, Kulseng-Hanssen S. Surgical strategies for women with pelvic organ prolapse and urinary stress incontinence. Int Urogynecol J. 2010;21(2):179–86.
30. Richter HE, Albo ME, Zyczynski HM, Kenton K, Norton PA, Sirls LT, et al. Retropubic versus transobturator midurethral slings for stress incontinence. N Engl J Med. 2010;362(22):2066–76.
31. Visco AG, Brubaker L, Nygaard I, Richter HE, Cundiff G, Fine P, et al. The role of preoperative urodynamic testing in stress-continent women undergoing sacrocolpopexy: the Colpopexy and Urinary Reduction Efforts (CARE) randomized surgical trial. Int Urogynecol J. 2008;19(5):607–14.
32. Serati M, Bogani G, Sorice P, Braga A, Torella M, Salvatore S, et al. Robot-assisted sacrocolpopexy for pelvic organ prolapse: a systematic review and

meta-analysis of comparative studies. Eur Urol. 2014;66(2):303–18.

33. Goldman HB. Occult stress urinary incontinence: what have clinical trials taught us? AUA News. 2015;20(9):1–4.

34. Kraus SR. Occult stress urinary incontinence: what have clinical trials taught us? AUA News. 2015;20(9):4–7.

35. King AB, Goldman HB. Stress incontinence surgery at the time of prolapse surgery: mandatory or forbidden? World J Urol. 2015;33(9):1257–62.

36. Elkadry EA, Kenton KS, FitzGerald MP, Shott S, Brubaker L. Patient-selected goals: a new perspective on surgical outcome. Am J Obstet Gynecol. 2003;189(6):1551–7.

37. Hullfish KL, Bovbjerg VE, Steers WD. Patient-centered goals for pelvic floor dysfunction surgery: long-term follow-up. Am J Obstet Gynecol. 2004;191(1):201–5.

38. Al-Mandeel H, Ross S, Robert M, Milne J. Incidence of stress urinary incontinence following vaginal repair of pelvic organ prolapse in objectively continent women. Neurourol Urodyn. 2011;30(3):390–4.

39. Lensen EJ, Withagen MI, Kluivers KB, Milani AL, Vierhout ME. Urinary incontinence after surgery for pelvic organ prolapse. Neurourol Urodyn. 2013;32(5):455–9.

40. Costantini E, Lazzeri M, Bini V, Del Zingaro M, Zucchi A, Porena M. Burch colposuspension does not provide any additional benefit to pelvic organ prolapse repair in patients with urinary incontinence: a randomized surgical trial. J Urol. 2008;180(3):1007–12.

41. Chermansky CJ, Krlin RM, Winters JC. Selective management of the urethra at time of pelvic organ prolapse repair: an assessment of postoperative incontinence and patient satisfaction. J Urol. 2012;187(6):2144–8.

42. Wolters JP, King AB, Rapp DE. Satisfaction in patients undergoing concurrent pelvic floor surgery for stress urinary incontinence and pelvic organ prolapse. Female Pelvic Med Reconstr Surg. 2014;20(1):23–6.

43. Nygaard I, Brubaker L, Zyczynski HM, Cundiff G, Richter H, Gantz M, et al. Long-term outcomes following abdominal sacrocolpopexy for pelvic organ prolapse. JAMA. 2013;309(19):2016–24.

44. Ballert KN, Biggs GY, Isenalumhe A, Rosenblum N, Nitti VW. Managing the urethra at transvaginal pelvic organ prolapse repair: a urodynamic approach. J Urol. 2009;181(2):679–84.

45. Daneshgari F, Kong W, Swartz M. Complications of mid urethral slings: important outcomes for future clinical trials. J Urol. 2008;180(5):1890–7.

46. Brubaker L, Nygaard I, Richter HE, Visco A, Weber AM, Cundiff GW, et al. Two-year outcomes after sacrocolpopexy with and without burch to prevent stress urinary incontinence. Obstet Gynecol. 2008;112(1):49–55.

47. Digesu GA, Salvatore S, Chaliha C, Athanasiou S, Milani R, Khullar V. Do overactive bladder symptoms improve after repair of anterior vaginal wall prolapse? Int Urogynecol J. 2007;18(12):1439–43.

48. Nager CW. Role of urodynamics in the evaluation of urinary incontinence and prolapse. Curr Obstet Gynecol Rep. 2013;2(3):139–46.

49. Svenningsen R, Borstad E, Spydslaug AE, Sandvik L, Staff AC. Occult incontinence as predictor for postoperative stress urinary incontinence following pelvic organ prolapse surgery. Int Urogynecol J. 2012;23(7):843–9.

50. Serati M, Giarenis I, Meschia M, Cardozo L. Role of urodynamics before prolapse surgery. Int Urogynecol J. 2015;26(2):165–8.

51. Anger JT, Scott VC, Kiyosaki K, Khan AA, Sevilla C, Connor SE, et al. Quality-of-care indicators for pelvic organ prolapse: development of an infrastructure for quality assessment. Int Urogynecol J. 2013;24(12):2039–47.

52. Jelovsek JE, Chagin K, Brubaker L, Rogers RG, Richter HE, Arya L, et al. A model for predicting the risk of de novo stress urinary incontinence in women undergoing pelvic organ prolapse surgery. Obstet Gynecol. 2014;123(2 Part 1):279–87.

53. Richardson ML, Elliott CS, Shaw JG, Comiter CV, Chen B, Sokol ER. To sling or not to sling at time of abdominal sacrocolpopexy: a cost-effectiveness analysis. J Urol. 2013;190(4):1306–12.

54. Raman SV, Raker CA, Sung VW. Concomitant apical prolapse repair and incontinence procedures: trends from 2001-2009 in the United States. Am J Obstet Gynecol. 2014;211(3):222.e1–5.

55. Glazener C, Cooper K. Anterior vaginal repair for urinary incontinence in women. Cochrane Database Syst Rev. 2001;1(1):CD001755.

56. Kammerer-Doak DN, Cornella JL, Magrina JF, Stanhope CR, Smilack J. Osteitis pubis after Marshall-Marchetti-Krantz urethropexy: a pubic osteomyelitis. Am J Obstet Gynecol. 1998;179(3):586–90.

57. Colombo M, Milani R, Vitobello D, Maggioni A. A randomized comparison of Burch colposuspension and abdominal paravaginal defect repair for female stress urinary incontinence. Am J Obstet Gynecol. 1996;175(1):78–84.

58. Groutz A, Gordon D, Wolman I, Jaffa AJ, Kupferminc MJ, David MP, et al. The use of prophylactic Stamey bladder neck suspension to prevent postoperative stress urinary incontinence in clinically continent women undergoing genitourinary prolapse repair. Neurourol Urodyn. 2000;19(6):671–6.

59. Barnes NM, Dmochowski RR, Park R, Nitti VW. Pubovaginal sling and pelvic prolapse repair in women with occult stress urinary incontinence: effect on postoperative emptying and voiding symptoms. Urology. 2002;59(6):856–60.

60. Rouprêt M, Misraï V, Vaessen C, Cardot V, Cour F, Richard F, et al. Laparoscopic approach for artificial urinary sphincter implantation in women with intrinsic sphincter deficiency incontinence: a single-centre preliminary experience. Eur Urol. 2010;57(3):499–505.

61. Ogah J, Cody J, Rogerson L. Minimally invasive synthetic suburethral sling operations for stress urinary incontinence in women: a short version Cochrane review. Neurourol Urodyn. 2011;30(3):284–91.
62. Ford A, Rogerson L, Cody J, Ogah J. Midurethral sling operations for stress urinary incontinence in women. Cochrane Database Syst Rev. 2015;(7):CD006375. doi:10.1002/14651858. CD006375.pub3.
63. Ford AA, Ogah JA. Retropubic or transobturator mid-urethral slings for intrinsic sphincter deficiency-related stress urinary incontinence in women: a systematic review and meta-analysis. Int Urogynecol J. 2016;27(1):19–28.
64. Siegel AL. Vaginal mesh extrusion associated with use of Mentor transobturator sling. Urology. 2005;66(5):995–9.
65. Schimpf MO, Rahn DD, Wheeler TL, Patel M, White AB, Orejuela FJ, et al. Sling surgery for stress urinary incontinence in women: a systematic review and metaanalysis. Am J Obstet Gynecol. 2014;211(1):71. e1–e27.
66. Botros C, Lewis C, Culligan P, Salamon C. A prospective study of a single-incision sling at the time of robotic sacrocolpopexy. Int Urogynecol J. 2014;25(11):1541–6.
67. Ulmsten U, Henriksson L, Johnson P, Varhos G. An ambulatory surgical procedure under local anesthesia for treatment of female urinary incontinence. Int Urogynecol J. 1996;7(2):81–6.
68. Suskind AM, Kaufman SR, Dunn RL, Stoffel JT, Clemens JQ, Hollenbeck BK. Population-based trends in ambulatory surgery for urinary incontinence. Int Urogynecol J. 2013;24(2):207–11.
69. Francis SL, Agrawal A, Azadi A, Ostergard DR, Deveneau NE. Robotic Burch colposuspension: a surgical case and instructional video. Int Urogynecol J. 2015;26(1):147–8.
70. Marschall J, Carpenter CR, Fowler S, Trautner BW, CDC Prevention Epicenters Program. Antibiotic prophylaxis for urinary tract infections after removal of urinary catheter: meta-analysis. BMJ. 2013;346:f3147. doi:10.1136/bmj.f3147. Review. Erratum in: BMJ. 2013;347:f5325.
71. Albo ME, Richter HE, Brubaker L, Norton P, Kraus SR, Zimmern PE, et al. Burch colposuspension versus fascial sling to reduce urinary stress incontinence. N Engl J Med. 2007;356(21):2143–55.
72. Anger JT, Litwin MS, Wang Q, Pashos CL, Rodríguez LV. The effect of concomitant prolapse repair on sling outcomes. J Urol. 2008;180(3):1003–6.
73. Osmundsen B, Gregory WT, Denman MA, Adams K, Edwards R, Clark A. Tension-free vaginal tape failure after robotic sacrocolpopexy and tension-free vaginal tape for concomitant prolapse and stress incontinence. Female Pelvic Med Reconstr Surg. 2015;21(5):244–8.

Katarzyna Bochenska and Sarah Collins

Introduction

Pelvic organ prolapse (POP) is a prevalent condition affecting millions of women worldwide. In the United States, over 5.6 million inpatient procedures for POP were performed between 1979 and 2006 [1]. It is estimated that the number of American women with at least one pelvic floor disorder will increase from 28.1 million in 2010 to 43.8 million in 2050, resulting in a 47% increase in the number of women undergoing surgery for their conditions [2]. Management options for symptomatic POP include observation, pelvic floor physical therapy, pessary use, and surgery via abdominal, vaginal, laparoscopic, or robotic approaches.

Restoring apical support is recognized as an important component of any surgical procedure for POP. The abdominal sacrocolpopexy (ASC) technique involves suspension of the vagina through attachment to the anterior longitudinal ligament on the sacral promontory using a bridging material. Sacrocolpopexy has superior anatomic outcomes compared to a variety of vaginal procedures including sacrospinous colpopexy, uterosacral colpopexy, and transvaginal mesh repairs [3]. Minimally invasive approaches to ASC carry several advantages over traditional open techniques including shorter hospital stays, decreased intraoperative blood loss, and less postoperative pain [4, 5]. Both laparoscopic and robotic ASC approaches have similar anatomic and functional outcomes, as well as low complication rates [6, 7].

Utilization of the robotic approach specifically has increased in recent years [8]. Robotic technology offers enhanced three-dimensional visualization, improved dexterity, and wrist-like manipulation of instruments with increased freedom of movement and elimination of tremor. It also offers the ability to use telestration for teaching by allowing a member of the surgical team to draw on a touchscreen or in the robotic console. Additionally, surgeon comfort may be improved given the seated position and ergonomic positioning of the console [9].

As with most surgical procedures, patient selection and positioning, precise operative entry, operating room and equipment considerations, and a cohesive surgical team are pivotal to successful robotic sacrocolpopexy.

K. Bochenska, M.D. (✉) • S. Collins, M.D.
Division of Female Pelvic Medicine and
Reconstructive Surgery, Department of Obstetrics and
Gynecology, Northwestern University, Prentice
Women's Hospital, 250 East Superior Street,
Chicago, IL 60611, USA
e-mail: katarzyna.bochenska@nm.org;
sarah.collins@nm.org

© Springer International Publishing AG 2018
J.T. Anger, K.S. Eilber (eds.), *The Use of Robotic Technology in Female
Pelvic Floor Reconstruction*, DOI 10.1007/978-3-319-59611-2_5

Patient Selection

All patients should undergo a targeted urogyneco-logic history and physical examination, including assessment of POP in the standing position prior to treatment. Initial counseling should include a directed conversation to identify the patient's bothersome pelvic symptoms and treatment goals. Non-surgical (pessary, observation, physical therapy) and surgical options for treating symptomatic POP should be reviewed in detail. Surgical risks including, but not limited to, organ injury (urinary tract, bowel, nerve, discs, blood vessels, muscles), recurrent prolapse, urinary incontinence, voiding dysfunction, prolonged catheterization, reoperation, and infection should be discussed. Durability and perioperative course associated with abdominal (open, laparoscopic, and robotic) and vaginal prolapse repairs with and without mesh as well as vaginal closure procedures (colpocleisis) should be reviewed. Additionally, the surgeon should discuss the role of concomitant anti-incontinence procedures, if warranted, with the patient.

Medical conditions may preclude a minimally invasive approach, as patients must be able to tolerate pneumoperitoneum and the Trendelenburg position for an extended period of time [10]. Moreover, patient preferences, surgeon skill and comfort level, and availability of the surgical robot may factor into surgical route planning.

Patient Positioning

Unlike open or vaginal surgery, where bowel packs are used to assist with retraction and visualization of the operative field, robotic ASC relies heavily on gravity. Steep intraoperative Trendelenburg positioning is essential to clear both small and large bowel from the pelvis and facilitate access to the presacral space. Unlike hysterectomy alone, which can be accomplished with lesser degrees of Trendelenburg, maximum Trendelenburg is required to safely perform the presacral dissection during a robotic ASC.

Because steep Trendelenburg is critical to procedure completion, it is important to position and secure the patient appropriately on the operating table to prevent slipping toward the head of the bed. Multiple strategies have been reported, including positioning patients on a disposable piece of egg crate foam that is secured to the operating table under the patient's torso [11]. Similarly, gel pads (AliGel or Overlay Pad, AliMed, Inc., Dedham, MA) or a bean bag (Olympic Vac-Pac, Marlin Medical, Bayswater North, VIC, Australia or Bean Bag Positioner, AliMed, Inc., Dedham, MA) are used successfully (Fig. 5.1).

We recommend the Hug-U-Vac Steep Trend Positioner (Allen Medical Systems Inc., Acton, MA) as it is quick, easy to use, and provides excellent support to the patient's head, neck,

Fig. 5.1 Example of gel pad used to secure patient on the operating table

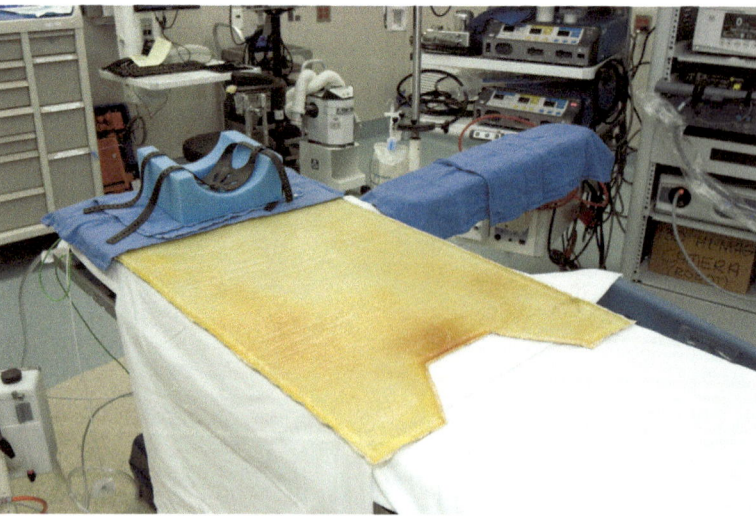

Fig. 5.2 Patient is in dorsal lithotomy and steep Trendelenburg and secured to the operating table using a bean bag device

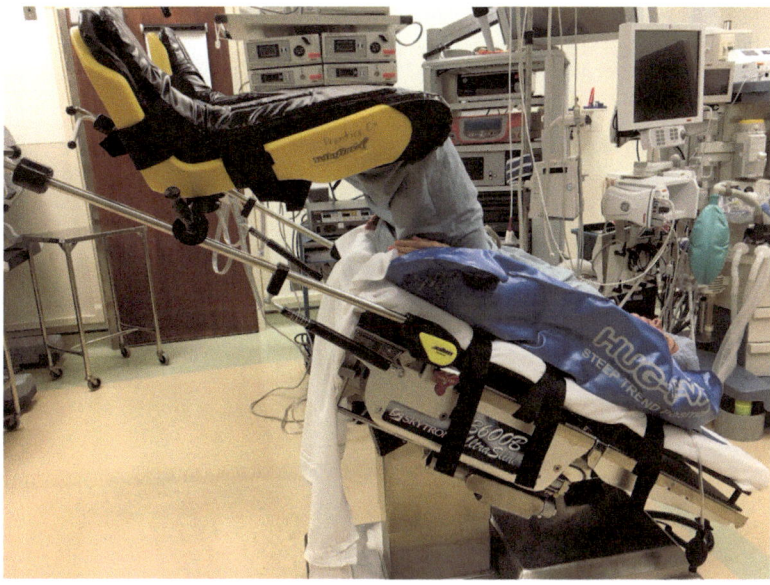

shoulders, and arms (Fig. 5.2). There are also several commercially available, disposable memory-foam systems (The Pink Pad, Xodus Medical, New Kensington, PA or Devon, Medtronic, Minneapolis, MN). Other devices utilize the patient's posterior neck as a point of stability (Trengard, DA Surgical, Chagrin Falls, OH). A padded strap can be placed across the chest to further secure the patient to the operating table (Alistrap, AliMed, Inc., Dedham, MA). Older techniques, such as those that utilize shoulder bolsters secured to the head of the operating table, are also available, but may increase the risk of brachial plexus injuries [12].

Patients should be placed in the dorsal lithotomy position with their bilateral lower extremities secured into supportive stirrups. Care should be taken to avoid pressure on the popliteal fossa or lateral knee, and the patient's heels should be firmly secured in the boot of the stirrup (Fig. 5.3). The patient's arms should be tucked at their sides with their arms, wrists, and hands in a neutral position and a "thumbs-up" orientation to avoid ulnar and radial nerve injury. Care should be taken to ensure that no undue pressure is placed on the extensor surfaces of the upper extremities. This can be accomplished using disposable foam, though many commercially available devices such as the Hug-U-Vac Steep Trend Positioner (Allen

Medical Systems Inc., Acton, MA) do not require additional padding. The patient's occiput should also be appropriately padded using foam material.

Prior to sterile preparation, the patient should be carefully examined to ensure all pressure points are appropriately padded. Additionally, the patient should be placed in maximum Trendelenburg to test that she is adequately supported and does not move excessively on the operating room table. Her vital signs should be briefly monitored in this position to ensure appropriate cardiopulmonary adaptation. Once patient stability and positioning are assured, sterile preparation can be performed. Intraoperatively, care should be taken to avoid extreme flexion, extension, or abduction of the lower extremities to help minimize the risk of neuromuscular injuries.

Port Placement

Abdominal port placement is an essential component of performing a robotic sacrocolpopexy. Visualization and access to the sacral promontory may be compromised if the robotic camera port is inserted too caudally on the anterior abdominal wall. Additionally, if robotic ports are placed too close to one another, arm collisions can occur. A variety of port configurations are reported in the

Fig. 5.3 Patient's bilateral lower extremities are secured in supportive stirrups

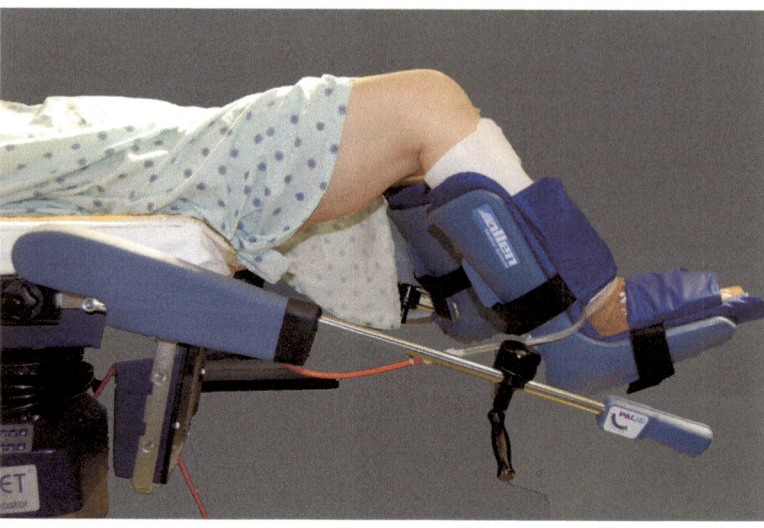

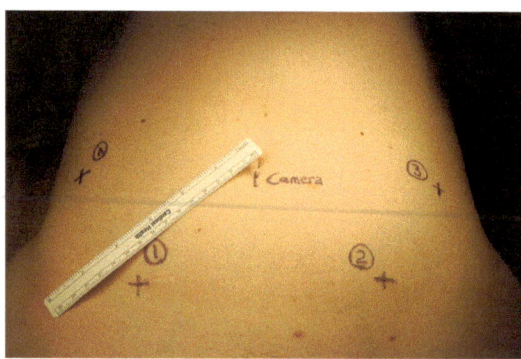

Fig. 5.4 A "W" robotic port configuration

literature, especially to accommodate variations in body habitus. In our experience, different configurations work best for different surgical robotic platforms.

For the da Vinci Si robotic system (Intuitive Surgical, Sunnyvale, CA), we utilize a "W" configuration to facilitate access to the lower pelvis and sacral promontory (Fig. 5.4). After pneumoperitoneum is obtained using a Veress needle and appropriate insufflation is confirmed, the robotic camera is placed through an 8 mm laparoscopic port in the umbilicus. Two additional 8 mm robotic ports are inserted under direct visualization inferior to the umbilicus approximately 10 cm lateral to the umbilical port to maximize access to the pelvis and movement of the robotic

arms. The final 8 mm robotic port is placed on the patient's left side. This port is located 10 cm lateral to the umbilicus. An optional 8 mm accessory port can be placed on the patient's right side, mirroring the third robotic port. By only using 8 mm ports, we anticipate that short-term increases in postoperative pain associated with robotic surgery, compared to laparoscopy, will be reduced [13].

If an accessory port is not used, the sacrocolpopexy mesh can be rolled and passed into the abdominal cavity through an empty robotic trocar using a laparoscopic needle driver. Newer suture management devices (StitchKit, Origami Surgical) obviate the need to pass needles into and out of the abdomen during stitching. These devices can be passed into the peritoneal cavity vaginally before cuff closure or through an 8 mm port incision before trocar placement. They can be removed at the conclusion of the procedure through one of the robotic port site incisions.

The da Vinci Xi (Intuitive Surgical, Sunnyvale, CA) surgical platform includes several technological enhancements over its predecessor, the da Vinci Si. The da Vinci Xi patient cart has four robotic arms that are mounted on a mobile overhead boom (Fig. 5.5). These arms are thinner than previous platform models and the robotic arm joints can be manipulated to provide greater patient clearance, allowing for closer placement

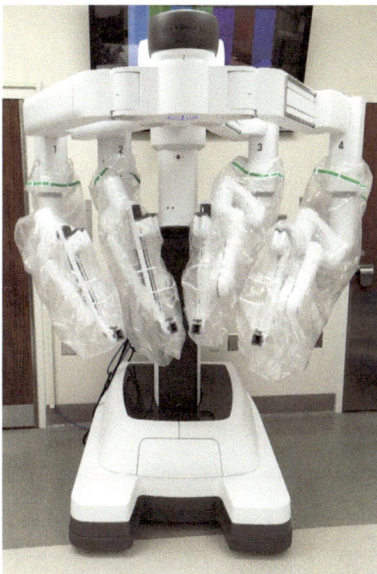

Fig. 5.5 Da Vinci Xi with four robotic arms that are mounted on a mobile overhead boom

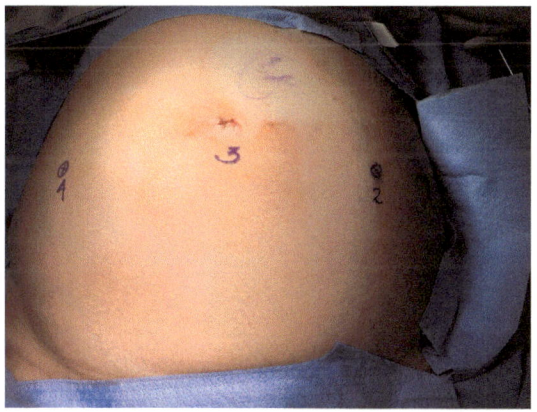

Fig. 5.6 An "arc" robotic port configuration

of robotic arms with fewer collisions. For this system, we have adopted a modified "arc" configuration for port placement (Fig. 5.6). After pneumoperitoneum is obtained using a Veress needle and insufflation has been confirmed, the robotic camera is placed through an 8 mm laparoscopic port in the umbilicus. An 8 mm robotic port is initially inserted on the patient's right side 10 cm lateral and 1 cm caudal to the umbilicus. A second 8 mm port is placed on the patient's left side located 10 cm lateral and 1 cm caudal to the umbilicus, symmetrically mirroring the port on

the patient's right side. Finally, an additional 8 mm port is inserted on the patient's left side, lateral to the previously placed left-sided port.

Robotic Docking

The robotic arms are attached to the robotic ports in a process called "docking." It is important to place the patient in maximum Trendelenburg position prior to docking the surgical robot as this is what allows the bowels to shift out of the pelvis, facilitating access to the presacral space. On the Da Vinci Si system, it is not possible to move the operating table after the surgical robot is docked. If it is discovered that the operating table is not optimally positioned after docking, the patient cart must be undocked before positioning adjustments can be made.

Various docking techniques are described in pelvic surgery. Center-docking, or placing the patient cart between the patient's legs, is simplest to perform but leads to limited access to the patient's vagina or rectum for manipulation and hinders cystoscopy. Therefore, we suggest a parallel docking approach, which places the leading edge of the patient cart in direct line with the edge of the operating table (Fig. 5.7). The patient cart may then be advanced along the edge of the operating table until the camera arm reaches the umbilical port. This typically results in an overlap of 5–10 cm between the patient cart and operating table. The robotic arms may then be attached to the previously inserted ports.

The da Vinci Xi (Intuitive Surgical, Sunnyvale, CA) has streamlined the docking process compared to earlier models of the da Vinci system. Laser crosshairs on the robotic boom facilitate aligning the patient cart with the designated camera port (Fig. 5.8). After the robotic ports have been inserted, the camera port is docked first, and the camera is focused on the target anatomy, which in the case of sacrocolpopexy is the uterus or vagina. This "autotargeting" feature then allows the remaining robotic arms to autorotate on the boom to minimize clashing and optimize performance. The flexibility provided by mounting the robotic arms on a mobile overhead boom obviates the need for parallel docking.

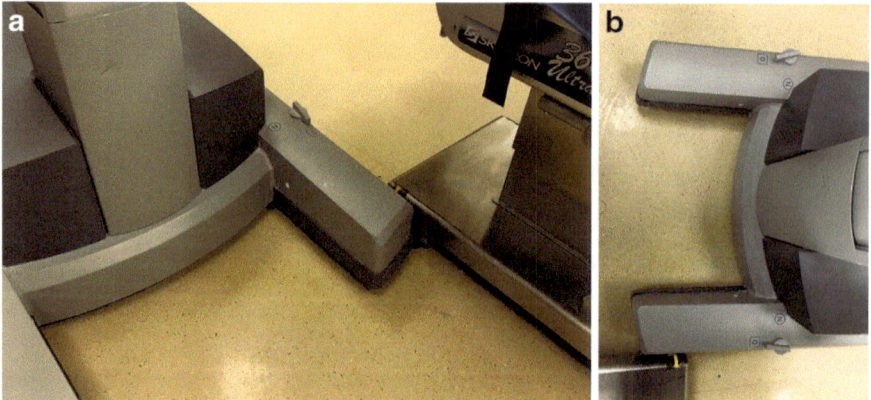

Fig. 5.7 (**a**, **b**) Parallel docking approach using the Da Vinci Si robotic platform

Fig. 5.8 (**a**, **b**) Laser crosshairs on the robotic boom facilitate aligning the patient cart with the designated camera port. Once autotargeting has been completed, the remaining robotic arms autorotate on the boom. This obviates the need for parallel docking

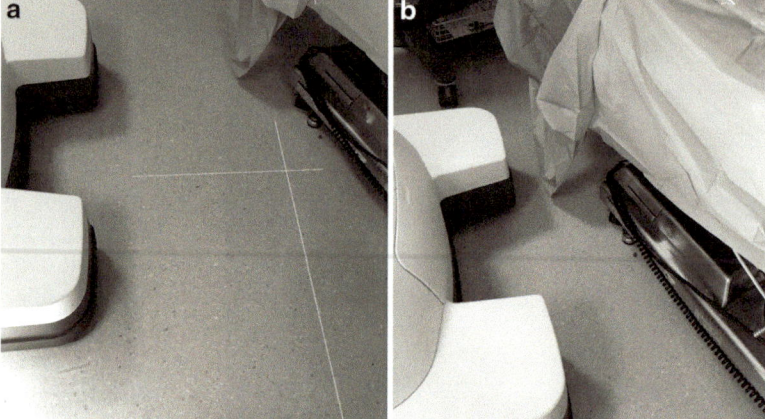

Both parallel docking and docking using the overhead da Vinci Xi boom allow easy access to the vagina or rectum for manipulation during hysterectomy, anterior and posterior vaginal dissections, and sacrocolpopexy graft attachment. Additionally, cystoscopy or concomitant anti-incontinence procedures can be performed while the robot is still docked, which promotes procedural efficiency.

Operating Room Considerations

While patient positioning, port placement, and subsequent docking are crucial for operative set up, several operating room considerations should also be taken into account. The positioning of the surgical robot, robotic console, scrub table, and anesthesia machines should be optimized to facilitate movement of the surgical robot and operating room staff as needed. Some surgical teams place markings on the operating room floor to indicate where each component of surgical equipment should be placed. Some have even marked the floor with tape to outline the path that the patient cart should take to dock at the optimal position at the operating table. At the console, the surgeon should adjust the stool, eyepiece, and armrest to allow for maximal ergonomic comfort (Fig. 5.9). These settings may be stored in the console memory for each surgeon who uses the surgical robot regularly.

Equipment

Prior to commencing the surgical procedure, a survey should be performed to ensure that all necessary equipment is present and available.

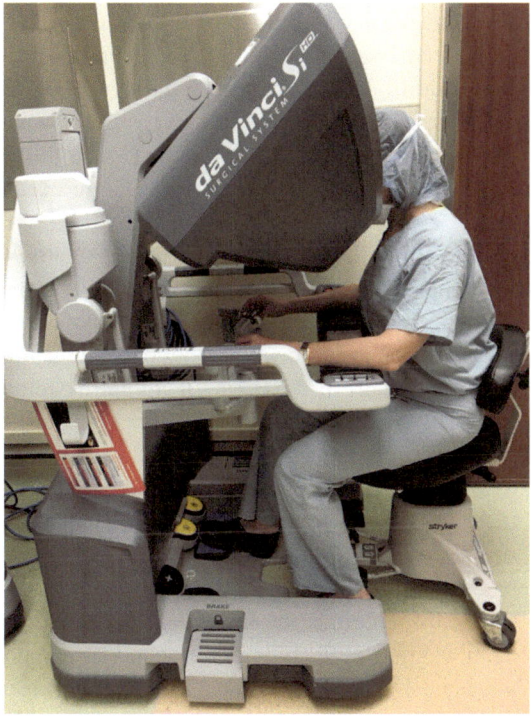

Fig. 5.9 Surgical console ergonomics

Most robotic ASC, with or without hysterectomy, can be accomplished using five or six robotic instruments, no accessory port, and only one instrument change (Fig. 5.10). A systematic approach that minimizes instrument changes and additional set-up will aid in reducing operative times. If a concomitant hysterectomy is planned, we recommend the following initial instrument configuration for right hand-dominant surgeons (robotic arms are described/numbered according to the da Vinci Xi system):

- Monopolar scissors in Arm 1
- Camera in Arm 2
- Bipolar Maryland or fenestrated bipolar grasper in Arm 3
- Tenaculum (or fenestrated grasper if no uterus) or Prograsp in Arm 4

The hysterectomy, anterior and posterior dissections, and presacral dissection can all be accomplished with this first set of instruments. We recommend performing the hysterectomy, except for the colpotomy, then sharply dissecting the bladder from the anterior vaginal wall and rectum from the posterior vaginal wall while applying upward traction on the uterus with the tenaculum. A lucite stent (Marina Medical, Sunrise, FL) placed in the vagina can facilitate hysterectomy, vaginal dissection, and

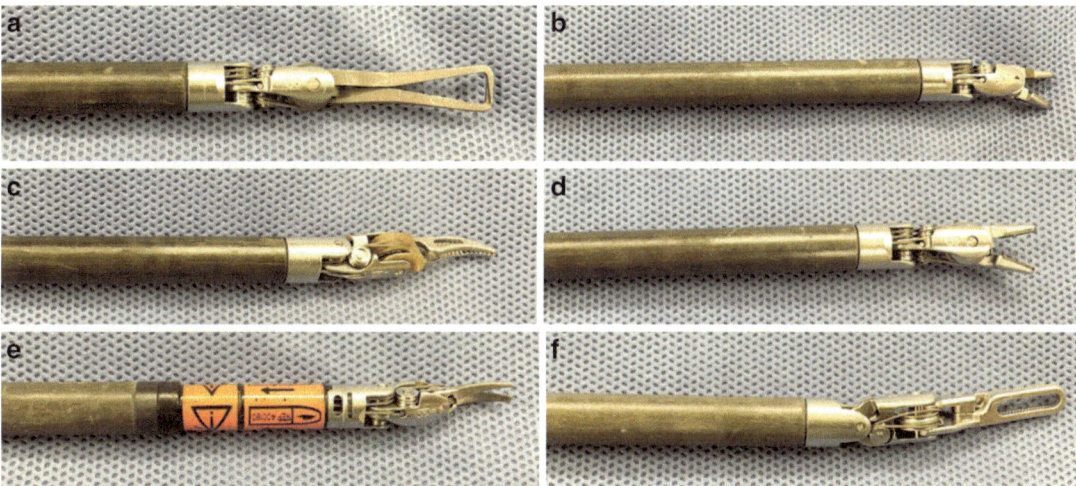

Fig. 5.10 (**a–f**) Robotic equipment including tenaculum

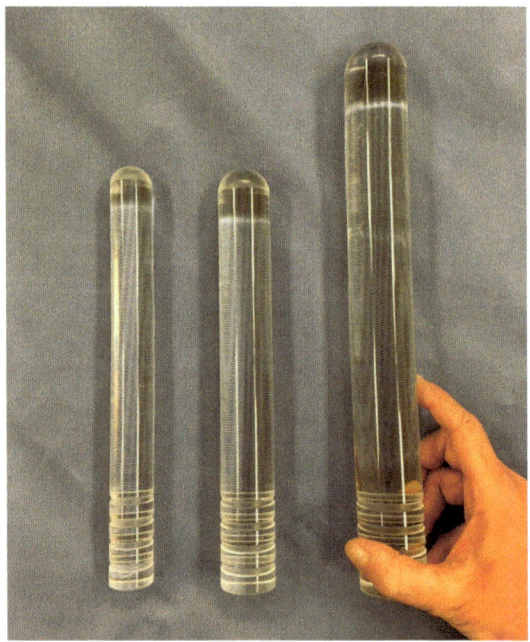

Fig. 5.11 Three different sizes of the lucite stent (Marina Medical, Sunrise, FL)

sacrocolpopexy mesh tensioning (Fig. 5.11). The robotic tenaculum may be used to grasp, elevate, and deviate the uterine fundus to perform a hysterectomy. If a supracervical hysterectomy is performed, the robotic tenaculum can grasp the remaining cervix to provide countertraction during vaginal dissection and mesh attachment. Once the colpotomy is made, the lucite stent can be placed in the vagina to maintain pneumoperitoneum until the vaginal cuff is closed. By using the lucite stent, a uterine manipulator is not necessary.

Because vaginal manipulation is critical to vaginal dissection, mesh attachment, and mesh tensioning, the use of stainless steel end-to-end anastomosis sizers (EEA, Covidien) in the vagina or rectum is also reported. We suggest the use of a lucite stent in the vagina because it fills the entire vaginal canal and facilitates delineating surgical planes. The stent can also be easily used to move the vagina in a cephalad direction during mesh attachment and tensioning. The bedside assistant should be educated on the use and optimal manipulation of the lucite stent to improve operative efficiency.

Finally, before exchanging the dissecting instruments, the presacral space is identified using appropriate bony and vascular landmarks. The peritoneum overlying the sacrum is carefully opened and the anterior longitudinal ligament is exposed below the sacral promontory, near the levels of S1–S2. We advise avoiding dissection below the level of S3, where entry into the venous plexus can result in catastrophic hemorrhage [14]. Additionally, we advise avoiding placement of suture directly on the sacral promontory, where the disc is present 73% of the time [15].

Once all spaces are dissected, a large needle driver is placed in Arm 3 and a large suture cut needle driver in Arm 1. This promotes operative efficiency by necessitating only one instrument change. We also place two 2-0 polydiaxone sutures through the open vaginal cuff and suture the vaginal cuff at this stage, if a total hysterectomy has been performed.

To minimize need for an accessory port, we recommend a canister suture delivery system (StitchKit, Origami Surgical), which contains six sutures of CV-4 polytetrafluoroethylene sutures in an enclosed container that can be placed in the body through either an 8 mm port or through an open vaginal cuff (Fig. 5.12). The sacrocolpopexy mesh may be successfully attached using these sutures, and the used needles may be returned to the canister, which may be removed intact from the abdominal cavity at the conclusion of the procedure.

Wide pore, lightweight polypropylene mesh is commonly used to suspend the vaginal apex. The mesh may be configured into a "Y" shape prior to introduction into the body, or a premade "Y" shaped mesh may be purchased. A variety of sutures have been described to affix the mesh to the vagina including delayed absorbable monofilament suture (2-0 PDS, Ethicon) or polytetrafluoroethylene sutures (Gore-Tex, Gore Medical, Flagstaff, AZ), which we have adopted. Additionally, barbed suture may be a promising and efficient mode of mesh attachment [16]. The type, length, and number of sutures needed for the procedure should be communicated to the scrub technician and circulating nurse prior to starting the procedure to allow maximal preparation for suturing.

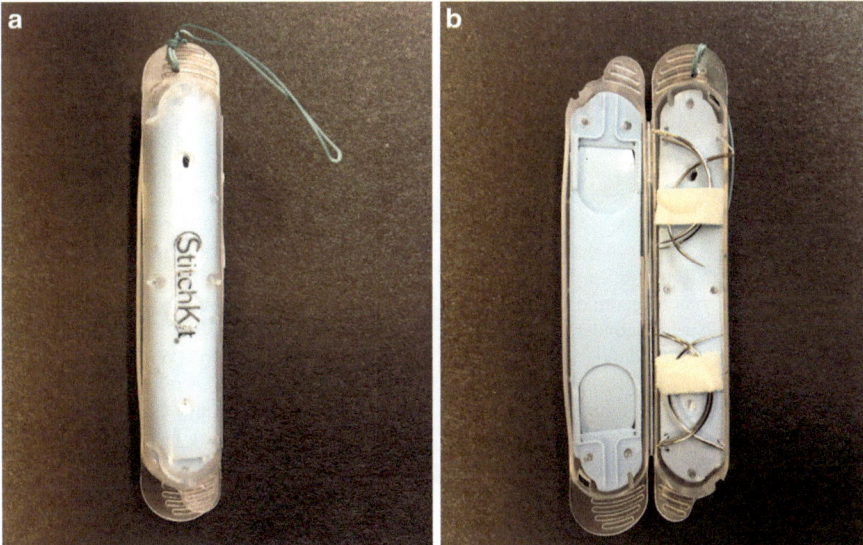

Fig. 5.12 A canister suture delivery system (StitchKit, Origami Surgical), which contains six sutures of CV-4 polytetrafluoroethylene sutures in an enclosed container

Teamwork

As with most surgical procedures, a cohesive surgical team facilitates operating room efficiency. Due to the specific nuances associated with robotic surgery, including port placement, docking, and surgical assistance at the bedside, the surgical team should be educated prior to the procedure on their assigned roles as well as the surgical steps of the procedure. In addition to the operating room technician, circulating nurse, and anesthesia staff, an experienced surgical assistant is necessary to provide vaginal manipulation as well as a bedside assistance through the accessory port (if used). Finally, using a standard protocol will expedite the case and allow for the staff to anticipate the next step in the procedure.

Conclusions

Preparation prior to initiating a robotic sacrocolpopexy is paramount to surgical success. With careful patient selection and positioning, precise operative entry, operating room and equipment considerations, and a cohesive surgical team, the robotic sacrocolpopexy can be performed efficiently.

References

1. Jones KA, Shepherd JP, Oliphant SS, Wang L, Bunker CH, Lowder JL. Trends in inpatient prolapse procedures in the United States, 1979-2006. Am J Obstet Gynecol. 2010;202(5):501.e1–7.
2. Wu JM, Kawasaki A, Hundley AF, Dieter AA, Myers ER, Sung VW. Predicting the number of women who will undergo incontinence and prolapse surgery, 2010 to 2050. Am J Obstet Gynecol. 2011;205(3):230.e1–5.
3. Maher C, Feiner B, Baessler K, Schmid C. Surgical management of pelvic organ prolapse in women. Cochrane Database Syst Rev. 2013;4:CD004014.
4. Freeman RM, Pantazis K, Thomson A, Frappell J, Bombieri L, Moran P, Slack M, Scott P, Waterfield M. A randomized controlled trial of abdominal versus laparoscopic sacrocolpopexy for the treatment of post-hysterectomy vaginal vault prolapse: LAS study. Int Urogynecol J. 2014;25:437–8.
5. Geller EJ, Siddiqui NY, Wu JM, Visco AG. Short-term outcomes of robotic sacral colpopexy compared with abdominal sacral colpopexy. Obstet Gynecol. 2008;112:1201–6.
6. Mueller MG, Jacobs KM, Mueller ER, Abernethy MG, Kenton KS. Outcomes in 450 women after minimally invasive abdominal sacrocolpopexy for pelvic organ prolapse. Female Pelvic Med Reconstr Surg. 2016;22(4):267–71.
7. Kenton K, Mueller ER, Tarney C, Bresee C, Anger JT. One-year outcomes after minimally invasive sacrocolpopexy. Female Pelvic Med Reconstr Surg. 2016;22(5):382–4.

8. Flack CK, Monn MF, Patel NB, Gardner TA, Powell CR. National trends in the performance of robot-assisted sacral colpopexy. J Endourol. 2015;29(7):777–83.

9. Schreuder HW, Verheijen RH. Robotic surgery. BJOG. 2009;116(2):198–213.

10. McLarney JT, Rose GL. Anesthetic implications of robotic gynecologic surgery. J Gynecol Endosc Surg. 2011;2(2):75–8.

11. Tarr ME, Paraiso MFR. Laparoscopic and robotic surgery for pelvic organ prolapse and stress urinary incontinence. In: Urogynecology and reconstructive pelvic surgery. 4th ed. Elsevier Saunders; 2015. p. 297.

12. Romanowski L, Reich H, McGlynn F, Adelson MD, Taylor PJ. Brachial plexus neuropathies after advanced laparoscopic surgery. Fertil Steril. 1993;60(4):729–32.

13. Paraiso MF, Jelovsek JE, Frick A, Chen CC, Barber MD. Laparoscopic compared with robotic sacrocolpopexy for vaginal prolapse: a randomized controlled trial. Obstet Gynecol. 2011;118(5):1005–13.

14. Good MM, Abele TA, Balgobin S, Montoya TI, McIntire D, Corton MM. Vascular and ureteral anatomy relative to the midsacral promontory. Am J Obstet Gynecol. 2013;208(6):486.e1–7.

15. Abernethy M, Vasquez E, Kenton K, Brubaker L, Mueller E. Where do we place the sacrocolpopexy stitch? A magnetic resonance imaging investigation. Female Pelvic Med Reconstr Surg. 2013;19(1):31–3.

16. Tan-Kim J, Nager CW, Grimes CL, Luber KM, Lukacz ES, Brown HW, Ferrante KL, Dyer KY, Kirby AC, Menefee SA. A randomized trial of vaginal mesh attachment techniques for minimally invasive sacrocolpopexy. Int Urogynecol J. 2015;26(5):649–56.

Steps of Robotic-Assisted Sacrocolpopexy

Karyn S. Eilber and Juzar Jamnagerwalla

Introduction

The incidence of pelvic organ prolapse (POP) is increasing in parallel with the growth of the aging population and rates of obesity [1, 2]. The optimal treatment modality for POP is dependent on multiple factors including patient age, comorbidities, desire for preservation of sexual function, patient preference, and surgeon experience. Low stage POP can often be adequately addressed with a native tissue transvaginal repair; however, it has been shown that high stage prolapse is invariably associated with loss of apical support [3], and reoperation rates for POP at 10 years are significantly reduced when a concomitant apical suspension procedure is performed at the time of anterior colporrhaphy [4].

Commonly performed transvaginal apical suspension procedures include sacrospinous or uterosacral ligament fixation. Although these procedures have acceptable success rates (79–87%) [5, 6], abdominal sacrocolpopexy is the

gold standard for apical suspension with success rates in excess of 90% for both open [7, 8] and robotic-assisted laparoscopic approaches [9].

Open abdominal sacrocolpopexy was first described in 1962 by Lane [10]. Historically, this procedure was performed either through a Pfannenstiel or lower midline abdominal incision. In recent years, the robotic approach has gained popularity and is associated with significantly less blood loss and shorter length of stay compared to the open abdominal approach [11]. Although generally advantageous, robotic-assisted sacrocolpopexy (RASC) does have some disadvantages compared to both open and traditional laparoscopic approaches including longer operative times and increased cost. Furthermore, patients with morbid obesity (body mass index >35) or a significant history of previous abdominal surgery are often advised that RASC may not be feasible. In the authors' experience, patients often choose the open approach if they already have a previous abdominal incision.

Pre-procedure Setup

The setup for RASC has been described in the previous chapter; however, a few points regarding patient positioning and setup are worth reinforcing. To begin, patients are placed on the operating room table in low lithotomy position with their legs in adjustable pneumatic stirrups. Care should be taken to position the patient such

K.S. Eilber, M.D. (✉)
Department of Surgery, Division of Urology,
Cedars-Sinai Medical Center, 99 North La Cienega
Boulevard, Suite 307, Beverly Hills, CA, USA
e-mail: karyn.eilber@cshs.org

J. Jamnagerwalla, M.D.
Division of Urology, Department of Surgery,
Cedars-Sinai Medical Center, Los Angeles, CA, USA
e-mail: Juzar.Jamnagerwalla@cshs.org

© Springer International Publishing AG 2018
J.T. Anger, K.S. Eilber (eds.), *The Use of Robotic Technology in Female
Pelvic Floor Reconstruction*, DOI 10.1007/978-3-319-59611-2_6

Fig. 6.1 Positioning and identification of robotic arms

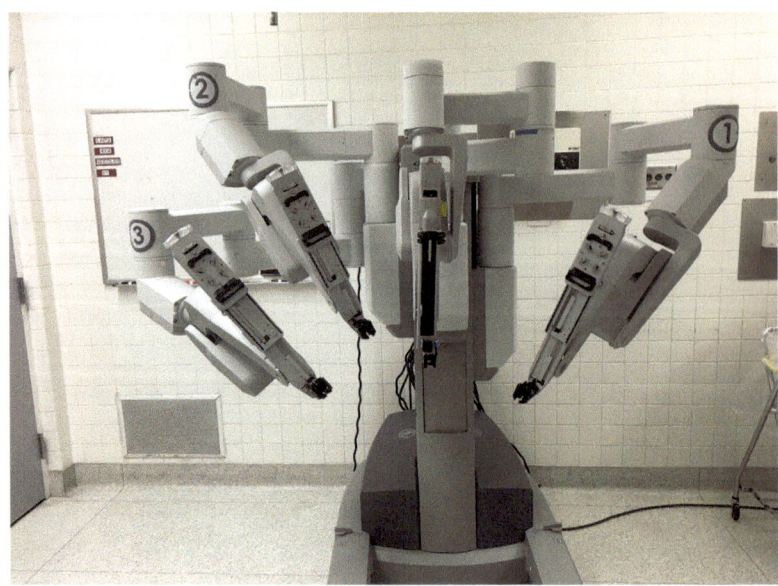

that a weighted speculum can be inserted for any transvaginal procedures following the RASC. The robot is positioned as such that arm #3 is positioned next to arm #2 (Fig. 6.1).

The abdomen and genital areas are prepped with surgical scrub, and prophylactic intravenous antibiotics are administered. The authors typically choose a first-generation cephalosporin unless a concomitant colorectal procedure is being performed, in which case a second- or third-generation cephalosporin is more appropriate. Pneumatic compression stockings or other anti-embolic prophylaxis are routinely used. In order to prevent facial trauma, a "butler" tray is placed with the edge of the tray aligned with the patient's nose. A separate half sheet is used to cover the butler and this also serves as a convenient location to place instruments (Fig. 6.2).

Surgical draping is vital to maintain sterility and organization of cords and tubing. When placing the initial sterile towels to outline the surgical field, the authors have found that using incision drapes with adhesive to secure the towels in place prevents inadvertent contamination during the remainder of draping and throughout the procedure. Once the towels have been placed, a standard laparoscopy drape is placed and the cords and tubes are inserted within a pocket

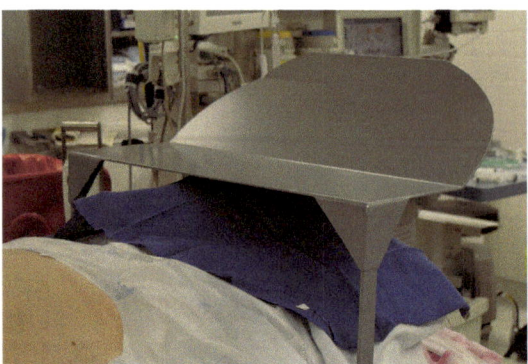

Fig. 6.2 "Butler" tray to prevent facial trauma

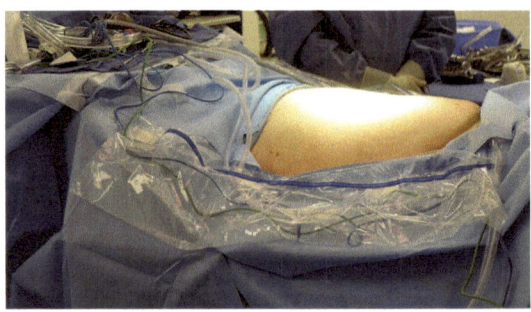

Fig. 6.3 Cords and tubing are placed inside the pocket of a laparoscopy drape

(Fig. 6.3). If the robot is side-docked, then the cords should be inserted in a pocket on the side opposite the robot.

After port placement (as described in Chap. 5), the authors prefer to place the patients in a steep Trendelenburg position. This can be accomplished by raising the operating room table as high as possible then placing the patient in Trendelenburg. Once the patient is at the desired angle, the operating room table is then lowered to desired height. In order to prevent the patient from sliding cephalad, the authors routinely place the patient on egg crate foam.

Exposure of Sacral Promontory

The authors routinely begin the procedure with exposure of the sacral promontory. If this cannot be achieved laparoscopically in a safe and timely fashion, then conversion to an open procedure should be considered. In order to visualize the sacral promontory, the small bowel must be retracted cephalad and the sigmoid colon must be mobilized out of the pelvis and retracted laterally (to the patient's left). Both the small bowel and colon are usually easily retracted unless there are adhesions preventing their mobilization. In this case, it may be necessary to perform lysis of adhesions until they can be adequately retracted out of the operative field. Once the sigmoid colon is retracted laterally, the sacral promontory is typically visualized. Robotic arm #3 can be used to retract the colon and maintain exposure of the promontory (Fig. 6.4a).

After the sacral promontory is identified, the anterior longitudinal ligament must be exposed. The authors use a fenestrated bipolar forceps in the left robotic arm (robotic arm #2) and an electrocautery scissors in the right robotic arm (robotic arm #1). The fenestrated bipolar forceps or a vessel sealing device are preferred for concomitant hysterectomy. The peritoneum overlying the sacral promontory is opened in both the cephalad and caudal directions. Invariably, there is adipose tissue covering the ligament. Obese patients can have significant adipose tissue overlying the ligament, so it may

be useful to periodically have the bedside assistant palpate the promontory to confirm its location. Care must be taken to maintain meticulous hemostasis during this dissection as presacral vessels can cause significant bleeding. If bleeding is encountered, the fenestrated bipolar forceps is well suited to hold pressure on the area while the assistant introduces a suction device. On occasion, a second assistant port must be inserted in the right upper quadrant to enable the bedside assistant to perform simultaneous suction while assisting the surgeon. In the authors' experience, it is extremely unusual to need to convert to an open procedure. The ligament is readily identifiable by its smooth, white appearance (Fig. 6.4b).

Opening of Peritoneum

The authors routinely cover the colpopexy mesh with peritoneum to reduce the risk of bowel obstruction, although data exists that may indicate otherwise [12]. In their series of 128 patients, Elneil et al. [12] reported no bowel complications following abdominal ASC without covering the mesh with peritoneum. However, we have witnessed bowel obstruction in the setting of mesh left uncovered, and reoperation revealed a closed loop bowel obstruction due to small bowel adhering to the mesh.

The peritoneal opening that originated at the sacral promontory is extended towards the pelvis in a "hockey stick" configuration (veering to the right of the sigmoid colon) directed at the posterior vagina. Care must be taken to visualize the right ureter during this dissection and to maintain adequate distance from the ureter when electrocautery is used in order to avoid thermal injury to the ureter.

The peritoneal edges should be separated as wide as possible to facilitate the subsequent peritoneal closure over the mesh. This is especially important as one dissects distally in the pelvis (at the location of the posterior vagina) as bringing the left edge of the peritoneal opening over the mesh can be difficult when the peritoneum is not well mobilized in this area (Fig. 6.5).

Fig. 6.4 (**a**) Robotic arm #3 is used to retract the sigmoid colon laterally to expose the sacral promontory. (**b**) The anterior longitudinal ligament is readily identified by its smooth, white appearance

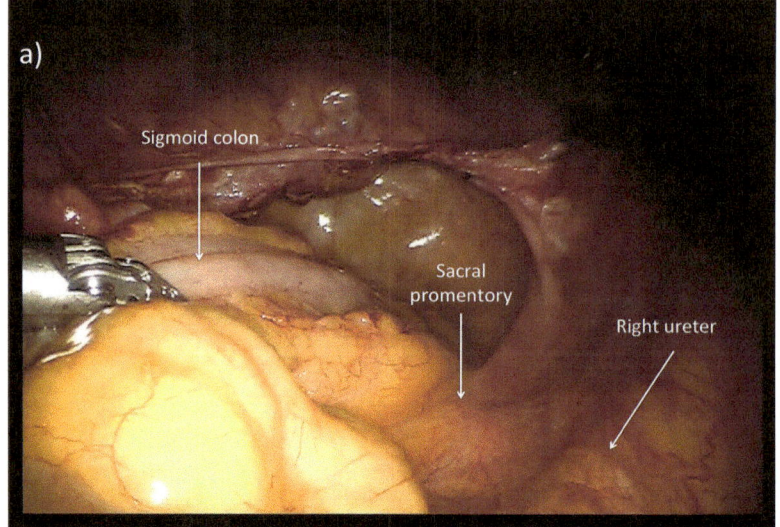

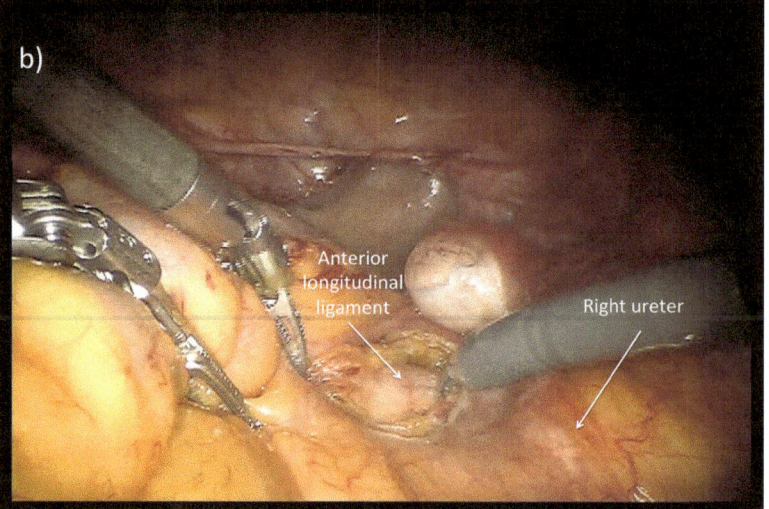

Fig. 6.5 The peritoneum is opened in a "hockey stick" fashion towards the posterior vagina

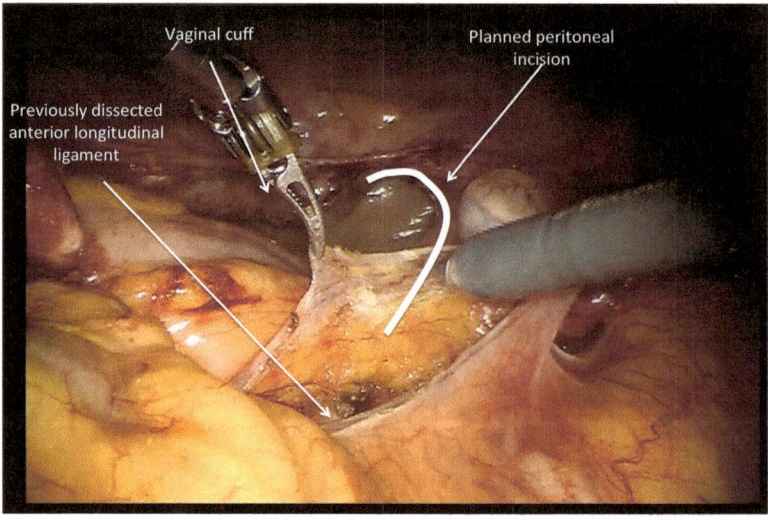

Dissection of the Vesicovaginal Space

Distal dissection of the vesicovaginal space is a key part of RASC as distal placement of mesh on the anterior vaginal wall can address associated cystocele and obviate the need for anterior colporrhaphy. If sacrocolpopexy is performed at the time of hysterectomy, this tissue plane will have already been partly dissected during the hysterectomy; however, when sacrocolpopexy is performed after prior hysterectomy, there can be significant adhesions making identification of the tissue plane more difficult. Often, the bladder completely covers the vaginal apex.

In order to facilitate dissection, the use of a vaginal stent is critical. A vaginal stent allows the bedside assistant to manipulate the vagina for dissection and aids in subsequent suture placement. The authors use an end to end anastomosis (EEA) sizer, but there are also commercially available stents specifically manufactured for this purpose including a lighted version and one that can be attached to the operating room table.

Exposure for dissection of the vesicovaginal space is achieved by retracting the bladder superiorly with robotic arm #3. The vaginal stent is then pushed cephalad and posteriorly. In doing so, the general location of the tissue plane is identified (Fig. 6.6). Sharp dissection in combination with electrocautery is usually necessary to initiate the

dissection, but once the tissue plane is identified, blunt dissection is often adequate to complete the dissection. When a significant cystocele is present, the vesicovaginal space needs to be dissected as far distally as possible to facilitate distal mesh placement. The authors have found that by placing the mesh as far distally as possible, even large cystoceles can be repaired without the need for additional transvaginal repair.

When dense adhesions are present such that the tissue plane is not readily identifiable, the bladder can be filled with fluid via a bladder catheter to aid in identification of the correct plane. Alternatively, a cystoscope can be inserted in the bladder and transillumination can outline the bladder. Any cystotomy that occurs during this dissection is typically small and repaired readily with an absorbable suture. In this scenario, a bladder catheter should remain postoperatively. The duration of catheter drainage and need for cystogram are at the surgeon's discretion and are dependent on the size of the defect repaired.

Dissection of the Rectovaginal Space

The rectovaginal space is dissected and extended distally in a similar fashion as the vesicovaginal space, and distal placement of the posterior vaginal mesh can address posterior compartment

Fig. 6.6 Dissection of the vesicovaginal space

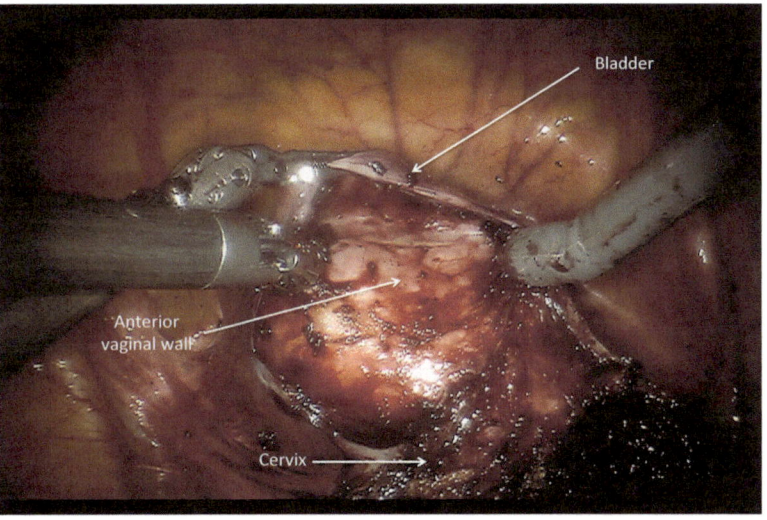

defects and obviate the need for concomitant posterior colporrhaphy. When this tissue plane is not readily apparent, a second EEA sizer can be inserted into the rectum to facilitate dissection. It is critical to assure that the rectum is completely dissected from the posterior vaginal wall to eliminate the risk of suturing mesh to rectum.

At completion of the rectovaginal dissection, the peritoneum previously covering the posterior vaginal wall is now mobilized and made in continuity with the peritoneal opening that originated at the sacrum. Maximal mobilization of the peritoneal edges in this area facilitates subsequent mesh coverage following the colpopexy.

Suturing of Mesh to the Anterior and Posterior Vaginal Walls

In the original description of robotic sacrocolpopexy, a permanent, synthetic mesh was used [13]. Although the Food and Drug Administration safety communications involving mesh specifically addressed vaginally placed mesh [14], some surgeons are still hesitant to use synthetic mesh and opt for biologic grafts such as autologous fascia or xenografts. If the former is used, open sacrocolpopexy should be considered as harvesting of rectus fascia and the colpopexy can be done through a single incision. The authors advocate use of synthetic mesh, as randomized controlled trials have shown objective cure rates significantly higher with mesh use compared with cadaveric fascia lata, 91% vs. 68%, respectively, $P = 0.007$ [15]. More recently, data has become available regarding use of autologous rectus fascia, but long-term results are lacking [16].

Polypropylene mesh is the most commonly used synthetic mesh. There are commercially available products that are specifically manufactured for POP repair. These products are provided as a sheet that can be cut to the desired size and configuration or as a prefabricated "Y" shape. Alternatively, a sheet of soft polypropylene mesh is an acceptable alternative. The authors use this type of mesh and cut the sheet of mesh into two separate strips as this allows for differential tensioning of the anterior and posterior compartments.

Cell ingrowth into mesh occurs within seven to 14 days [17], so based on this, an argument could be made to use absorbable suture when placing mesh; however, there is a dearth of data using absorbable suture. Since the initial descriptions of RASC included polytetrafluoroethylene (PTFE) suture [13], the authors use Gore-tex® suture, which is a monofilament nonabsorbable suture made of expanded PTFE. The authors also prefer Gore-tex® suture as its texture facilitates knot tying without slippage.

For placement of mesh on the anterior vaginal wall, one strip of polypropylene mesh is placed as far distally as previously dissected, and secured in place with a suture (Fig. 6.7). Use of the vaginal stent to provide countertraction during suture placement is invaluable. Five subsequent sutures are placed to create three rows of two sutures. Care should be taken not to place the sutures too deep as this could result in suture or mesh exposure into the vaginal canal. Most reports indicate use of six sutures although the actual number likely varies based on surgeon preference. The authors routinely suture the mesh to the cervix if present, as this provides strong tissue onto which the mesh can be secured. The same is repeated on the posterior vagina.

Tensioning of the Mesh

After both strips of mesh are sutured to the anterior and posterior vaginal walls, they are then sutured to the anterior longitudinal ligament overlying the sacral promontory. Robotic arm #3 is used to retract the peritoneum overlying the promontory to expose the ligament. The assistant grasps both strips of mesh and, together with the surgeon, each strip is adjusted to desired tension. If a "Y" mesh is used and there is asymmetric tension on the vaginal walls, the mesh can be plicated with a polypropylene suture to correct the asymmetry. The vaginal stent should be removed, or at least retracted to the mid-vagina, while tensioning the mesh to avoid overcorrection of the prolapse. Unfortunately, an objective measure of mesh tension does not exist; however, the authors release tension if the mesh appears distorted once the vaginal stent is removed.

Fig. 6.7 The mesh is placed as far distally as possible and sutured in place

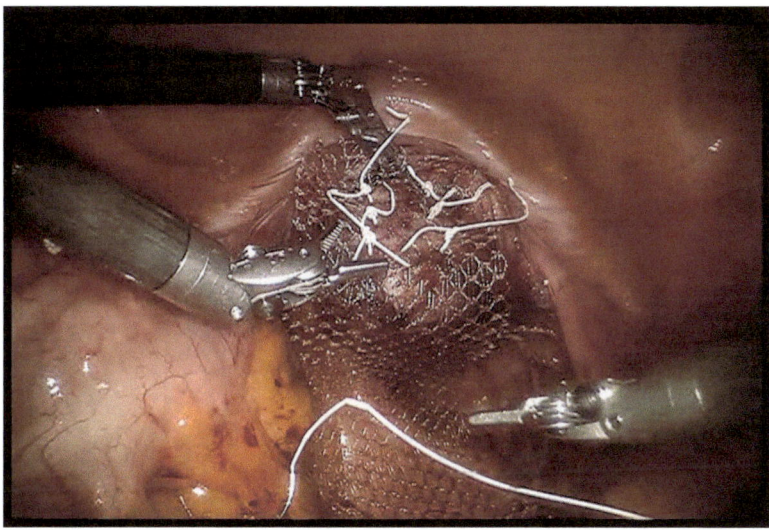

Suturing Mesh to the Anterior Longitudinal Ligament

Once the desired tension is established, the assistant securely holds the mesh near the promontory and the vaginal stent is reintroduced to reduce tension on the mesh while it is sutured in place. Typically, two sutures are placed into the anterior longitudinal ligament to secure the mesh in place. The surgeon can secure the mesh strips to the ligament in one of two ways: (1) placing both sutures through the mesh and ligament then tying them down after both sutures have been placed, or (2) placing one suture through the mesh and ligament and immediately tying it down before placing the second suture. The advantages of the former are full exposure of the ligament while placing both sutures without interference by the mesh (Fig. 6.8). An advantage of the latter is that once the first suture is tied down, the assistant no longer needs to hold the mesh near the promontory and is able to assist in other ways. Regardless of technique, the suture should be placed through the mesh *before* it is placed into the ligament so that the suture can be tied down immediately if any bleeding is encountered. Ideally, any presacral vessels in the vicinity of the dissection were cauterized previously so bleeding at the time of mesh suturing rarely occurs.

White et al. recommended that sutures be placed in a horizontal fashion to maximize tensile strength and reduce the risk of suture pullout [18]; however, when necessary, the authors do not hesitate to place sutures in a vertical fashion in order to avoid vessels in the vicinity. A common occurrence during suture placement is placing the sutures too deep and entering the periosteum of the sacrum. Properly placed sutures in the anterior longitudinal ligament alone have adequate tensile strength to avoid suture pullout. Cadaver studies have shown that the depth of the anterior longitudinal ligament measures 1.4–2.3 mm at the sacrum [19]. Risks of deep suture placement into the sacrum include pain and increased risk of osteomyelitis.

Closure of the Peritoneum

After the mesh is secured to the anterior longitudinal ligament, any excess mesh is excised. Closure of the peritoneum increases operative time, but it may reduce the risk of bowel complications via adhesion of small bowel to the exposed mesh. The peritoneum is closed using a running, locking Vicryl suture, starting from the sacral promontory and heading towards the vaginal cuff. The closure is tension free secondary to

Fig. 6.8 Sutures are placed in a horizontal fashion through the anterior longitudinal ligament. The suture is first placed through the mesh and then through the ligament

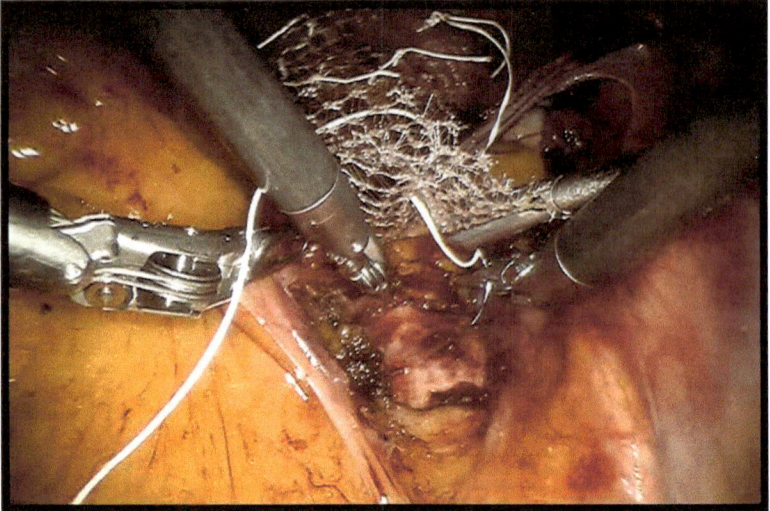

the dissection performed earlier. A barbed type suture (V-lock™) can also be used to close the peritoneum.

Closure of Trocar Sites

Once the peritoneum is closed, the robot is undocked. The camera trocar site and the assistant trocar site (if a 12 mm trocar is used) are closed under direct vision using a Carter-Thomason® laparoscopic port closure device. We prefer this over the use of a traditional suture, especially in obese patients, as it allows excellent reapproximation of the fascia under direct vision. The epithelium of all trocar sites is closed with a subcuticular suture.

Cystoscopy

Cystoscopy is performed at the conclusion of the procedure at the discretion of the surgeon. If there is any concern for ureteral or bladder injury, then cystoscopy is imperative. The incidence of ureteral injury after abdominal sacrocolpopexy has been reported to be 1% in both open and minimally invasive series [20]. To aid in identifying ureteral efflux, different agents can be used including a preoperative oral dose of phenazopyridine or intraoperative intravenous administra-

tion of indigotindisulfonate sodium, methylene blue, or sodium fluorescein. Cystoscopy will also confirm that no suture was inadvertently placed in the bladder.

Vaginal Examination

Postoperative vaginal examination is performed to confirm appropriate apical support, evaluate for any exposed mesh or suture, and determine if additional transvaginal anterior or posterior colporrhaphy is necessary. It has been our experience that appropriate apical support almost always results in significant anatomic improvement of anterior prolapse and concomitant anterior colporrhaphy is rarely needed. Posterior defects, however, often require concomitant repair as distal rectoceles may not be adequately addressed by sacrocolpopexy.

Other procedures such as a urethral sling or other reconstructive procedures are reviewed elsewhere in this textbook.

Postoperative Care

At the conclusion of the procedure, a vaginal packing is placed if any vaginal procedures were performed and is removed along with the urinary catheter on the morning of postoperative day number one. Patients are encouraged to ambulate on the evening of surgery. Analgesia is achieved with 30 mg of ketorolac around the clock (renal function permitting) and oral narcotics for breakthrough pain. Patients are allowed to advance their diet as tolerated immediately postoperatively. The majority of patients are discharged home on postoperative day number one.

Conclusion

Robotic-assisted sacrocolpopexy has revolutionized the treatment of vault prolapse by providing a safe, effective, and minimally invasive approach for abdominal sacrocolpopexy.

References

1. Chow D, Rodriguez LV. Epidemiology and prevalence of pelvic organ prolapse. Curr Opin Urol. 2013;23(4):293–8. doi:10.1097/MOU.0b013e3283619ed0.
2. Hendrix SL, Clark A, Nygaard I, Aragaki A, Barnabei V, McTiernan A. Pelvic organ prolapse in the Women's Health Initiative: gravity and gravidity. Am J Obstet Gynecol. 2002;186(6):1160–6.
3. Rooney K, Kenton K, Mueller ER, FitzGerald MP, Brubaker L. Advanced anterior vaginal wall prolapse is highly correlated with apical prolapse. Am J Obstet Gynecol. 2006;195(6):1837–40. doi:10.1016/j.ajog.2006.06.065.
4. Eilber KS, Alperin M, Khan A, Wu N, Pashos CL, Clemens JQ, et al. Outcomes of vaginal prolapse surgery among female Medicare beneficiaries: the role of apical support. Obstet Gynecol. 2013;122(5):981–7. doi:10.1097/AOG.0b013e3182a8a5e4.
5. van Raalte HM, Lucente VR, Molden SM, Haff R, Murphy M. One-year anatomic and quality-of-life outcomes after the Prolift procedure for treatment of posthysterectomy prolapse. Am J Obstet Gynecol. 2008;199(6):694.e1–6. doi:10.1016/j.ajog.2008.07.058.
6. Elmer C, Altman D, Engh ME, Axelsen S, Vayrynen T, Falconer C, et al. Trocar-guided transvaginal mesh repair of pelvic organ prolapse. Obstet Gynecol. 2009;113(1):117–26. doi:10.1097/AOG.0b013e3181922164.
7. Occelli B, Narducci F, Cosson M, Ego A, Decocq J, Querleu D et al. [Abdominal colposacroplexy for the treatment of vaginal vault prolapse with or without urinary stress incontinence]. Ann Chir. 1999;53(5):367–77.
8. Snyder TE, Krantz KE. Abdominal-retroperitoneal sacral colpopexy for the correction of vaginal prolapse. Obstet Gynecol. 1991;77(6):944–9.
9. Siddiqui NY, Geller EJ, Visco AG. Symptomatic and anatomic 1-year outcomes after robotic and abdominal sacrocolpopexy. Am J Obstet Gynecol. 2012;206(5):435.e1–5. doi:10.1016/j.ajog.2012.01.035.
10. Lane FE. Repair of posthysterectomy vaginal-vault prolapse. Obstet Gynecol. 1962;20:72–7.
11. Geller EJ, Siddiqui NY, Wu JM, Visco AG. Short-term outcomes of robotic sacrocolpopexy compared with abdominal sacrocolpopexy. Obstet Gynecol. 2008;112(6):1201–6. doi:10.1097/AOG.0b013e31818ce394.
12. Elneil S, Cutner AS, Remy M, Leather AT, Toozs-Hobson P, Wise B. Abdominal sacrocolpopexy for vault prolapse without burial of mesh: a case series. BJOG. 2005;112(4):486–9. doi:10.1111/j.1471-0528.2004.00426.x.
13. Di Marco DS, Chow GK, Gettman MT, Elliott DS. Robotic-assisted laparoscopic sacrocolpopexy for treatment of vaginal vault prolapse. Urology. 2004;63(2):373–6. doi:10.1016/j.urology.2003.09.033.
14. Togami JM, Brown E, Winters JC. Vaginal mesh—the controversy. F1000 Med Rep. 2012;4:21. doi:10.3410/M4-21.
15. Culligan PJ, Blackwell L, Goldsmith LJ, Graham CA, Rogers A, Heit MH. A randomized controlled trial comparing fascia lata and synthetic mesh for sacral colpopexy. Obstet Gynecol. 2005;106(1):29–37. doi:10.1097/01.AOG.0000165824.62167.c1.
16. Abraham N, Quiroret A, Goldman HB. Transabdominal sacrocolpopexy with autologous rectus fascia graft. Int Urogynecol J. 2016;27(8):1273–5. doi:10.1007/s00192-016-2987-7.
17. LeBlanc KA, Bellanger D, Rhynes KV 5th, Baker DG, Stout RW. Tissue attachment strength of prosthetic meshes used in ventral and incisional hernia repair. A study in the New Zealand White rabbit adhesion model. Surg Endosc. 2002;16(11):1542–6. doi:10.1007/s00464-001-8271-y.
18. White AB, Carrick KS, Corton MM, McIntire DD, Word RA, Rahn DD, et al. Optimal location and orientation of suture placement in abdominal sacrocolpopexy. Obstet Gynecol. 2009;113(5):1098–103. doi:10.1097/AOG.0b013e31819ec4ee.
19. Graham E, Akl A, Brubaker L, Dhaher Y, Fitzgerald C, Mueller ER. Investigation of sacral needle depth in minimally invasive sacrocolpopexy. Female Pelvic Med Reconstr Surg. 2016;22(4):214–8. doi:10.1097/SPV.0000000000000261.
20. Nygaard IE, McCreery R, Brubaker L, Connolly A, Cundiff G, Weber AM, Zyczynski H, Pelvic Floor Disorders Network. Abdominal sacrocolpopexy: a comprehensive review. Obstet Gynecol. 2004;104(4):805–23.

Janine L. Oliver and Christopher M. Tarnay

The Role of Hysterectomy at the Time of Abdominal Apical Repair

Is the Uterus Just a Passenger or a Driving Factor of Prolapse?

In 1934, Bonney suggested a passive role of the uterus in uterovaginal prolapse stating "I would postulate that prolapse is purely a vaginal phenomenon, in the causation of which the uterus does not play any direct part but acts more or less a deterrent" [1]. The need for hysterectomy at the time of prolapse repair has never been proven and, even in rare cases of isolated uterine prolapse, hysterectomy alone is rarely an adequate treatment, as it fails to address the underlying deficiency causing prolapse. Additionally, removal of the uterus disrupts the uterosacral-cardinal ligament complex, which may further weaken support. Nonetheless,

J.L. Oliver, M.D.
Division of Urology, Department of Surgery,
University of Colorado Hospital,
12605 E. 16th Avenue, Aurora, CO 80045, USA
e-mail: janine.oliver@ucdenver.edu

C.M. Tarnay, M.D. (✉)
Department of Obstetrics & Gynecology and
Urology, Ronald Reagan UCLA Medical Center,
UCLA 100 Medical Plaza, Suite 383, Los Angeles,
CA 90095, USA
e-mail: ctarnay@mednet.ucla.edu

hysterectomy has historically been, and will likely remain, a mainstay in the surgical treatment of uterovaginal prolapse. In fact, while overall the number of hysterectomies performed annually in the United States has declined over recent years, the approximately 15–18% performed for pelvic organ prolapse has remained relatively stable.

Rationale and Advantages of Concomitant Hysterectomy with Sacrocolpopexy or Sacrocervicopexy

Fundamentally, the main rationale for hysterectomy at the time of prolapse repair is improved durability of the repair compared with a uterine-sparing procedure. Long-term comparative data on obviating hysterectomy, for example with abdominal sacrohysteropexy (Fig. 7.1a), in particular utilizing the laparoscopic or robotic approach, is lacking. Women with stage IV uterovaginal prolapse or cervical elongation may not be ideal candidates for hysteropexy, although data to support this is sparse. The issue of uterine preservation is further complicated by wide variations in technique. A small study of supracervical hysterectomy with sacrocervicopexy (Fig. 7.1b), however, showed superior subjective outcomes compared with sacrohysteropexy in symptomatic women [2]. Of note, this study was

© Springer International Publishing AG 2018
J.T. Anger, K.S. Eilber (eds.), *The Use of Robotic Technology in Female Pelvic Floor Reconstruction*, DOI 10.1007/978-3-319-59611-2_7

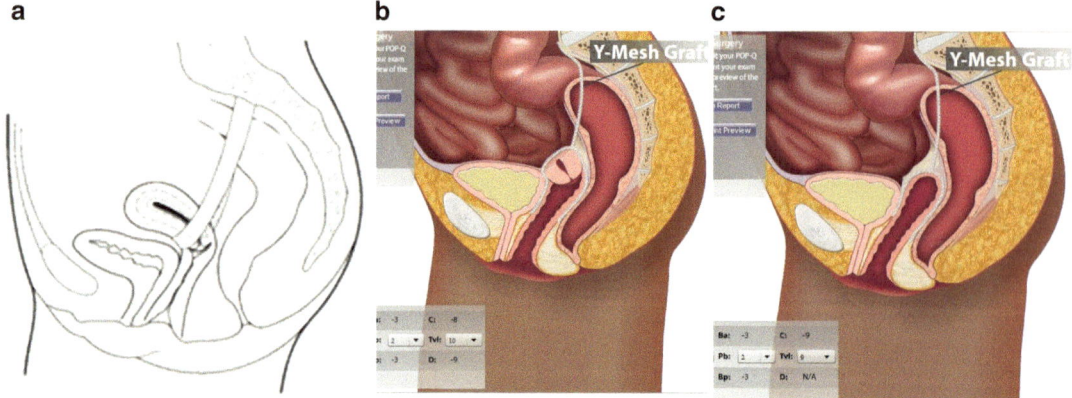

Fig. 7.1 Hysteropexy (**a**) vs. cervicopexy (**b**) vs. sacrocolpopexy (**c**)

not randomized and selection bias may have been a confounding variable in postoperative patient satisfaction.

More recently, a retrospective study of 34 patients who underwent total laparoscopic hysterectomy with laparoscopic sacrocolpopexy (TLH with LSC) compared with 65 patients who underwent laparoscopic sacrohysteropexy by the same group of surgeons found significantly higher subjective patient satisfaction and impact on quality of life based on validated questionnaires in the TLH with LSC cohort [3]. The rate of recurrent vaginal vault or uterine prolapse ≥stage 2 was significantly higher in the laparoscopic sacrohysteropexy group. Ten women (15.4%) in this cohort had recurrent, symptomatic prolapse, while no patients in the TLH with LSC cohort experienced recurrent, symptomatic prolapse.

Aside from the issues of increased durability, other potential advantages of hysterectomy for the patient include elimination of the need for further contraceptive use for those of reproductive age, eradication of menses, and discontinuation of ongoing gynecologic surveillance of the endometrium and cervix if a total hysterectomy is performed. It is also now standard to perform salpingectomy at the time of hysterectomy, thereby reducing the patient's risk not only of endometrial and cervical, but also ovarian malignancy in a single operation.

When to Consider Uterine Preservation

As overall hysterectomy rates decline, hysteropexy is gaining attention. While it remains not as well-studied as hysterectomy-based repairs for the treatment of prolapse and additional research is needed to assess long-term outcomes, there are patients for whom a uterine-sparing procedure such as sacrohysteropexy may be better suited. Compared with hysterectomy and prolapse repair, hysteropexy is associated with a shorter operative time, less blood loss, and a faster return to work [4, 5]. Other advantages include patient preference for retaining a healthy organ and maintenance of fertility. There have been several reports of cesarean section delivery following hysteropexy [6, 7].

Importantly, however, there are several contraindications to uterine-sparing procedures. Women who have uterine abnormalities, endometrial hyperplasia, or neoplasia are not appropriate candidates. Other considerations for uterine preservation include current or recent cervical dysplasia, familial cancer syndromes such as BRCA 1 and 2 or hereditary nonpolyposis colonic cancer syndrome, tamoxifen therapy, large fibroids, adenomyosis, and inability to comply with routine gynecologic surveillance.

A more detailed discussion of sacrohysteropexy can be found elsewhere in this textbook.

Preoperative Considerations in Patients Undergoing Hysterectomy

Preoperative Evaluation and Informed Consent

Pregnancy must always be ruled out in women of reproductive age on the day of surgery. A recent normal Papanicolaou test (Pap smear) should be documented before performing a hysterectomy. A transvaginal ultrasound examination should be performed if a pelvic mass or any other abnormality, such as an enlarged or globular uterus, is palpated during the bimanual pelvic examination. Sampling of the endometrium or pelvic ultrasound should be performed in patients with irregular or intermenstrual vaginal bleeding, postmenopausal bleeding, and those who have risk factors for malignancy such as polycystic ovarian syndrome (PCOS). In women with abnormal uterine bleeding (AUB), it is generally recommended that all women older than 45 years of age and women 45 years or younger with a risk of unopposed estrogen exposure (such as seen in obesity or PCOS), failed medical management, persistent AUB, or other risk factors for endometrial malignancy undergo endometrial biopsy (after excluding pregnancy) [8, 9]. If there are any suspicious findings, consultation with a gynecologic oncologist is recommended prior to surgery.

As many have stated, informed consent for hysterectomy is not a single event but a process. Documentation must clearly state that the patient has completed childbearing. If mesh is going to be used for concomitant sacrocolpopexy, the risks and benefits of mesh use for this application as well as alternative non-mesh procedures should be thoroughly discussed.

Risk of Unanticipated Uterine Malignancy

While the uterus is the most common site of gynecologic malignancy in the United States, several studies have examined the risk of unanticipated uterine malignancy and demonstrate the overall rate is low, approximately 0.3–0.6% [10–12]. While routine screening of all asymptomatic postmenopausal women with endometrial evaluation via endometrial biopsy or transvaginal ultrasound improves the preoperative detection of endometrial cancer, universal preoperative screening is not cost-effective given the low overall risk [13]. Screening methods also have poor sensitivity, with most cases of occult malignancy following hysterectomy for prolapse being found in asymptomatic women [10]. Thus, currently, there is no strong evidence to support performing routine preoperative endometrial assessment in asymptomatic women undergoing hysterectomy for prolapse.

Total vs. Subtotal Hysterectomy

A total hysterectomy refers to removal of the uterus and cervix. A subtotal hysterectomy (supracervical hysterectomy) indicates uterine corpus removal only. The cervix is preserved. The ovaries and fallopian tubes are not a part of the term hysterectomy. Terms such as "partial" hysterectomy are imprecise; however, these terms are often used by patients to imply that the uterus was removed but ovaries were left in situ.

Impact of Choice on Outcomes

Risk of Prolapse Recurrence
The effect of leaving the cervix in situ on 1-year prolapse recurrence rates following total robotic hysterectomy (TRH) vs. supracervical robotic hysterectomy (SRH) at the time of robotic sacrocolpopexy has been examined [14]. In a retrospective analysis of 83 women presenting with preoperative stage II or greater uterovaginal prolapse, women who underwent an SRH were 2.8 times more likely to have a recurrent prolapse, defined as ≥stage II in any compartment, at 1 year, compared with those who underwent a TRH. When a composite score was used, however, with success defined as no mesh exposure, no prolapse at or beyond point 0 on the Pelvic Organ Prolapse Quantification System (POP-Q),

and an answer of "no" to the prolapse-specific questions in the Pelvic Organ Prolapse Distress Inventory 6 (POPDI-6), there was no difference between the groups. More women in the SRH group reported feeling or seeing a bulge at 1 year after surgery and described it as "somewhat bothersome," although this difference was not statistically significant (18.6% vs. 10.3%, $p = 0.29$).

As the main difference in postoperative POP-Q score was seen in the mean values of point Ba, the authors of this study postulate their observations may be due to differences in technique of anterior and apical vaginal wall dissection, and that this may be more challenging when the cervix remains in situ. While in this study, as is the case in the authors' practice, the extent of the anterior dissection was reportedly carried down to the level of the trigone, it may be theorized that redundant or an excessively long anterior vaginal wall may be more difficult to affix to the mesh with the additional length of the cervix in situ. In other words, those patients with greater anterior vaginal wall length, or predominantly anterior prolapse, may be at greater risk of recurrence.

Others, however, have suggested that retention of the cervix may be beneficial as it allows continuity between DeLancey level 2 and level 1 apical support. Regardless of the potential role in recurrence, which needs further study, retention of the cervix has the important benefit of reducing the risk of postoperative mesh exposure, which will be discussed further in this chapter.

Sexual Function

Small studies in the past have suggested improvements in sexual function for women undergoing supracervical hysterectomy compared to those undergoing total hysterectomy. These improvements have been attributed to less vaginal vault pain, less vaginal shortening, potential advantages in cervicovaginal innervation, and continued production of cervical mucus in patients undergoing supracervical hysterectomy [15–17]. More recent and robust studies have not shown a difference in sexual function [18, 19]. In a cohort of 237 premenopausal women undergoing total

laparoscopic, supracervical laparoscopic, or total vaginal hysterectomy for benign uterine pathology, hysterectomy in general, regardless of technique, had significant positive effects on postoperative sexual function and quality of life as measured by Female Sexual Function Index (FSFI) and EuroQol five dimensions questionnaire (EQ-5D) scores, but postoperative scores did not differ among those women who retained their cervix versus those who did not [20]. One benefit worth mentioning, however, is that patients may return to vaginal intercourse more quickly following supracervical hysterectomy.

Risk of Mesh Complications

The risk of mesh exposure following sacrocolpopexy with poly-propylene mesh is significant, ranging from 3.4 to 27% [21–24]. Development of mesh exposure is likely multifactorial, as reflected in the wide variation in these reported rates. However, several consistent risk factors have emerged from the available data including the use of non-Type I polypropylene mesh (those with microporous or multi-filamentous structure) and smoking, both of which increase the risk of mesh exposure [22, 25].

Most relevant to the discussion in this chapter, however, is that concomitant hysterectomy increases the risk of mesh exposure. Based on multiple retrospective studies, it is now widely accepted that performing total hysterectomy at the time of sacrocolpopexy with mesh increases the risk of mesh-related complications following surgery compared with supracervical hysterectomy [23, 24, 26–28]. In a retrospective study of 102 women who underwent hysterectomy and sacrocolpopexy, a significantly higher mesh exposure rate of 14% was observed in the women who underwent total hysterectomy and sacrocolpopexy compared to a rate of 0% when supracervical hysterectomy was performed with sacrocolpopexy at 3 months follow-up [23]. In a similar retrospective analysis, total hysterectomy was associated with a sevenfold increase in mesh exposure rates compared to concomitant supracervical hysterectomy and sacrocolpopexy [28].

Therefore, if mesh sacrocolpopexy is indicated at time of hysterectomy, and presuming patient factors allow, it is recommended that a supracervical hysterectomy and sacrocervicopexy be performed. Despite the lessened risk of mesh complications with cervical preservation, it is still imperative that the surgeon has a thorough discussion of the risks of mesh placement and alternative native tissue repair options. Lastly, if the cervix cannot be spared and total hysterectomy must be performed, the patient must be informed of the elevated risk of mesh-related complications. Common-sense attention to technique, such as avoiding vaginotomy and avoiding mesh placement in a manner that overlaps the colpotomy suture line, may help minimize this risk.

Vaginotomy also increases the risk of mesh complications during sacrocolpopexy. Attention to preserving the integrity of the vaginal wall during dissection, particularly of the bladder off the anterior vagina, is paramount. Any defects or areas of devitalized tissue can result in vaginal mesh exposures.

Patient Selection and Evaluation

Candidates for cervical preservation include those with no history of abnormal cervical cytology and those with a remote history of abnormal cervical cytology, but recent normal screening. Regardless of history of cervical dysplasia, patients undergoing supracervical hysterectomy should be clearly counseled regarding the need to continue cervical cancer screening and only patients who are reliable for follow-up should be selected.

For those patients with a history of abnormal cervical cytology or high-risk human papillomavirus (HPV), the risk of cervical cancer or need to undergo future cervical excision must be assessed and considered when contemplating sacrocolpopexy with hysterectomy. The potential ramifications of not removing the cervix in a patient with prior abnormal cytology history should be thoroughly discussed with the patient including that

subsequent surgery to remove the cervix may be challenging. The decision whether or not to perform total hysterectomy, and therefore the risk of mesh exposure, should be weighed against the risk of recurrent or progressive cervical dysplasia. Non-mesh, native tissue-based approaches to prolapse repair, both vaginal and laparoscopic, should also be considered and discussed with all patients.

Technique of Robotic Hysterectomy and Sacrocervicopexy

Principles of the Laparoscopic Approach

The benefits of laparoscopic surgery with regard to length of hospital stay and patient recovery across surgical disciplines are now well-established. Although the laparoscopic approach is associated with favorable outcomes and minimal morbidity, the use of rigid laparoscopic instruments can constrain accessing and suturing in the deep pelvis. The surgical robot and its articulating instruments clearly provide an advantage in this setting. Nevertheless, many of the same principles first used for the laparoscopic approach can be applied to robotic hysterectomy. Many descriptions of the technique exist in the literature [29]. Here we will briefly describe our technique and tips for this approach.

Key Technical Steps

Surgical Team, Patient Positioning, and Port Placement

At least one proficient bedside assistant is needed. The use of steep Trendelenburg position is key to optimize exposure. Limited bowel preparation prior to surgery is routinely performed to minimize rectosigmoid distension, which may impact visualization of the sacral promontory. It is our practice to use enemas on the day prior to surgery. For women with chronic constipation, a magnesium citrate bowel cleansing regimen may

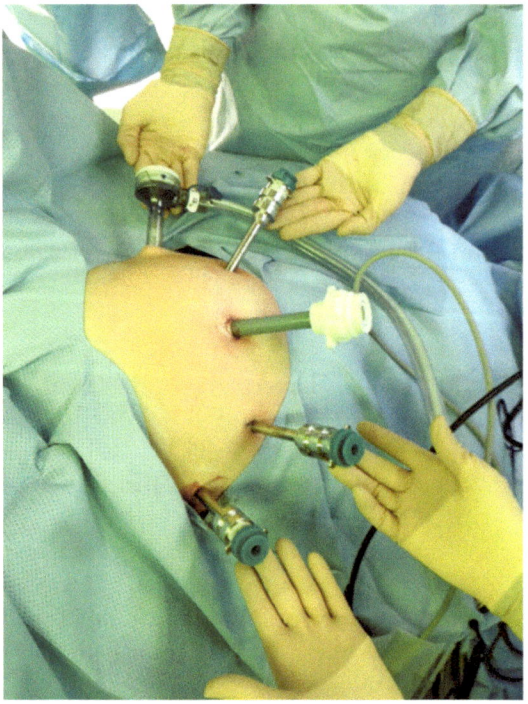

Fig. 7.2 Port placement (CT)

be more effective. After preparing and draping the patient, a Foley catheter is inserted. The uterine manipulator is then placed at this time (based on surgeon's preference). To maximize efficiency, this can be done by the surgeon or qualified assistant, while another member of the surgical team is setting up the required instruments and accessories for laparoscopy. Pneumoperitoneum is established. Ports are placed in a radial fashion as shown in Fig. 7.2.

After confirming the feasibility of the procedure laparoscopically, the robot is docked. We prefer a parallel (side) docking approach, which has the advantage of providing more space for the assistant to manipulate the uterus more comfortably. The robotic cart (the patient-side component with the arms) is positioned just medial to the patient's left lower extremity, which allows full range of motion of the robotic instruments as well as allowing the bedside surgeon access to the vaginal manipulator and right lateral port for assistance using laparoscopic instruments. This configuration may be reversed based on surgeon

preference and/or handedness. Monopolar scissors are then typically placed in the surgeon's dominant hand to facilitate dissection. ProGrasp™ forceps are then placed in the left lateral port, presuming the setup described above, and a bipolar energy device is placed in the remaining port.

Ureteral Identification

The ureters should be identified early and the course of each ureter should be clearly delineated prior to surgical management of the adnexa and the uterine vessels. A careful incision in the peritoneum overlying the ureter in the ovarian fossa bilaterally is made and extended to follow the course of the ureter toward the cardinal ligament (Fig. 7.3). This provides ready identification of the ureters during dissection for the remainder of the case. We find this is best performed as one of the first steps in the case to avoid challenges that may be posed by anatomical distortion and visualization as the case proceeds.

Consideration for Salpingectomy

Recent studies have suggested that high-grade serous ovarian cancer predominantly arises within the fallopian tubes [30, 31]. This data are strongly supported by observations of a decreased risk of ovarian cancer in women with a history of bilateral salpingectomy (BS) [32]. Therefore, risk reduction may theoretically be achieved by salpingectomy. In fact, although mainly based on data from three studies, a recent meta-analysis observed a 49% reduction in ovarian cancer risk among women who had undergone BS compared with those who had not [33].

These research findings are mainly applicable to two patient populations: those with genetic risk factors for ovarian cancer, and of interest to pelvic reconstructive surgeons, those women at population risk undergoing routine pelvic surgery for benign indications, who may benefit from incidental salpingectomy.

Salpingectomy is favorable to salpingo-oophorectomy at the time of hysterectomy for premenopausal women because it avoids the subsequent health risks associated with iatrogenic

Fig. 7.3 Creation of peritoneal window over left ureter near cardinal ligament

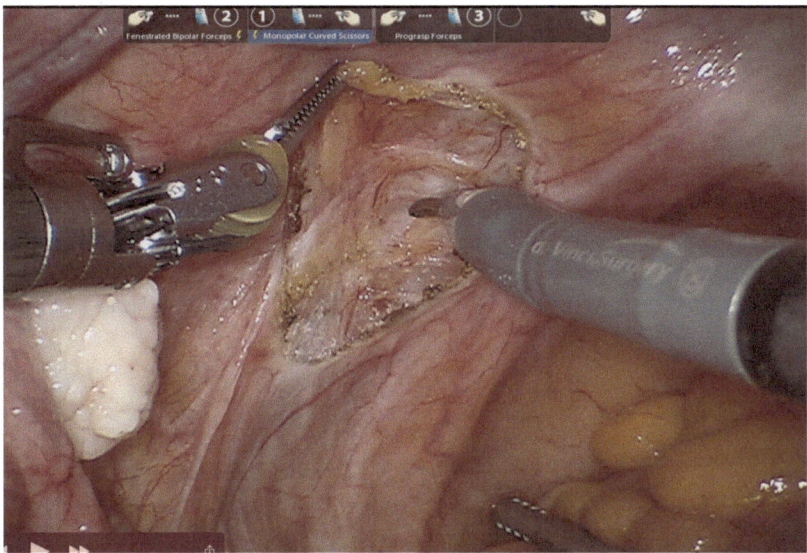

premature menopause after oophorectomy, including coronary artery disease and osteoporosis [34]. Recent studies have indicated that BS performed simultaneously with hysterectomy does not lead to impaired ovarian function and, aside from a minimal increase in operative time, does not increase surgical morbidity [35–37].

Thus, based on the available evidence, after thorough counseling of the risks and benefits of performing this procedure, it is the authors' practice to recommend prophylactic salpingectomy to patients undergoing hysterectomy at the time of sacrocolpopexy. This practice is also supported by recently published opinions from the American Congress of Obstetricians and Gynecologists and the Society of Gynecologic Oncology [38, 39].

Technique of Bilateral Salpingectomy

Salpingectomy requires only a minor change in surgical technique, yet does require meticulous attention in order to preserve ovarian vasculature. Salpingectomy should remove the tube completely from its fimbriated end up to the utero-tubal junction. Any fimbrial attachments on the ovary should be dessicated or removed. Care should be taken not to interrupt blood supply to the ovary through the infundibulopelvic ligament because the collateral vasculature from the tubal mesosalpinx is occluded during the tubal removal.

Technique of Hysterectomy

An energy device is typically used to desiccate and divide the round ligament, utero-ovarian ligament, and the fallopian tube. After the round ligament is transected, the incision is continued over the anterior leaf of the broad ligament toward the vesicouterine fold. The bladder is dissected from the lower uterine segment, at least 2 cm distal to the cervix. The bladder flap is created using monopolar cautery. The energy source is used to divide the broad ligament down to the cardinal ligament, and then to skeletonize the uterine artery, which is desiccated at the level of the uterocervical junction. The uterine artery is divided high on the uterocervical junction and medially hugging the "cup" of the uterine manipulator to avoid the ureter (Fig. 7.4). Identification of the uterocervical junction can also be done in cases without a manipulator by visualization and assistant port palpation of the small bulk of the proximal surface that creates an identifiable "knuckle" on the anterior surface of the utero-vaginal interface.

Fig. 7.4 Relative position of uterine vessels and ureter on left. Distance between uterine artery and ureter is increased cephalad displacement of uterine manipulator

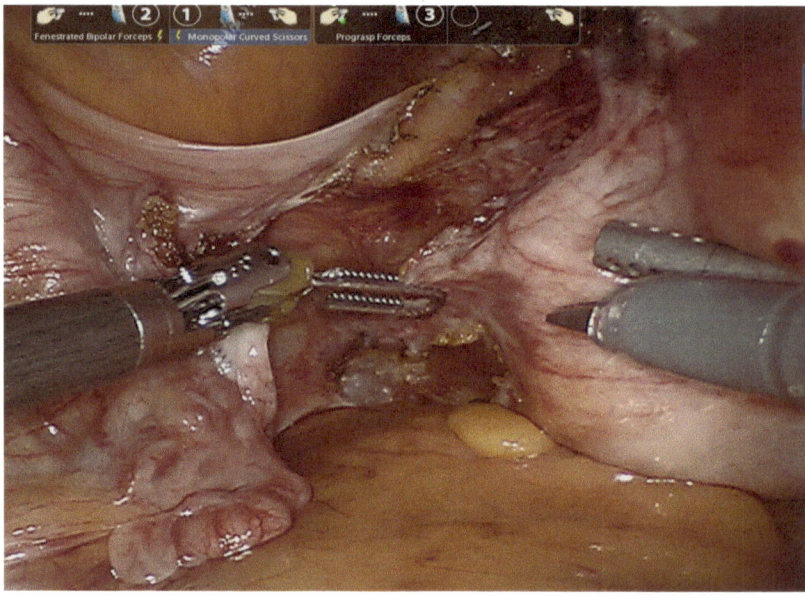

Removal of the Uterine Corpus

Many approaches have been described for retrieval of the uterine corpus including simple mechanical, manual, and electromechanical morcellation [40–43]. Techniques have been described to extract tissue fragments through an extended abdominal port incision, posterior colpotomy, transcervically, through an abdominal port, or through the morcellator itself [44–46].

The role of power morcellation and the recent controversy surrounding this technique will be discussed in detail in another chapter. In brief, it is the authors' practice to have a thorough discussion of the current evidence and risks of morcellation, including power morcellation, and the risks associated with underlying malignancy, which allows the patient to make an informed decision. In general, it is the authors' belief that the risk of occult uterine malignancy in the form of a leiomyosarcoma in women undergoing hysterectomy has been overestimated, particularly in women without suspected uterine myomas. However, the recent practice of contained morcellation is an enhancement as it reduces risk of the spread of benign myometrial and endometrial tissue, which can seed and become problematic for the patient. At the time

of this writing, it is currently our practice to perform contained manual morcellation with a scalpel through the midline abdominal port incision after placing the uterus in a specimen pouch, using Lahey clamps to stabilize the uterus as it is morcellated. This allows for controlled morcellation and requires minimal extension of the midline port incision. It further removes the requirement for the application of a power morcellator device and its negative connotation, deserved or otherwise.

Modifications for Sacrocervicopexy

Uterine Amputation

The technique of robotic sacrocolpopexy has been discussed in a previous chapter, so this discussion will be limited to modifications of the standard sacrocolpopexy technique and considerations when a sacrocervicopexy is being performed following supracervical hysterectomy. As in a sacrocolpopexy procedure, one should start at the sacral promontory and expose the anterior longitudinal ligament. If the necessary exposure cannot be accomplished robotically, then time should not be wasted on pursuing the other steps of the procedure robotically.

Fig. 7.5 After uterine amputation, anterior distension with vaginal manipulator assists dissection of anterior vagina and bladder

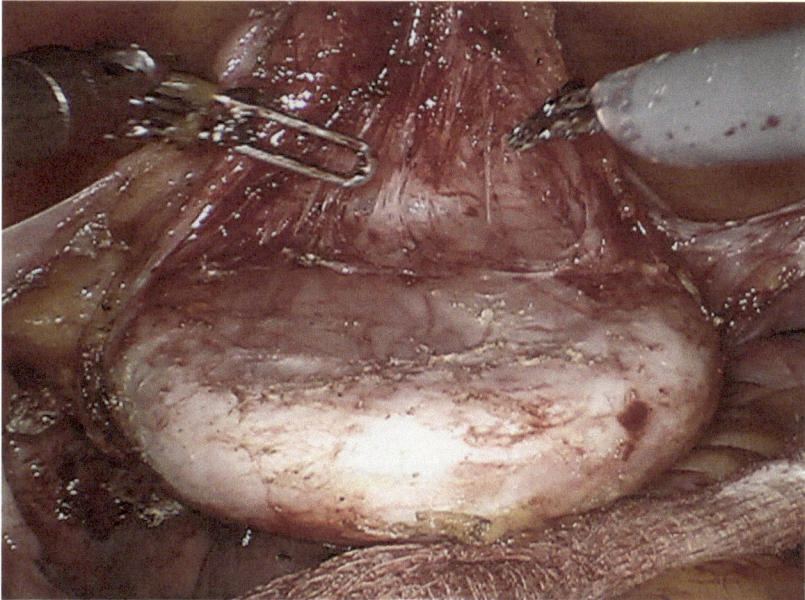

As discussed above, leaving the cervix in situ reduces the risk of mesh exposure and provides a solid platform for mesh fixation. A dissection of the anterior and posterior vaginal walls is key (Fig. 7.5). This is most easily performed prior to uterine amputation, as traction on the uterine corpus can be used to improve visualization of the surgical planes. However, this dissection can be completed after uterine corpus amputation. After the vessels are secured, the uterus is transected at or just below the level of the internal os, the presumed junction between endometrium and cervical columnar epithelium. An important technique during division of the uterine vasculature is to ensure cephalad displacement of the uterus by the bedside assistant. This maneuver will increase the distance between the ureter and the uterine artery. After division of the uterine vasculature, the uterus is amputated from the cervix. Though there are devices for this procedure (LiNA Loop Gold™, Lina Medical, Norcross GA), it is the authors' preference to use monopolar scissors. The pelvic sidewall makes a poor "work bench;" therefore, use of an instrument to provide a backboard for the cervix during amputation is suggested (Fig. 7.6). Cephalad traction on the fundus will help expedite the process. If a uterine manipulator has been used, it is generally removed after the midpoint or two thirds of the cervical width has been reached. The authors do not find it necessary to oversew the cervix, but care must be taken to ensure adequate hemostasis prior to mesh placement.

Management of the Endocervix

Cauterization or excision of the remaining endocervix is often performed with the goal of decreasing post-hysterectomy cyclic bleeding. In a randomized study of 140 women who underwent laparoscopic supracervical hysterectomy either with or without "reverse cervical conization," no differences in intermittent postoperative vaginal bleeding were observed at 12-month follow-up, occurring in 37% with conization and 33% without conization [47]. It remains the authors' practice to perform reverse conization by cauterization of the endocervical canal with monopolar scissor electrocautery (Fig. 7.7). This procedure adds minimally to the operative time, has little to no associated risks, and has been shown by others in a larger retrospective series to have a much lower postoperative intermittent vaginal bleeding rate of 2% [47, 48].

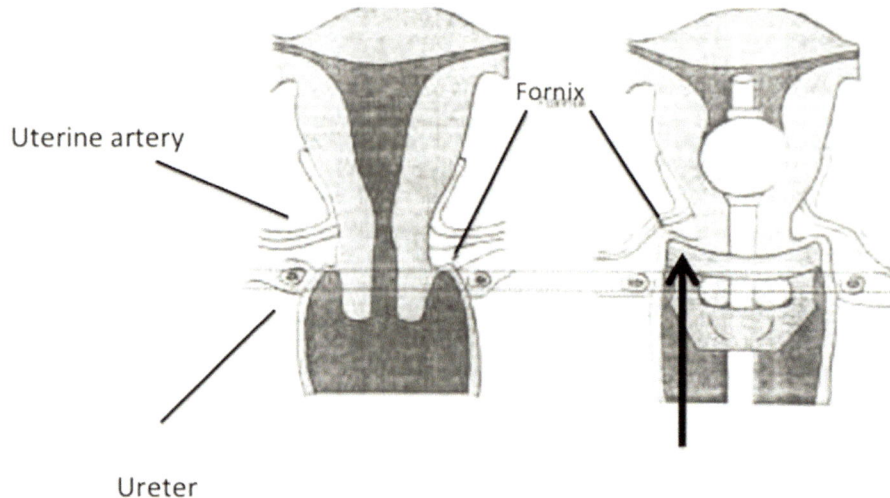

Fig. 7.6 Use of accessory instrument to serve as 'backboard' during amputation of uterine corpus to protect sidewall

Fig. 7.7 Cauterization of endocervix (reverse cone) after supracervical hysterectomy

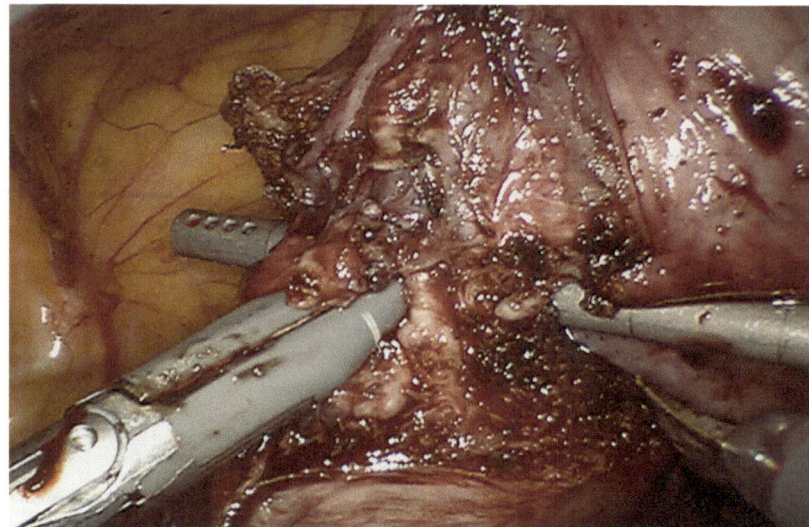

Vaginal Manipulation

Once the cervix is amputated, vaginal manipulation can be challenging. Many methods have been described such as using a robotic tenaculum to apply traction to the cervix or using malleable retractors or an EEA sizer to delineate the vaginal fornices, but devices such as the Colpassist™ vaginal fornix manipulator (Boston Scientific, Marl-borough, MA) are also very useful for this purpose (Fig. 7.8). This device is specifically designed for this purpose and provides a strong

suturing platform. Following these steps, sacrocervicopexy proceeds in a similar fashion to sacrocolpopexy.

Tips and Tricks

Selection of Uterine Manipulator Device

Uterine manipulators are useful tools to help expose anatomy during robotic/laparoscopic hysterectomy. Evidence is limited and there are

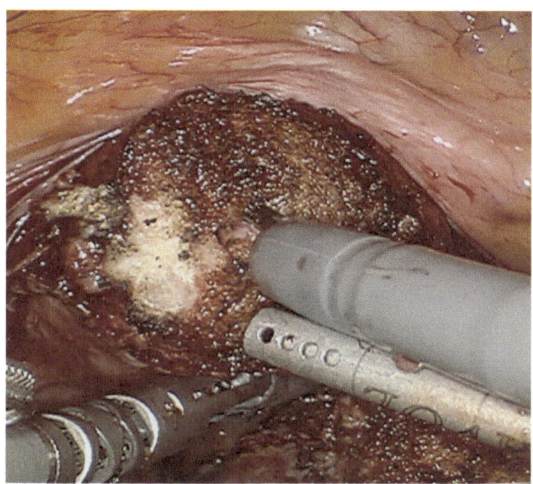

Fig. 7.8 (**a, b**) Vaginal positioning devices to assist in sacrocolpopexy and sacrocervicopexy. Source: http://www.bostonscientific.com/en-US/products/pelvic-floor-reconstruction/upsylon-y-mesh.html

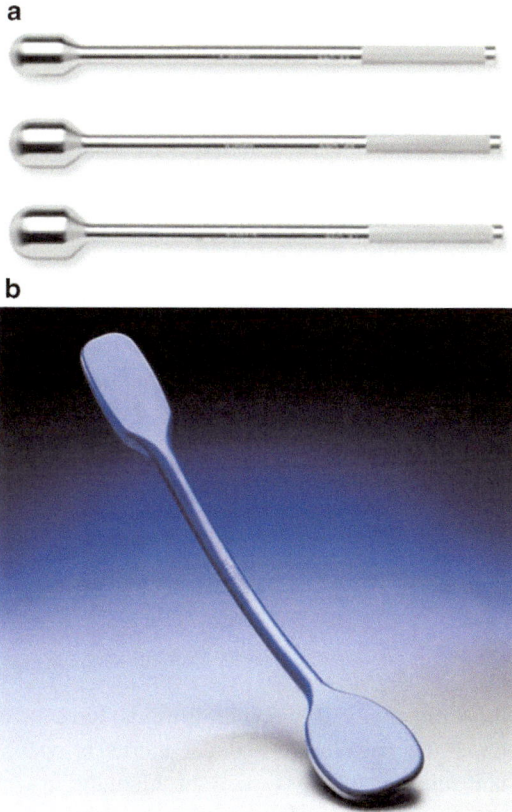

Fig. 7.9 Uterine manipulation devices to assist in uterine positioning during hysterectomy. (**a–c**) VCare® Uterine Manipulator/Elevator (ConMed Endosurgery, Utica, NY) http://www.conmed.com/endomechanical-instrumentation/vcare.php Vcare®. (**d**) Advincula Delineator™. VCare® Uterine Manipulator/Elevator (ConMed Endosurgery, Utica, NY). http://www.conmed.com/endomechanical-instrumentation/vcare.php

likely confounding factors in the available evidence, but use of a uterine manipulator may lessen the risk of ureteral injury [49, 50]. This is proposed to occur by allowing for improved lateral and cephalad movement of the uterus, increasing the distance between the cervix and ureter and facilitating dissection of the uterine artery and around the cervix. Uterine manipulators also allow for improved exposure of the cul-de-sac by providing a mechanism to elevate the uterus and provide delineation of the vaginal fornices, while maintaining pneumoperitoneum.

Data on the safety of these devices, in general, is limited and in need of further investigation. Yet, while alternative techniques for handling the uterus during laparoscopy have been published, it is currently the author's practice and opinion that using a uterine manipulator offers the most efficient method of uterine movement during surgery. It should be noted, however, that many FPMRS surgeons, in particular urologists who did not use a uterine manipulator in residency, do not use a manipulator for robotic supracervical hysterectomy.

The Vcare® manipulator (ConMed Corporation, Utica, New York) is a lightweight disposable instrument (Fig. 7.9a). It does not offer independent motion of the intrauterine tip, rather it uses leverage to manipulate the uterus. The Vcare handles easily, has a wide range of motion, offers good delineation, and maintains pneumoperitoneum well. However, the lightweight design may be less suitable to manipulate larger uteri. In the setting of an enlarged uterus (>12 cm), the authors also find the Advincula Delineator™ (CooperSurgical, Inc., Trumbull, Connecticut) useful (Fig. 7.9b). While similar to other disposable manipulators like the Vcare, no studies have examined its safety and efficacy.

Several other devices are available for uterine manipulation during robotic hysterectomy. A full discussion of all available devices is outside the scope of this text, so the authors would suggest the recent review by van den Haak et al. for the interested reader [51]. Considerations in selecting a device may include cost, surgeon preference, and device-specific complications. Surgeons should be aware of the risks unique to partly disposable or disposable lightweight uterine manipulators that require assembly, including the risk of adverse events due to disintegration of the instrument or retained parts. The goal is to use a device that is safe, user-friendly for the assistant, and appropriate for the surgical plan and patient's anatomy.

Handling Anatomical Abnormalities

Fibroids

Fibroids are present in over 60% of women. In most menopausal women, fibroids have often undergone involution and the uterus is smaller and subsequently less likely problematic in contributing to surgical management. However, in the patient where fibroids are still large, preoperative planning is relevant. Size and location of the fibroids can impact the feasibility of the laparoscopic approach (as fibroid location may limit access to the uterine pedicles), need for morcellation, type of uterine manipulator required, and location of port placement. While bimanual exam may be used to estimate uterine size, a more detailed anatomic assessment with ultrasound or MRI can be helpful to determine fibroid anatomy, guide patient counseling, and more certainly determine the operative plan. For these reasons, for women with prolapse selected to undergo the laparoscopic approach, it is the authors' practice to utilize MRI so that the number, size, and location of the fibroids can be determined. Intraoperative modifications, as mentioned above, are required for large myomas, particularly ones that are located in the broad ligament that may limit access to or distort the uterine vasculature.

Previous Cesarean Delivery

In women with previous cesarean deliveries, the lower uterine segment and vesicouterine plane will be scarred. This can lead to challenges in dissection of this potential space, increased bleeding, and an elevated risk of bladder injury during mobilization. For this portion of the hysterectomy, sharp dissection without excessive desiccation can help with visualization of the proper plane. Retrograde filling of the bladder can help with identification of the proper plane of dissection. If there is concern for a cystotomy, technical considerations for identification and repair are discussed later in this chapter.

Choice of Energy Device for Robotic Hysterectomy

The use of energy devices can be implemented using the assistant port and hand-held instruments. The robotic system also has options for integrated energy devices including monopolar and bipolar cautery instruments (electrical energy), the da Vinci Harmonic™ ACE (mechanical energy), and the da Vinci PK™ Dissecting Forceps (advanced bipolar).

All energy devices used in robotic/laparoscopic surgery have distinct thermal spreads depending on the power setting and application time. Few studies have examined the effect of different energy devices on outcomes of robotic/laparoscopic hysterectomy. Variability in surgeon technique and application of these devices as well as variation in patient anatomy can complicate studying the impact of energy device choice. In a small randomized study of 45 patients undergoing total laparoscopic hysterectomy, choice of device did not affect operative time, blood loss during surgery, or length of hospitalization [52].

It is the authors' opinion that an important consideration in selection of an energy device for use during robotic hysterectomy is thermal spread (lateral temperature changes which occur during use of the device). Devices with wide thermal spread may increase the risk of thermal injury to surrounding viscera, such as bowel, bladder, and particularly the ureter. Injuries may be either immediate or delayed. In an independent evaluation of thermal spread of robotic monopolar, bipolar, and ultrasonic instruments, among the worst performers were the robotic scissors, the automatic robotic PKS™, and LigaSure™ instruments [53]. These three devices, when activated for 1 s at 30 W (the most common clinical setting), showed lateral temperature increases above 45 °C as far as 2.6, 2.5, and 2.8 mm, respectively, from the instrument tip. The Maryland bipolar instrument had a 1.5 mm spread, and the Harmonic® scalpel had the lowest spread at 1.1 mm. A useful clinical tip from this study is that thermal spread can be mitigated by placing a second instrument alongside the energy device and touching the tissue to act as a heat sink. The thermal spread decreased by 0.5–1.0 mm for the instruments tested using this maneuver.

Other factors to consider in choosing an energy device include its utility as a grasping, dissecting, and dessicating instrument. Costs and operative time can be minimized with the use of fewer robotic instruments and less frequent instrument changes during the case.

Complications

Several potential complications specific to laparoscopic hysterectomy, robotic or otherwise, should be considered when selecting and counseling patients. Particularly for hysterectomy performed for benign indications, complications such as bleeding requiring transfusion or vascular or bowel injury are low [54]. Among lower urinary tract injuries, cystotomy is the most common. Women who have undergone prior cesarean deliveries are at an increased risk of bladder injury at the time of hysterectomy [55–57]. Cystotomy is most often successfully managed with primary closure and prolonged bladder drainage; however, cystotomy does carry a small risk of subsequent fistula formation [56]. Ureteral injury or stricture and uretero or vesicovaginal fistula remain among the most feared

complications. While some fistulas may be managed conservatively, a significant percentage will require reoperation to repair. Large uterine size, longer operative time, and bladder injury have been associated with vesicovaginal fistula formation [56].

If there is any concern for cystotomy, use of a diluted dye such as methylene blue to retrograde fill the bladder can help identify an injury. Fistulas can best be avoided by a multi-layered, water-tight, and tension-free cystotomy closure that is totally separated from the vaginal cuff. If a cystotomy occurs, and closure fulfills these requirements, one can continue safely with the procedure. Interposition tissue such as omentum can be considered to separate the cystotomy from the underlying mesh.

The sequelae of a ureteral injury are greatest when the injury is missed intraoperatively. These may be avoided by intraoperative cystoscopy with IV dye to assure ureteral efflux. IV infusion of either indigo carmine, methylene blue, or sodium fluorescein or preoperative administration of oral phenazopyridine are all excellent means to allow for cystoscopic visualization of ureteral efflux. However, cystoscopy is not 100% sensitive for detecting ureteral injury, particularly those of delayed thermal nature.

Of specific concern with the rise in robotic hysterectomy is an associated increase in the rate of urinary tract injury with this approach compared to vaginal hysterectomy. In a recent systematic review and meta-analysis of 79 studies of benign gynecologic surgeries, the rates of intra- and postoperative urinary tract injury per 1000 hysterectomies in which cystoscopy was not routinely used were highest for robotic procedures [58]. Intraoperatively detected rates of ureteral and bladder injury were markedly higher with routine intraoperative cystoscopy, but cystoscopy did not significantly impact the rate of postoperatively detected urinary tract injury (i.e., missed intraoperative injury) when all types of surgical approaches were considered. The studies examined in this meta-analysis are potentially limited by underreporting when routine cystoscopy was not used because of undiagnosed injuries and patients lost to follow-up. Data may reflect an ongoing learning curve for robotic hysterectomy, as some studies suggest these rates may be decreasing with time and increased surgeon experience, but this observation is nevertheless concerning and requires further follow-up.

Other rare but serious complications of total hysterectomy include vaginal cuff dehiscence with evisceration [59, 60], which has a variable timeframe of presentation and unfortunately has seen disproportionately higher rates following adoption of the laparoscopic and robotic approach. Hur et al. reported a vaginal cuff dehiscence rate of 0.11% with the vaginal approach versus 0.75% with total laparoscopic hysterectomy [61]. More recently in a study of 2382 total hysterectomies, there was a 0.96% rate of cuff dehiscence, and robotic approach was associated with increased odds of cuff dehiscence in a multivariate analysis [62]. The reason for this remains unclear, but the cause is likely multifactorial. Use of thermal energy may contribute [63, 64]. Sexual intercourse may be a triggering event [65], so it is important to examine patients and ensure complete cuff healing before permitting them to return to sexual activity. Not unexpectedly, most evidence at this point, however, points toward the technique of vaginal cuff suturing as the main factor likely driving this concerning trend [62, 66, 67]. While further studies are certainly needed, it is the authors' opinion, as well as others [66], that the magnified view of the robotic laparoscope, by giving a false sense of the depth of suture placement, leads the surgeon to include an insufficient amount of tissue when suturing the cuff closed. Inadequate (i.e., loose) tensioning may also play a role, facilitated by the lack of haptic feedback.

Conclusions

Hysterectomy is likely to remain a mainstay in the treatment of pelvic organ prolapse, particularly as an adjunct to sacrocolpopexy.

Supracervical hysterectomy with bilateral salpingectomy should be performed when patients allow. This will decrease the risk of mesh-related complications from cervix removal and the development of ovarian cancer from retained fallopian tubes. Robotic technology has expanded access to the laparoscopic approach for pelvic surgeons and allowed this procedure to be performed with less patient discomfort and shorter hospital stay, but is not without risks associated with adoption of a new approach. Thoughtful preoperative planning and the technical considerations discussed in this chapter can help minimize the risk of complications and achieve a good outcome for the patient.

References

1. Bonney V. The principles that should underlie all operations for prolapse*. BJOG. 1934;41:669–83. doi:10.1111/j.1471-0528.1934.tb08799.x.
2. Gracia M, Perelló M, Bataller E, et al. Comparison between laparoscopic sacral hysteropexy and subtotal hysterectomy plus cervicopexy in pelvic organ prolapse: a pilot study. Neurourol Urodyn. 2015;34:654–8. doi:10.1002/nau.22641.
3. Pan K, Cao L, Ryan NA, et al. Laparoscopic sacral hysteropexy versus laparoscopic sacrocolpopexy with hysterectomy for pelvic organ prolapse. Int Urogynecol J. 2016;27:93–101. doi:10.1007/s00192-015-2775-9.
4. Maher CF, Cary MP, Slack MC, et al. Uterine preservation or hysterectomy at sacrospinous colpopexy for uterovaginal prolapse? Int Urogynecol J Pelvic Floor Dysfunct. 2001;12:381–4.
5. Maher CF, Carey MP, Murray CJ. Laparoscopic suture hysteropexy for uterine prolapse. Obstet Gynecol. 2001;97:1010–4.
6. Lewis CM, Culligan P. Sacrohysteropexy followed by successful pregnancy and eventual reoperation for prolapse. Int Urogynecol J. 2012;23:957–9. doi:10.1007/s00192-011-1631-9.
7. Zucchi A, Lazzeri M, Porena M, et al. Uterus preservation in pelvic organ prolapse surgery. Nat Rev Urol. 2010;7:626–33. doi:10.1038/nrurol.2010.164.
8. Committee on Practice Bulletins—Gynecology. Practice bulletin no. 128: diagnosis of abnormal uterine bleeding in reproductive-aged women. Obstet Gynecol. 2012;120:197–206. doi:10.1097/AOG.0b013e318262e320.
9. Committee on Practice Bulletins—Gynecology. Practice bulletin no. 136: management of abnormal uterine bleeding associated with ovulatory dysfunction. Obstet Gynecol. 2013;122:176–85. doi:10.1097/01.AOG.0000431815.52679.bb.
10. Ramm O, Gleason JL, Segal S, et al. Utility of preoperative endometrial assessment in asymptomatic women undergoing hysterectomy for pelvic floor

dysfunction. Int Urogynecol J. 2012;23:913–7. doi:10.1007/s00192-012-1694-2.

11. Frick AC, Walters MD, Larkin KS, Barber MD. Risk of unanticipated abnormal gynecologic pathology at the time of hysterectomy for uterovaginal prolapse. Am J Obstet Gynecol. 2010;202:507.e1–4. doi:10.1016/j.ajog.2010.01.077.

12. Bogani G, Serati M, Cromi A, Ghezzi F. Risk of undiagnosed uterine malignancies at the time of robotic supracervical hysterectomy and sacrocolpopexy. Eur Urol. 2015;67:352. doi:10.1016/j.eururo.2014.08.058.

13. McPencow AM, Erekson EA, Guess MK, et al. Cost-effectiveness of endometrial evaluation prior to morcellation in surgical procedures for prolapse. Am J Obstet Gynecol. 2013;209:22.e1–9. doi:10.1016/j.ajog.2013.03.033.

14. Myers EM, Siff L, Osmundsen B, et al. Differences in recurrent prolapse at 1 year after total vs supracervical hysterectomy and robotic sacrocolpopexy. Int Urogynecol J. 2015;26:585–9. doi:10.1007/s00192-014-2551-2.

15. El-Mowafi D, Madkour W, Lall C, Wenger J-M. Laparoscopic supracervical hysterectomy versus laparoscopic-assisted vaginal hysterectomy. J Am Assoc Gynecol Laparosc. 2004;11:175–80.

16. Lieng M, Qvigstad E, Istre O, et al. Long-term outcomes following laparoscopic supracervical hysterectomy. BJOG. 2008;115:1605–10. doi:10.1111/j.1471-0528.2008.01854.x.

17. Lyons T. Laparoscopic supracervical versus total hysterectomy. J Minim Invasive Gynecol. 2007;14:275–7. doi:10.1016/j.jmig.2006.10.032.

18. Flory N, Bissonnette F, Amsel RT, Binik YM. The psychosocial outcomes of total and subtotal hysterectomy: a randomized controlled trial. J Sex Med. 2006;3:483–91. doi:10.1111/j.1743-6109.2006.00229.x.

19. Pouwels NSA, Brito LGO, Einarsson JI, et al. Cervix removal at the time of hysterectomy: factors affecting patients' choice and effect on subsequent sexual function. Eur J Obstet Gynecol Reprod Biol. 2015;195:67–71. doi:10.1016/j.ejogrb.2015.09.040.

20. Radosa JC, Meyberg-Solomayer G, Kastl C, et al. Influences of different hysterectomy techniques on patients' postoperative sexual function and quality of life. J Sex Med. 2014;11:2342–50. doi:10.1111/jsm.12623.

21. Nygaard IE, McCreery R, Brubaker L, et al. Abdominal sacrocolpopexy: a comprehensive review. Obstet Gynecol. 2004;104:805–23. doi:10.1097/01.AOG.0000139514.90897.07.

22. Cundiff GW, Varner E, Visco AG, et al. Risk factors for mesh/suture erosion following sacral colpopexy. Am J Obstet Gynecol. 2008;199:688.e1–5. doi:10.1016/j.ajog.2008.07.029.

23. Osmundsen BC, Clark A, Goldsmith C, et al. Mesh erosion in robotic sacrocolpopexy. Female Pelvic Med Reconstr Surg. 2012;18:86–8. doi:10.1097/SPV.0b013e318246806d.

24. Culligan PJ, Murphy M, Blackwell L, et al. Long-term success of abdominal sacral colpopexy using synthetic mesh. Am J Obstet Gynecol. 2002;187:1473–82. doi:10.1067/mob.2002.129160.

25. Visco AG, Weidner AC, Barber MD, et al. Vaginal mesh erosion after abdominal sacral colpopexy. Am J Obstet Gynecol. 2001;184:297–302. doi:10.1067/mob.2001.109654.

26. Deffieux X, Letouzey V, Savary D, et al. Prevention of complications related to the use of prosthetic meshes in prolapse surgery: guidelines for clinical practice. Eur J Obstet Gynecol Reprod Biol. 2012;165:170–80. doi:10.1016/j.ejogrb.2012.09.001.

27. Akyol A, Akca A, Ulker V, et al. Additional surgical risk factors and patient characteristics for mesh erosion after abdominal sacrocolpopexy. J Obstet Gynaecol Res. 2014;40:1368–74. doi:10.1111/jog.12363.

28. Bensinger G, Lind L, Lesser M, et al. Abdominal sacral suspensions: analysis of complications using permanent mesh. Am J Obstet Gynecol. 2005;193:2094–8. doi:10.1016/j.ajog.2005.07.066.

29. Kho RM, Hilger WS, Hentz JG, et al. Robotic hysterectomy: technique and initial outcomes. Am J Obstet Gynecol. 2007;197:113.e1–4. doi:10.1016/j.ajog.2007.05.005.

30. Kim J, Coffey DM, Creighton CJ, et al. High-grade serous ovarian cancer arises from fallopian tube in a mouse model. Proc Natl Acad Sci U S A. 2012;109:3921–6. doi:10.1073/pnas.1117135109.

31. Erickson BK, Conner MG, Landen CN. The role of the fallopian tube in the origin of ovarian cancer. Am J Obstet Gynecol. 2013;209:409–14. doi:10.1016/j.ajog.2013.04.019.

32. Falconer H, Yin L, Grönberg H, Altman D. Ovarian cancer risk after salpingectomy: a nationwide population-based study. J Natl Cancer Inst. 2015. doi:10.1093/jnci/dju410.

33. Yoon S-H, Kim S-N, Shim S-H, et al. Bilateral salpingectomy can reduce the risk of ovarian cancer in the general population: a meta-analysis. Eur J Cancer. 2016;55:38–46. doi:10.1016/j.ejca.2015.12.003.

34. Parker WH, Feskanich D, Broder MS, et al. Long-term mortality associated with oophorectomy compared with ovarian conservation in the nurses' health study. Obstet Gynecol. 2013;121:709–16. doi:10.1097/AOG.0b013e3182864350.

35. Findley AD, Siedhoff MT, Hobbs KA, et al. Short-term effects of salpingectomy during laparoscopic hysterectomy on ovarian reserve: a pilot randomized controlled trial. Fertil Steril. 2013;100:1704–8. doi:10.1016/j.fertnstert.2013.07.1997.

36. Morelli M, Venturella R, Mocciaro R, et al. Prophylactic salpingectomy in premenopausal low-risk women for ovarian cancer: primum non nocere. Gynecol Oncol. 2013;129:448–51. doi:10.1016/j.ygyno.2013.03.023.

37. McAlpine JN, Hanley GE, Woo MMM, et al. Opportunistic salpingectomy: uptake, risks, and com-

plications of a regional initiative for ovarian cancer prevention. Am J Obstet Gynecol. 2014;210:471. e1–11. doi:10.1016/j.ajog.2014.01.003.

38. Walker JL, Powell CB, Chen L-M, et al. Society of Gynecologic Oncology recommendations for the prevention of ovarian cancer. Cancer. 2015;121:2108–20. doi:10.1002/cncr.29321.

39. Committee on Gynecologic Practice. Committee opinion no. 620: salpingectomy for ovarian cancer prevention. Obstet Gynecol. 2015;125:279–81. doi:10.1097/01.AOG.0000459871.88564.09.

40. Brucker S, Solomayer E, Zubke W, et al. A newly developed morcellator creates a new dimension in minimally invasive surgery. J Minim Invasive Gynecol. 2007;14:233–9. doi:10.1016/j.jmig.2006.10.004.

41. Donnez O, Jadoul P, Squifflet J, Donnez J. A series of 3190 laparoscopic hysterectomies for benign disease from 1990 to 2006: evaluation of complications compared with vaginal and abdominal procedures. BJOG. 2009;116:492–500. doi:10.1111/j.1471-0528.2008.01966.x.

42. Morrison JE, Jacobs VR. Outpatient laparoscopic hysterectomy in a rural ambulatory surgery center. J Am Assoc Gynecol Laparosc. 2004;11:359–64.

43. Phillips DR, Nathanson HG, Milim SJ, Haselkorn JS. 100 laparoscopic hysterectomies in private practice and visiting professorship programs. J Am Assoc Gynecol Laparosc. 1995;3:47–53.

44. De Grandi P, Chardonnens E, Gerber S. The morcellator knife: a new laparoscopic instrument for supracervical hysterectomy and morcellation. Obstet Gynecol. 2000;95:777–8.

45. Kresch AJ, Lyons TL, Westland AB, et al. Laparoscopic supracervical hysterectomy with a new disposable morcellator. J Am Assoc Gynecol Laparosc. 1998;5:203–6.

46. Rosenblatt PL, Apostolis CA, Hacker MR, DiSciullo A. Laparoscopic supracervical hysterectomy with transcervical morcellation and sacrocervicopexy: initial experience with a novel surgical approach to uterovaginal prolapse. J Minim Invasive Gynecol. 2012;19:749–55. doi:10.1016/j.jmig.2012.06.009.

47. Berner E, Qvigstad E, Langebrekke A, Lieng M. Laparoscopic supracervical hysterectomy performed with and without excision of the endocervix: a randomized controlled trial. J Minim Invasive Gynecol. 2013;20:368–75. doi:10.1016/j.jmig.2013.01.003.

48. Erian J, Hassan M, Pachydakis A, et al. Efficacy of laparoscopic subtotal hysterectomy in the management of menorrhagia: 400 consecutive cases. BJOG. 2008;115:742–8. doi:10.1111/j.1471-0528.2008.01698.x.

49. Janssen PF, Brölmann HAM, Huirne JAF. Recommendations to prevent urinary tract injuries during laparoscopic hysterectomy: a systematic Delphi procedure among experts. J Minim Invasive Gynecol. 2011;18:314–21. doi:10.1016/j. jmig.2011.01.007.

50. Janssen PF, Brölmann HAM, Huirne JAF. Causes and prevention of laparoscopic ureter injuries: an analysis of 31 cases during laparoscopic hysterectomy in the Netherlands. Surg Endosc. 2013;27:946–56. doi:10.1007/s00464-012-2539-2.

51. van den Haak L, Alleblas C, Nieboer TE, et al. Efficacy and safety of uterine manipulators in laparoscopic surgery: a review. Arch Gynecol Obstet. 2015;292:1003–11. doi:10.1007/s00404-015-3727-9.

52. Aytan H, Nazik H, Narin R, et al. Comparison of the use of LigaSure, HALO PKS cutting forceps, and ENSEAL tissue sealer in total laparoscopic hysterectomy: a randomized trial. J Minim Invasive Gynecol. 2014;21:650–5. doi:10.1016/j. jmig.2014.01.010.

53. Hefermehl LJ, Largo RA, Hermanns T, et al. Lateral temperature spread of monopolar, bipolar and ultrasonic instruments for robot-assisted laparoscopic surgery. BJU Int. 2014;114:245–52. doi:10.1111/bju.12498.

54. Aarts JW, Nieboer TE, Johnson N, et al. Surgical approach to hysterectomy for benign gynaecological disease. Cochrane Database Syst Rev. 2015. doi:10.1002/14651858.CD003677.pub5.

55. Rooney CM, Crawford AT, Vassallo BJ, et al. Is previous cesarean section a risk for incidental cystotomy at the time of hysterectomy? A case-controlled study. Am J Obstet Gynecol. 2005;193:2041–4. doi:10.1016/j.ajog.2005.07.090.

56. Duong TH, Taylor DP, Meeks GR. A multicenter study of vesicovaginal fistula following incidental cystotomy during benign hysterectomies. Int Urogynecol J. 2011;22:975–9. doi:10.1007/s00192-011-1375-6.

57. Duong TH, Patterson TM. Lower urinary tract injuries during hysterectomy in women with a history of two or more cesarean deliveries: a secondary analysis. Int Urogynecol J. 2014;25:1037–40. doi:10.1007/s00192-013-2324-3.

58. Teeluckdharry B, Gilmour D, Flowerdew G. Urinary tract injury at benign gynecologic surgery and the role of cystoscopy: a systematic review and meta-analysis. Obstet Gynecol. 2015;126:1161–9. doi:10.1097/AOG.0000000000001096.

59. Patravali N, Kulkarni T. Bowel evisceration through the vaginal vault: a delayed complication following hysterectomy. J Obstet Gynaecol. 2007;27:211. doi:10.1080/01443610601157695.

60. Walsh CA, Sherwin JRA, Slack M. Vaginal evisceration following total laparoscopic hysterectomy: case report and review of the literature. Aust N Z J Obstet Gynaecol. 2007;47:516–9. doi:10.1111/j.1479-828X.2007.00793.x.

61. Hur H-C, Donnellan N, Mansuria S, et al. Vaginal cuff dehiscence after different modes of hysterectomy. Obstet Gynecol. 2011;118:794–801. doi:10.1097/AOG.0b013e31822f1c92.

62. Fuchs Weizman N, Einarsson JI, Wang KC, et al. Vaginal cuff dehiscence: risk factors and associated morbidities. JSLS. 2015. doi:10.4293/JSLS.2013.00351.

63. Hur H-C, Guido RS, Mansuria SM, et al. Incidence and patient characteristics of vaginal cuff dehiscence after different modes of hysterectomies. J Minim Invasive Gynecol. 2007;14:311–7. doi:10.1016/j.jmig.2006.11.005.

64. Lawlor ML, Rao R, Manahan KJ, Geisler JP. Electrosurgical settings and vaginal cuff complications. JSLS. 2015. doi:10.4293/JSLS.2015.00088.

65. Ceccaroni M, Berretta R, Malzoni M, et al. Vaginal cuff dehiscence after hysterectomy: a multi-center retrospective study. Eur J Obstet Gynecol Reprod Biol. 2011;158:308–13. doi:10.1016/j.ejogrb.2011.05.013.

66. Uccella S, Ghezzi F, Mariani A, et al. Vaginal cuff closure after minimally invasive hysterectomy: our experience and systematic review of the literature. Am J Obstet Gynecol. 2011;205:119.e1–12. doi:10.1016/j.ajog.2011.03.024.

67. Rettenmaier MA, Abaid LN, Brown JV, et al. Dramatically reduced incidence of vaginal cuff dehiscence in gynecologic patients undergoing endoscopic closure with barbed sutures: a retrospective cohort study. Int J Surg. 2015;19:27–30. doi:10.1016/j.ijsu.2015.05.007.

The Role of Power Morcellation and Controversies

A. Lenore Ackerman

Introduction

In female pelvic floor reconstruction, hysterectomy is frequently performed at the time of concurrent colpopexy for pelvic organ prolapse. Robotic-assisted sacrocolpopexy (RASC), the laparoscopic version of the gold-standard approach to uterine prolapse repair, offers many benefits, such as less post-operative pain, a quicker recovery, fewer wound complications, less post-operative morbidity, and a shorter hospital stay. Frequently, the uterus is too large to be removed from the abdominal cavity through either the vaginal outlet or trocar incisions. When this is the case, as in patients with uterine leiomyomas ("fibroids"), either a larger incision must be made ("mini-laparotomy") or the specimen needs to be reduced in size by morcellation. This can be done by hand, as with a scissors or scalpel, or using an electromechanical surgical instrument commonly called a "power morcellator." This instrument uses a rotating cylindrical knife inserted through a laparoscopic trocar incision to divide large tissues into smaller pieces that can be removed through the blade's cylindrical core

(Fig. 8.1). Such devices are absolutely necessary to allow patients with very large uterine fibroids to enjoy the benefits of minimally invasive surgery.

Prior to the adoption of power morcellation, more than 80% of gynecologic surgeons reported significant hand fatigue and even carpal tunnel syndrome associated with hand morcellation, with increasing severity correlating with greater caseloads [1]. Power morcellation was first introduced by Steiner in 1993 [2] and approved by the US Food and Drug Administration (FDA) in 1995. The technology greatly improved the capacity to morcellate large tissues, such as the uterus or prostate, which previously required open surgery, made minimally invasive surgical techniques practical for a larger number of women, particularly obese patients, and reduced surgeon strain and injury. Such perceived benefits led to the rapid adoption of laparoscopic hysterectomy with power morcellation as the most common procedure performed for uterine fibroids.

Power Morcellation and the FDA

In April of 2014, however, the FDA issued a safety communication [3] discouraging the use of power morcellators due to the risk of potential upstaging of uterine sarcoma in undiagnosed patients. The report was prompted by the case of a Boston anesthesiologist who underwent

A. Lenore Ackerman, M.D., Ph.D. (✉)
Department of Surgery, Division of Urology,
Cedars-Sinai Medical Center, 99 N. La Cienega
Blvd., Suite 307, Beverly Hills, CA 90211, USA
e-mail: a.lenore.ackerman@cshs.org

© Springer International Publishing AG 2018
J.T. Anger, K.S. Eilber (eds.), *The Use of Robotic Technology in Female Pelvic Floor Reconstruction*, DOI 10.1007/978-3-319-59611-2_8

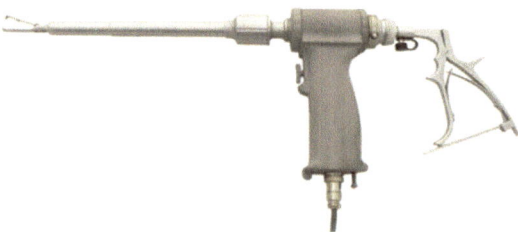

Fig. 8.1 Power morcellation device. The toothed grasper is used to deliver the tissue to be morcellated to the rotating cylindrical blade housed by the external beveled sheath

laparoscopic hysterectomy with morcellation for presumed fibroids in 2013. Pathologic review revealed uterine leiomyosarcoma (ULMS). At re-intervention, the sarcoma was found to have spread in the abdominal cavity, and she required aggressive treatment for this advanced stage cancer. Attributing her poor outcome to the use of morcellation during her surgery, she and her husband, a cardiothoracic surgeon, then called for an "immediate moratorium on intracorporeal morcellation during minimally invasive hysterectomy" in an open letter to President Barrack Obama, Senator Elizabeth Warren of Massachusetts, the FDA Commissioner, and the leadership of multiple professional medical organizations. Interestingly, they gave special mention to robotic-assisted surgery, criticizing Intuitive Surgical, Inc., for the absence of a "readily available warning label advising against its use to morcellate tumors with malignant potential inside the body" [4] despite concessions that the da Vinci robot is not itself a "morcellator." This petition prompted a review of power morcellation by the FDA. In their meta-analysis of 18 studies, the FDA reported a risk of 0.28% and 0.2% for undiagnosed uterine sarcoma (any histology) and ULMS, respectively, in patients with presumed fibroids. Explaining that this risk was higher than previously estimated, the "FDA is warning against the use of laparoscopic power morcellators in the majority of women undergoing myomectomy or hysterectomy for treatment of fibroids" [3]. In November 2014, the FDA warning was upgraded to a black-box warning stating that morcellation was contraindicated in perimenopausal or postmenopausal women and

in any "candidates for en-bloc tissue removal" [5], which could be literally interpreted to include all women.

While not specifically calling for a ban of power morcellators, this announcement spawned a heated debate throughout the medical and lay community. The news media has fanned the flames of public fear over the use of power morcellation with features such as "When Hysterectomy is a Death Sentence" (*USA Today*, February 2014), "A Surgical Procedure's Risks, Unmentioned" (*New York Times*, March 2014), and "Deadly Medicine: A Common Surgery for Women and the Cancer It Leaves Behind" (*Wall Street Journal*, September 2014). Overall, several themes emerged from the reporting on this issue in the popular press, including the impressions that the risk of dying from cancer is high when power morcellation is used, that morcellation is directly responsible for the spread of cancer, that patient outcomes would be better if other surgical techniques are used, and that device manufacturers, hospitals, and doctors were aware of this risk and sought to cover it up.

This portrayal of the debate has resulted in a powerful community backlash. Hundreds of lawsuits against physicians and device manufacturers are pending trial in state and federal courts. The Federal Bureau of Investigation is reportedly investigating power morcellators and whether manufacturers were aware of the risk of cancer spread. Many hospitals and hospital systems across the country have halted or limited the use of power morcellation. Some insurers have stopped covering the procedure, while others, like UnitedHealth Group Inc., the nation's largest health insurer, have begun to require prior authorizations. Johnson & Johnson, the parent company of Ethicon, Inc., manufacturer of the Gynecare Morcellex power morcellator, pulled the device from the market in July 2014. All of these restrictions have caused the vast majority of gynecologic surgeons to change their method of fibroid removal after the FDA report. One study reported that 84% of surgeons had switched methods of fibroid removal after the FDA warning from laparoscopic surgery with morcellation to mini-laparotomy [6].

The medical community overall has been frustrated by the drastic change induced by this public outcry. A recent commentary by Lisa Rosenbaum in the *New England Journal of Medicine* expressed this sentiment well, stating that "our capacity to speak science to emotion seems to be collapsing" [7]. Statements from gynecologists have echoed again and again the lack of solid scientific evidence to support a ban on the use of power morcellation, reiterating that minimally invasive surgery and morcellation have benefitted hundreds of thousands of women, and it would be a "disservice to deny these women this option" [8]. Statements from multiple professional societies have stressed the importance of informed consent in shared decision making for the treatment of presumed benign fibroids. While the FDA cannot control the quality of the data available, they have been harshly criticized for the choice of data included in their meta-analysis. The FDA report did not address conflicting data from multiple meta-analyses documenting cancer incidences more than an order of magnitude lower than that documented in the warning [9]. In addition, the exclusion of studies in which no cancer was diagnosed and the inclusion of cases in which morcellation should probably not have been offered may have drastically overestimated the cancer risk [10, 11]. The American Association of Gynecologic Laparoscopists' Tissue Extraction Task Force [12] emphasized that the studies examined by the FDA were not stratified by risk factors for sarcoma and did not reflect data for reproductive-age women. The reports were retrospective, representing data from referral centers or single institutions, spanned several decades with various histopathologic criteria, and even included women with preoperative diagnoses of sarcoma. A *Position Statement* from the Society of Gynecologic Oncology [13] echoes these points and recognizes that ULMS and endometrial stromal sarcomas, for which there are no reliable methods to differentiate from fibroids, have a very poor prognosis even when removed intact.

While many practitioners believe that there is a tremendous benefit in continuing to allow morcellation to be used in appropriately selected patients, the choice to do so is disappearing. While there is no denying that individuals with occult aggressive malignancies have suffered greatly from their disease, it is our responsibility to evaluate the data behind the claims in the FDA warning and determine if the conclusions are well-founded and benefit our patients and society.

"Many women choose to undergo laparoscopic hysterectomy or myomectomy because these procedures are associated with benefits such as a shorter post-operative recovery time and a reduced risk of infection compared to abdominal hysterectomy and myomectomy." [3]

Overall, there are significant benefits to patients who undergo minimally invasive surgeries compared to open techniques [14]. Patients have smaller incisions, less post-operative pain, and shorter hospital stays [15]. In the case of hysterectomy, these benefits are even more pronounced with the assistance of the operative robot [16]. In addition to improved recovery for patients, there are fewer complications, such as wound infections, bleeding requiring transfusion, deep vein thrombosis, nerve injury, and genitourinary and gastrointestinal tract injuries [17], many of which will require readmission and reoperation. Patients undergoing open abdominal hysterectomy have a threefold greater risk of mortality than those who undergo laparoscopic hysterectomy [18].

While generally associated with improved patient outcomes, there are complications unique to the use of power morcellation devices. Direct injuries to the bowel and large vessels, while uncommon, can occur. A review of the Manufacturer and User Facility Device Experience (MAUDE) database in 2014 revealed 66 reports of direct injuries, six of which were fatal [19]. These included injuries to the small and large bowel (31/66), large blood vessels (27/66), kidney (3/66), ureter (3/66), bladder (1/66), and diaphragm (1/66). Given the millions of procedures performed, these injury rates remain very low.

An additional concern with intracorporeal morcellation of any type is the development of parasitic fibroids or iatrogenic endometriosis, which can require repeat surgical treatment. Small chips or tissue fragments released from the specimen during morcellation can implant on the peritoneum and grow to cause symptoms such as pain, gastrointestinal or ureteral obstruction, or local organ dysfunction by exerting a mass effect [20, 21]. Even if asymptomatic, identification of an unknown abdominal mass frequently necessitates additional workup and surgical removal. The risk of such masses developing after uterine fibroid removal appears to increase significantly with the use of morcellation, with an overall incidence of 0.12–0.9% [22–24]. Exposure to gonadal steroid hormones increases this risk, with both premenopausal status and hormone replacement therapy promoting parasitic fibroid development and growth.

The most concerning of the complications attributed to morcellation, however, is the risk that an unrecognized malignancy could be spread in the abdomen and pelvis, leading to poor oncologic outcomes. This is the focus of the FDA safety warning and the main target of activism opposing the use of power morcellation.

> "If laparoscopic power morcellation is performed in women with unsuspected uterine sarcoma, there is a risk that the procedure will spread the cancerous tissue within the abdomen and pelvis, significantly worsening the patient's long-term survival." [3]

Obviously, the disruption of a tumor through morcellation is contrary to central oncologic principles. Histologically, the destruction of specimen architecture abolishes many of the anatomic features that allow a meaningful gross description, such as its dimensions, orientation, adjacency, borders, and margins [25]. As these specimens are often quite large, loss of these characteristics could affect the selection of parts of the tumor for histology that could be suspicious for malignancy, leading to a delayed or missed diagnosis [26, 27]. Even if a focus of cancer is discovered, tissue separation may prevent adequate determination of margins or adjacent spread, leading to suboptimal staging and over- or under-treatment.

The heart of this debate, however, is the question of whether morcellation specifically, particularly power morcellation, results in the upstaging of malignant disease by directly spreading cancerous tissue in the surgical field or not. The significance of upstaging is particularly important for ULMS, as the 5-year survival for stage IV cancers is very low (16–18%) in comparison to that for stage I cancers (57–95%) [28].

Multiple case reports have reiterated the risk of intraperitoneal seeding of sarcomatous tissue not seen at the initial surgery of laparoscopic myomectomy or hysterectomy using power morcellation [29, 30], which has been corroborated by larger case series that give overall upstaging rates of 15–64% [31–34]. In one such analysis at multiple institutions in Boston, eight cases of ULMS inadvertently morcellated during surgery for presumed fibroids underwent restaging procedures. Of these, three (37.5%) were upstaged. Of the five that were not upstaged, all were alive without disease more than 2 years later. Of the three that were upstaged, two died and the third was alive with signs of disease [33]. In the most widely cited study addressing ULMS upstaging risk [34], the authors retrospectively reviewed 1,091 cases of uterine morcellation. Seven cases of ULMS were identified, only one of which was initially treated at the study institution. This case did not demonstrate any dissemination at restaging surgery. The remaining six represented referrals from other institutions after various intervals, four of whom had visible reseeding at restaging surgery. Three of these patients died, two of whom were referred more than one year after their initial surgery, making it unclear if the peritoneal findings represented true dissemination or recurrence of aggressive disease. Both this and the previous study are derived from a single research group, including the same institutions over the same time period. It is unclear if these results are independent or if there is significant overlap of the patients. While this study is frequently cited as demonstrating that 57% (4/7) of ULMS demonstrate dissemination of disease after morcellation, this conclusion is somewhat misleading given the substantial bias of the population involved.

Overall, the data regarding upstaging and the direct dissemination of tumor as a result of morcellation are poor. The majority of studies have very low numbers, and few of these studies have stratified outcomes with regard to the type of morcellation (power vs. hand) or the approach (vaginal vs. laparoscopic) used. A recent systematic review of the literature by Pritts et al. determined that upstaging at the time of completion surgery occurred for 11/27 (41%) occult ULMS in which morcellation (any type) had been used and for which staging information was available [9]. As only five of these completion surgeries were performed immediately after the initial surgery, the remaining six may represent recurrence, not seeding. As these numbers assume that all 27 patients were stage I at their initial resection, it remains unclear if these numbers overstate the true risk. It is worth noting that, while the review focused on morcellation and cancer outcomes, three of the articles they considered also included a small number of open myomectomies; six ULMS were identified from these operations, resulting in three recurrences and two deaths, a similar rate as that seen after morcellation [35–37]. From the available data, there is no definitive evidence to demonstrate that power morcellation confers worse oncologic outcomes than hand morcellation or even myomectomy [9]. This does not imply that morcellation is completely safe, but only serves to emphasize the fact that better data is needed before policy decisions are made that drastically change practice patterns affecting hundreds of thousands of women each year.

Perhaps, a better question is addressed by the second half of the FDA statement above: is morcellation associated with poorer long-term survival in uterine cancer patients? Multiple studies, all retrospective, have demonstrated worse oncologic outcomes when morcellation is used. A recent systematic review and meta-analysis demonstrated a correlation between uterine morcellation and increased intra-abdominal recurrence and mortality in patients with unsuspected ULMS [38]. Morcellation (any type) increased the overall (62% vs. 39%, Odds Ratio [OR]: 3.16) and intra-abdominal (39% vs. 9%, OR 4.11) recurrence rates as well as overall mortality (48% vs. 29%, OR 2.42). This data is difficult to interpret. Only three of the 11 studies contained in the analysis demonstrated survival differences. This included

two studies by Park et al. which examined 106 patients with uterine sarcomas (50 with low-grade endometrial stromal sarcoma and 56 with ULMS) [39, 40] and a single-institution study from Boston detailing the outcomes of 58 patients with ULMS [41]. All three of these studies are limited by their retrospective nature. In addition, as it would be unethical to recommend laparoscopic hysterectomy to a patient with a known sarcoma, it is almost certain that the morcellation and non-morcellation groups represent fundamentally different populations. None of the studies provided a discussion of the type of preoperative workup, risk stratification, reason for referral, or the timing of the referral to provide a sense of the selection bias. While these data are inconclusive, there remains the suggestion that morcellation may worsen outcomes for a subset of patients with occult sarcoma, making the next step to determine the magnitude of this risk in patients undergoing surgery for presumed fibroids.

> *"Based on an FDA analysis of currently available data, we estimate that approximately 1 in 350 women undergoing hysterectomy or myomectomy for the treatment of fibroids is found to have an unsuspected uterine sarcoma, a type of uterine cancer that includes leiomyosarcoma."* [3]

One of the most challenging knowledge gaps in this debate is the real risk of undiagnosed sarcoma in presumed fibroids. The true prevalence has been difficult to estimate from current studies, ranging over more than an order of magnitude, from 0.45 to 0.014% [11], depending on the methodology of the study. The incidence quoted in the FDA report is derived from the analysis of a large insurance database review that identified 99 cases of uterine cancer (all histologies) in over 200,000 minimally invasive hysterectomies, only 36,000 of which used morcellation [42]. This translates to an incidence of one uterine cancer discovered in every 350 (0.28%) women undergoing minimally invasive hysterectomy for benign indications, not all of which were for fibroids. In addition, this study population was much older than that typically treated for fibroids: 67 of the 99 identified cancers were in patients over 50, so these numbers are likely not representative of the overall population seeking treatment for fibroids.

It is difficult to know what to make of this wide range of estimates. All of these studies lack risk stratification of the populations, frequently with no distinction in the types of uterine cancers, no specification of which cases utilized morcellation, and the outcomes of these cases. In the largest, most comprehensive systematic review addressing this question, Pritts et al. [9] identified 17 studies with outcomes data for patients undergoing hysterectomy or myomectomy for *presumed fibroids*, excluding in-bag morcellation or bag extraction. This pooled analysis of 29,877 fibroid patients provided a 0.014% rate of occult uterine malignancy. This difference likely results from multiple differences in methodology, among them is the inclusion of prospective studies, which typically describe lower rates of occult cancer. The predominant difference, however, is the restriction of this analysis to patients with presumed fibroids. While differences in methodology make this discrepancy understandable, it also makes clear the importance of asking the right questions when assessing and understanding the real risks to patients.

The vast majority of cases documenting mortality or cancer upstaging after morcellation occurred with ULMS, a disease carrying a poor prognosis even when discovered preemptively. Survival ranges from 15 to 55% depending on the number of mitoses per ten high power fields (hpf); a high-grade cancer with >10 hpf has a 5-year survival of only 15%. When embedded and confined to a uterus that is removed "en bloc," patients have a better prognosis, increasing the best survival rates up to 83% [36, 43]. ULMS, however, is incredibly rare, with an overall incidence of only 0.64/100,000 women [44]. While ULMS comprises 70% of all uterine sarcomas, these are only 2–7% of all uterine malignancies [43, 45]. Sarcomas typically spread hematogenously or lymphatically, not usually by direct extension, which has led several groups to propose that the poor oncologic outcomes after morcellation may also result from any approach that does not isolate the uterine vasculature before manipulation by enhancing hematogenous spread [9]. This may be supported by documentation of dissemination after open myomectomy [35–37].

The risk of sarcoma in a presumed fibroid in a patient younger than 40 is incredibly rare and is highest in women over 65 [46]. As the majority of fibroid symptoms begin to regress after menopause, the population of postmenopausal women seeking surgical treatment for presumed fibroids is a fundamentally different population than a premenopausal patient with heavy menstrual bleeding or pelvic pressure. Thus, a debate about the risk and benefits of morcellation needs to address population risk stratification and the impact of treatment on already poor disease outcomes.

"While the specific estimate of this risk [of unsuspected sarcoma] may not be known with certainty, the FDA believes that the risk is higher than previously understood." [3]

The majority of studies detailed above addressed the overall incidence of sarcoma in patients with presumed benign disease. Many surgeons, however, already perform individualized risk assessment, steering the higher risk patients away from morcellation-based procedures. To understand the danger that morcellation truly poses for unsuspecting patients, perhaps the better question to ask is: what is the risk of a patient desiring treatment for presumed fibroids who undergoes unintended morcellation of an undiagnosed ULMS with current practice patterns? In a recent retrospective study, the incidence of ULMS in women referred for treatment of fibroids was 0.54% (1:183), but rate of unintended morcellation was only 0.02% (1:4791). Of the 26 ULMS cases identified, six were diagnosed preoperatively, 14 underwent abdominal hysterectomy for suspicious risk factors, and five underwent laparotomy due to tumor size. Only one tumor was subjected to unintended morcellation in more than a decade [47]. In a retrospective cohort study of 1,004 women undergoing laparoscopic myomectomy or hysterectomy with power morcellation over more than 10 years at two institutions, two endometrial carcinomas, but no cases of ULMS, were identified [48]. In a retrospective cohort of 10,731 patients who underwent laparoscopic supracervical hysterectomy with power morcellation, an overall occult malignancy rate of 0.13% was noted, with individual incidences of 0.04% for endometrial stromal sarcoma, 0.02% (1:5365) for ULMS, and 0.07% for endometrial cancer. At a mean follow-up of 65.6 months, no recurrences were noted in 13/14 patients with malignancy: one of the two patients with occult ULMS died 13 months after surgery from peritoneal carcinomatosis and bone metastases [49].

These data are consistent across studies, but quite different from the numbers quoted in studies examined in the FDA meta-analysis. At the heart of this difference are the fundamentally different populations examined. While 0.28% of women undergoing surgery for presumed fibroids may have an undiagnosed malignancy, the risk of such a woman undergoing morcellation for her condition appears to be much lower, approximately 0.02% or less. These data are not mutually exclusive, but are answers to completely different questions. When framed in this light, the data support equally well the possibility that a better-defined patient risk assessment would prevent at least some of the cancer morbidity and mortality due to morcellation. So the claims from practitioners that minimally invasive surgery "employing morcellation remains safe when performed by experienced, high-volume surgeons in select patients who have undergone an appropriate preoperative evaluation" [12] appear valid.

> "At this time, there is no reliable method for predicting or testing whether a woman with fibroids may have a uterine sarcoma."

Preoperative Identification of Malignancy

While there is no pathognomonic set of features that can accurately rule out an unsuspected ULMS prior to hysterectomy, there are certain features that, if present in aggregate, may caution against the use of morcellation or minimally invasive removal. If there is any suspicion of malignancy, multiple evaluation methods, including assessment of individual patient risk factors,

imaging, and laboratory testing, can be used to inform the surgical decision making process before intervention.

As older, postmenopausal women undergoing surgery for presumed fibroids are at higher risk of ULMS, patient age and menopausal status must be central in the evaluation of a patient's preoperative risk of malignancy [46, 50]. Abnormal uterine bleeding in a postmenopausal woman should definitely prompt an evaluation for a malignant pathology, but the situation is more complex in a woman of childbearing age. Malignancy is more likely to be associated with non-cyclical bleeding, but this can have a myriad of causes in young, reproductive-age women. Given the relative rarity of sarcoma in this population, the pattern of bleeding is non-diagnostic. Women with specific histories of prior treatment for pelvic malignancies, particularly those who previously received tamoxifen or pelvic radiation [51], and those with certain hereditary conditions [52], such as Lynch syndrome or Hereditary Leiomyomatosis and Renal Cell Cancer (HLRCC), are at definitive higher risk of occult uterine malignancy and caution should be used in these patients when considering a minimally invasive surgical approach.

Ultrasound and Magnetic Resonance Imaging (MRI) are the most commonly used modalities to assess the uterus prior to hysterectomy. Ultrasound is more commonly used, likely due to its easy availability in the office, but MRI provides better three-dimensional spatial tissue discrimination and sensitivity [53–56]. While there are no diagnostic features for uterine sarcoma on either form of imaging [57, 58], several concerning features may raise suspicion if present. Presumed uterine fibroids containing occult malignancies tended to be larger on average than the average fibroid [59, 60], a feature that lacks clinical utility given the wide range of sizes of benign uterine leiomyomas. A rapid increase in size (within 3 months) can be concerning, but can occur with fibroids as well [61, 62], and there are at least case reports of presumed fibroids stable in size for many years that were found to contain a sarcomatous component [29]. Several reports have suggested that occult malignancies are more common in solitary presumed fibroids, with several studies showing more than 95% of cancers in solitary lesions [59, 63]. While recent studies have corroborated that occult uterine cancer is more common in solitary tumors, these overall rates are likely unrealistic. One recent case series of 15 sarcomas identified only 47% of occult ULMS in solitary lesions [60]. Certain imaging characteristics, such as irregular shape [64], "lacunes" (areas of hypointensity suggesting central necrosis in the absence of calcifications), increased peripheral and central vascularization [57, 59], and mixed echogenic and poorly echogenic regions [65] are associated with an increased risk of malignancy, but may also occur in degenerated fibroids. On MRI, regions of contrast enhancement have been helpful in distinguishing ULMS [66–68]; however, given the prevalence of fibroids, the false positive rate of approximately 15% given in these studies would misclassify tens of thousands of benign masses.

Computed tomography alone is unable to reliably distinguish occult uterine sarcoma from benign leiomyoma [69]. At the moment, there is limited utility for positron emission tomography (PET) with fluorodeoxyglucose (FDG) to assess the risk of occult malignancy. While FDG uptake is related to the presence of malignancy [70], it is also heavily influenced by estrogen status and overall cellularity [71], causing uptake levels to vary widely between tumors [72]. Alphafluorobeta-estradiol (FES) may be more sensitive than FDG in distinguishing LMS from fibroids [73], but further studies will be needed to establish its clinical utility.

There are no peripheral blood markers with any value in screening for occult uterine malignancy, but in patients with other risks factors, hematocrit, CA125, and lactate dehydrogenase (LDH) isoforms may have some limited utility. In a recent retrospective analysis of 15 patients who underwent inadvertent morcellation of ULMS for presumed fibroids in comparison to age-matched controls, a hematocrit less than 30 was independently associated with a diagnosis of ULMS [60]. As anemia is a common feature of women with symptomatic leiomyomas [74],

however, hematocrit may provide little additional information to guide clinical judgment. CA125 is elevated in some leiomyosarcomas, especially those that are of advanced stage [75, 76]. While increased, there is significant overlap of these levels with those seen in healthy patients, limiting the clinical utility of this testing. The most promising laboratory testing may be the assessment of total LDH and LDH isozyme type 3 elevation. In a prospective series of 227 patients, ten with ULMS had elevated enzymes, particularly in the relative fraction of isoform type 3, in comparison to patients with degenerated fibroids [68]. While total LDH elevation is quite nonspecific, measurement of the combined total and isozyme form provided a good discriminatory test. As the numbers in this study are still small, further studies will be needed to determine the reliability of LDH testing. In each of these laboratory tests, a positive result may add to a growing suspicion of cancer, but without that initial suspicion, laboratory testing provides little added information.

Several groups have also attempted to determine the benefit of histological analysis prior to surgery. While the benefit of endometrial sampling in the identification of endometrial carcinoma is well-described, less is known about any role for this procedure in the preoperative identification of uterine sarcoma. In one large retrospective series of almost 1,000 patients, 142 sarcomas were identified, 72 of which had undergone preoperative endometrial sampling. Sampling identified sarcoma in 62/72 (86%) cases, but the patient selection algorithm was not clear. If we assume that patients with abnormal uterine bleeding or other abnormal evaluation were preselected for screening, it is difficult to extrapolate what the utility of such testing would be in patients without risk factors (presumed uncomplicated fibroid) [77]. Needle biopsy without image guidance is of limited utility given frequent large areas of necrosis that could not distinguish leiomyosarcoma from degenerated fibroid; it is frequently difficult to make such distinctions, even in intact hysterectomy specimens [78, 79]. When performed in conjunction with image guidance, needle biopsy provides a negative predictive value. In a study of 435 patients, all seven patients with occult sarcomas were diagnosed by transcervical biopsy alone with a final sensitivity, specificity, positive, and negative predictive values of 100%, 98.6%, 58%, and 100.0%, respectively [80]. Use of such assessment in all patients, however, would result in high false positive rates, with significant fear, over-treatment, and cost, but might prove to be useful adjunctive testing in selected patients. There is no information on the possible local spread of sarcoma following puncture, however, and given the hematogenous pattern of spread for sarcomas, it is possible that this may outweigh the possible diagnostic benefit.

Prevention of Complications

While the data regarding outcomes is of poor quality, there is sufficient concern raised by many of these studies that morcellation may worsen outcomes for the small number of patients with an occult malignancy. Rather than banning minimally invasive approaches, it is reasonable first to consider what methods might be employed to improve outcomes and prevent the complications associated with morcellation.

While no surgery is completely risk-free, several simple techniques can be employed to minimize direct injury from power morcellation. During entry, enlargement of the skin and fascial incisions to the diameter of the morcellator reduces abdominal wall resistance and the force needed to manipulate the morcellator. The morcellator blade should be locked inside the protecting tube during insertion. Use of a midline trocar site minimizes the risk of ureteral and vessel injury at insertion and during morcellation. Sustaining adequate abdominal distension during morcellation as well as maintaining a constant awareness and direct visualization of close structures, particularly the intestines and blood vessels, decreases the risk of direct injury. It is crucial to keep the tip of the morcellator in sight, which is also facilitated by the use of a morcellator with a nozzle to promote continuous peeling rather than boring of the mass [81].

Even in a patient without malignancy, parasitic fibroids can develop after morcellation in a small number of patients; thus, the patient should be aware of this low risk when determining the benefits of different surgical approaches. Technical factors can also minimize this risk: stabilizing the specimen to prevent fast rotation during morcellation may reduce this risk. In addition, extensive irrigation of the abdomen and pelvis in reverse Trendelenburg and careful survey of the surgical field after irrigation, particularly in dependent areas, can prevent specimen loss. Before considering hormone replacement therapy, patients with fibroids who previously underwent surgical removal with morcellation should be aware of the increased risk of developing parasitic fibroids with gonadal hormone exposure.

The largest issue remains the prevention of poor oncologic outcomes, which realistically can never be completely eliminated. From the available data, pelvic ultrasound, both for operative planning as well as cancer screening, should be performed in all patients anticipating surgical management. MRI is a good alternative methodology if there is poor visualization by ultrasound, but would be prohibitively expensive if implemented for all patients. For suspicious lesions, adjuvant evaluation should be considered including the determination of vascularity parameters on ultrasound, total LDH and LDH isozyme 3 laboratory assessment, and possibly histologic analysis via endometrial sampling if there is abnormal bleeding or a high level of suspicion of sarcoma from imaging. While growth rates alone are not helpful, presumed fibroid growth on GnRH treatment or after menopause may raise serious concerns. But as any one of these assessments can be abnormal in the absence of malignancy, no single result can predict the presence of occult uterine sarcoma. In the end, the clinical judgment of the surgeon remains crucial in risk assessment and the determination of the appropriate surgical approach. Given that some risk will always be present for any surgeries for presumed fibroids, regardless of the approach, shared decision making and informed consent must remain important foci of fibroid treatment.

The development of new technologies to minimize the risk of spread of occult malignancy when using morcellation may also significantly improve the outcomes of those unfortunate patients who, despite our best attempts at screening, undergo suboptimal resection. Contained morcellation, such as "in-bag" morcellation (Supplemental Video), is currently under evaluation by multiple groups for use in uterine morcellation to prevent dissemination of occult sarcoma. While the details of each method differ, the specimen is placed in a bag and then morcellated using a power morcellator under direct vision away from the bowel and vessels (Fig. 8.2) [82, 83]. In early studies, the techniques appear to work well with comparable early outcomes to hand morcellation and myomectomy. Given the rarity of ULMS and the lack of long-term follow-up, it remains too soon to tell if this method significantly improves oncologic outcomes over uncontained power morcellation [21, 84–86]. Studies using in-bag morcellation for the vaginal removal of known endometrial cancer have demonstrated good outcomes without evidence of local spread or distant metastases [87, 88]. This technique has been used for low-grade Renal Cell Carcinoma (RCC) for decades without differences in survival compared to open nephrectomy [89, 90]. As ULMS can be a much more aggressive tumor than low-grade RCC, concerns over tumor spillage with bag rupture have remained an issue; such events are thought to be rare, but possible, and of uncertain clinical significance [86, 91]. Further information and longer follow-up is needed before this method can be validated to improve the safety of power morcellation.

The drastically different rates of occult malignancy in different series might suggest that these rates could also be influenced by the training and experience of the practitioners selecting appropriate patients and performing these advanced surgical techniques. One practical approach to improving outcomes may be as simple as limiting the use of morcellation devices to those with appropriate training, experience, and documented current competency [92, 93].

Overall, Is Abandonment of Morcellation a Good Decision?

Unfortunately, there is still insufficient data to make a concrete determination as to whether the use of morcellation poses an increased risk to all patients undergoing surgical treatment for symptomatic presumed fibroids. The majority of the available information is based on case histories and retrospective studies with low numbers of patients, typically without discrimination between types of morcellation, patient risk stratification, or selection biases, making interpretation and

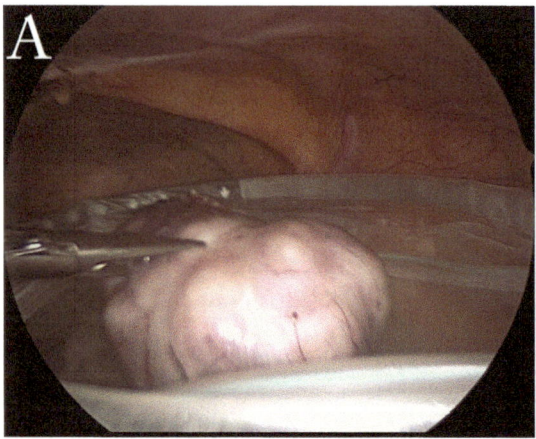 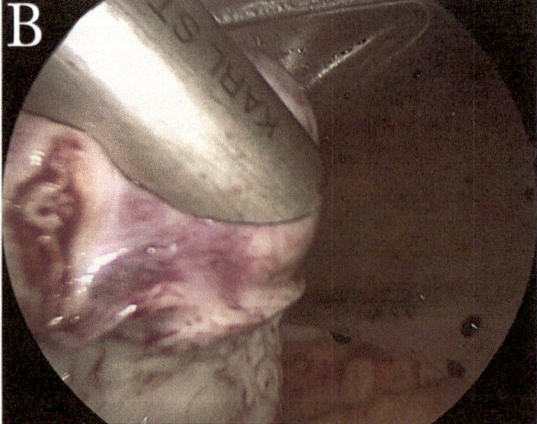

Fig. 8.2 Contained ("in-bag") morcellation. The specimen is first placed in a laparoscopic retrieval bag (**a**) and then morcellated using a power morcellator under direct vision away from the bowel and vessels (**b**)

comparison of the available studies challenging. Prospectively acquired data has tended to demonstrate lower risks than those reported in the retrospective studies [11], which is one of the many reasons why professionals have called for additional data before policy decisions are made. There is reasonable evidence, however, suggesting that morcellation may worsen the disease-free and overall survival of patients with unsuspected ULMS who undergo surgical removal. As such a negative outcome for some patients may be preventable, the discussion addressing whether morcellation should be used is an important one. But as a ban on the device itself is not the only way to prevent complications and improve outcomes, a more productive approach would be to focus on the acquisition of better data with prospective studies, identification of methods to improve appropriate patient selection, and development of techniques for containment to facilitate safer morcellation.

While it is our duty as surgeons to continue attempting to improve patient outcomes and minimize the potential for morbidity and mortality, we must also acknowledge that all procedures have some risk that can never be completely eliminated. While no one can deny the pain and suffering of those harmed, it is our obligation to consider rationally the impact of emotionally driven policy on the whole of society. The question then becomes, should we treat all presumed fibroids as potential cancers? While less than 0.5% of patients may be at risk of an occult malignancy, abandonment of morcellation as a possible tool in our treatment armamentarium will prevent a large subset of patients from benefitting from a minimally invasive approach. The advantages to minimally invasive surgery are many [14], providing patients with reduced morbidity and mortality rates, faster recoveries, and reduced pain in comparison to open surgery, even mini-laparotomy. With these benefits comes the risk of a poor oncologic outcome for those rare occult malignancies. A conservative approach treating all fibroids as potential malignancy, however, is not without cost and risk. This has already begun to become apparent. A study of patterns of care from the Michigan

Surgical Quality collaborative recently demonstrated the rates of minimally invasive hysterectomy have decreased since the FDA warning regarding morcellation, with concomitant increases in the rates of major surgical non-transfusion complications and readmissions as well as in the cost of care [94]. Given the rarity of occult malignancy, this study was not adequately powered to determine if there were any changes in the outcomes of occult malignancy in patients undergoing hysterectomy for presumed fibroids.

Additional analyses have attempted to answer this question through modeling, with the caveat that the assumptions made in the generation of these models are limited by the poor quality of the data previously reported. A team from the University of North Carolina recently sought to compare the relative risks, morbidity, and mortality from hysterectomy as well as the cost of treatment and mortality from ULMS in a comprehensive decision analysis utilizing a hypothetical cohort of 100,000 patients with symptomatic fibroids not amenable to vaginal removal [95]. The authors specified several assumptions, primarily that occult ULMS was always stage I or II and would be always upgraded to stage III when removed laparoscopically and that abdominal hysterectomy would always remove the specimen en bloc, conditions that likely overestimate the risk of morcellation and bias the results in favor of open hysterectomy. Regardless, the model predicted that, overall, there would be five additional deaths per 100,000 if all procedures were done abdominally and would result in lower global quality of life outcomes. Laparoscopic hysterectomy resulted in fewer costly complications with an overall increased quality of life years. A recent cost-effectiveness analysis determined that, under a wide range of probability and cost assumptions, non-morcellation hysterectomy via laparotomy cost more than minimally invasive hysterectomy with morcellation by almost $10,000 [96]. Even when the incidence of ULMS in the model was doubled from even the highest published estimates, a shift in care towards open hysterectomy still proved costly.

Similarly, a state transition Markov cohort simulation model compared the relative risks, morbidity and mortality from hysterectomy, and death from unsuspected ULMS. Several underlying assumptions limit the utility of this model, the largest of which is that laparoscopic hysterectomy can be performed in all patients without morcellation with an intact specimen. With those conditions, laparoscopic hysterectomy without morcellation provided the fewest complications and best outcomes. Laparoscopic hysterectomy with morcellation performed better than open hysterectomy in younger women, but worse in older women, reflecting the increased risk in these populations [97].

This conclusion reminds us of the dangers of dictating surgical approaches on a population-wide scale rather than considering the appropriate approach for each individual. In addition to traditional laparoscopy with or without morcellation, there are a myriad of surgical options to address symptomatic fibroids, including mini-laparotomy, laparotomy, myomectomy, colpotomy, total abdominal hysterectomy, vaginal hysterectomy, and laparoscopic-assisted vaginal hysterectomy with or without vaginal morcellation [98]. There are also several novel minimally invasive procedures to address fibroid symptoms, such as uterine artery embolization and high-intensity focused ultrasound (HIFU). While these techniques have preceded a diagnosis of malignancy in several case reports [99–102], the real risk of a negative impact on oncologic outcomes is unknown. Optimal approaches, determined by each patient's unique risk profile, may differ significantly for individual patients. As all procedures have risk, surgeons should be able to engage patients in the decision process to determine which approach may provide the most reasonable risk for that individual. Appropriate informed consent, not dictation of clinical practice, must be the centerpiece of surgical decision making.

One possible method to reduce the risk of unintended morcellation would be to perform imaging analysis, such as an office-based transvaginal ultrasound, prior to surgery. If any suspicious factors are identified at this screen, such as

irregular margins, high vascularity, or central necrosis, physicians could recommend additional evaluation prior to consideration of morcellation, such as measurement of hematocrit and LDH isoforms, additional imaging, or histological analysis. These results, coupled with the patient's age, presence or absence of abnormal uterine bleeding, and hormonal status, would generate an overall risk profile that could guide the choice of appropriate surgical approach. Brolmann et al. [11] proposed that the development of a standardized treatment algorithm that could be shared with patients (in which individual risk factors are considered in the decision-making process) might better aid patient understanding of the risks in each surgical approach.

Again, we must remember that no single risk factor is discriminatory and no pre-surgical evaluation can completely eliminate the risk of occult malignancy in a presumed uterine fibroid. Multiple suspicious findings, particularly in a postmenopausal patient, may raise concern about proceeding with morcellation. In a young woman without abnormal imaging characteristics, however, laparoscopic hysterectomy with morcellation remains a reasonable approach providing significant benefit to the patient with very low risk of occult malignancy. As it remains unclear whether power morcellation truly poses unique dangers to the small numbers of patients with occult uterine sarcomas, more extensive investigation is needed before system-wide policies are enacted. New techniques, such as contained (in-bag) morcellation, while still young, promise to make minimally invasive surgery and morcellation safer. Greater experience with these techniques in conjunction with appropriate training and credentialing at every level may also help improve the outcomes of minimally invasive approaches. As a field, our focus should be on participation in studies and registries to help better address these knowledge gaps and to evaluate objectively the individual and societal risks to these new techniques. But in the end, rather than dictating methods of care to all based on ambiguous data with unclear conclusions, the medical community needs to focus on a model of shared-decision making in which a complete and accurate discussion of the risks and benefits to each approach is balanced with each patient's personal goals for care.

References

1. Park A, Lee G, Seagull FJ, Meenaghan N, Dexter D. Patients benefit while surgeons suffer: an impending epidemic. J Am Coll Surg. 2010;210(3):306–13.
2. Steiner RA, Wight E, Tadir Y, Haller U. Electrical cutting device for laparoscopic removal of tissue from the abdominal cavity. Obstet Gynecol. 1993;81(3):471–4.
3. FDA discourages use of laparoscopic power morcellation for removal of uterus or uterine fibroids. Food Drug Adm. 2014;17(4).
4. Noorchashm H. Health alert: many women have died unnecessarily because dangerous cancers of the uterus and ovaries are being spread using MORCELLATORS. Stop MORCELLATION in minimally invasive gynecological surgery. 2014. https://www.change.org/p/women-s-health-alert-deadly-cancers-of-the-uterus-spread-by-gynecologists-stop-morcellating-the-uterus-in-minimally-invasive-and-robot-assisted-hysterectomy?source_location=update_footer&algorithm=promoted&grid_position=5)
5. Food and Drug Administration. Updated laparoscopic uterine power morcellation in hysterectomy and myomectomy: FDA safety communication. 2014 [updated 24 Nov 2014]. http://www.fda.gov/MedicalDevices/Safety/AlertsandNotices/ucm424443.htm
6. Desai VB, Guo XM, Xu X. Alterations in surgical technique after FDA statement on power morcellation. Am J Obstet Gynecol. 2015;212(5):685–7.
7. Rosenbaum L. N-of-1 policymaking—tragedy, trade-offs, and the demise of Morcellation. N Engl J Med. 2016;374(10):986–90.
8. Goff BA. SGO not soft on morcellation: risks and benefits must be weighed. Lancet Oncol. 2014;15(4):e148.
9. Pritts EA, Parker WH, Brown J, Olive DL. Outcome of occult uterine leiomyosarcoma after surgery for presumed uterine fibroids: a systematic review. J Minim Invasive Gynecol. 2015;22(1):26–33.
10. Adelman MR. The morcellation debate: the history and the science. Clin Obstet Gynecol. 2015;58(4):710–7.
11. Brolmann H, Tanos V, Grimbizis G, Ind T, Philips K, van den Bosch T, et al. Options on fibroid morcellation: a literature review. Gynecol Surg. 2015;12(1):3–15.
12. AAGL Advancing Minimally Invasive Gynecology Worldwide. AAGL practice report: morcellation during uterine tissue extraction. J Minim Invasive Gynecol. 2014;21(4):517–30.
13. Society of Gynecologic Oncology. SGO Position Statement: Morcellation 2013. https://www.sgo.org/newsroom/position-statements-2/morcellation/
14. Pitkin RM, Parker WH. Operative laparoscopy: a second look after 18 years. Obstet Gynecol. 2010;115(5):890–1.
15. Schlaerth AC, Abu-Rustum NR. Role of minimally invasive surgery in gynecologic cancers. Oncologist. 2006;11(8):895–901.
16. Shashoua AR, Gill D, Locher SR. Robotic-assisted total laparoscopic hysterectomy versus conventional total laparoscopic hysterectomy. JSLS. 2009;13(3):364–9.
17. Clarke-Pearson DL, Geller EJ. Complications of hysterectomy. Obstet Gynecol. 2013;121(3):654–73.
18. Wiser A, Holcroft CA, Tulandi T, Abenhaim HA. Abdominal versus laparoscopic hysterectomies for benign diseases: evaluation of morbidity and mortality. Gynecol Surg. 2013;10(2):117–22.
19. Milad MP, Milad EA. Laparoscopic morcellator-related complications. J Minim Invasive Gynecol. 2014;21(3):486–91.
20. Nezhat C, Kho K. Iatrogenic myomas: new class of myomas? J Minim Invasive Gynecol. 2010;17(5):544–50.
21. Kho KA, Nezhat CH. Evaluating the risks of electric uterine morcellation. JAMA. 2014;311(9):905–6.
22. Donnez O, Jadoul P, Squifflet J, Donnez J. A series of 3190 laparoscopic hysterectomies for benign disease from 1990 to 2006: evaluation of complications compared with vaginal and abdominal procedures. BJOG. 2009;116(4):492–500.
23. Cucinella G, Granese R, Calagna G, Somigliana E, Perino A. Parasitic myomas after laparoscopic surgery: an emerging complication in the use of morcellator? Description of four cases. Fertil Steril. 2011;96(2):e90–6.
24. Leren V, Langebrekke A, Qvigstad E. Parasitic leiomyomas after laparoscopic surgery with morcellation. Acta Obstet Gynecol Scand. 2012;91(10):1233–6.
25. Hagemann IS, Hagemann AR, LiVolsi VA, Montone KT, Chu CS. Risk of occult malignancy in morcellated hysterectomy: a case series. Int J Gynecol Pathol. 2011;30(5):476–83.
26. Rivard C, Salhadar A, Kenton K. New challenges in detecting, grading, and staging endometrial cancer after uterine morcellation. J Minim Invasive Gynecol. 2012;19(3):313–6.
27. Schneider A. Recurrence of unclassifiable uterine cancer after modified laparoscopic hysterectomy with morcellation. Am J Obstet Gynecol. 1997;177(2):478–9.
28. Zivanovic O, Leitao MM, Iasonos A, Jacks LM, Zhou Q, Abu-Rustum NR, et al. Stage-specific outcomes of patients with uterine leiomyosarcoma: a comparison of the international Federation of gynecology and obstetrics and American joint committee on cancer staging systems. J Clin Oncol. 2009;27(12):2066–72.

29. Anupama R, Ahmad SZ, Kuriakose S, Vijaykumar DK, Pavithran K, Seethalekshmy NV. Disseminated peritoneal leiomyosarcomas after laparoscopic "myomectomy" and morcellation. J Minim Invasive Gynecol. 2011;18(3):386–9.

30. Della Badia C, Karini H. Endometrial stromal sarcoma diagnosed after uterine morcellation in laparoscopic supracervical hysterectomy. J Minim Invasive Gynecol. 2010;17(6):791–3.

31. Morice P, Rodriguez A, Rey A, Pautier P, Atallah D, Genestie C, et al. Prognostic value of initial surgical procedure for patients with uterine sarcoma: analysis of 123 patients. Eur J Gynaecol Oncol. 2003;24(3–4):237–40.

32. Einstein MH, Barakat RR, Chi DS, Sonoda Y, Alektiar KM, Hensley ML, et al. Management of uterine malignancy found incidentally after supracervical hysterectomy or uterine morcellation for presumed benign disease. Int J Gynecol Cancer. 2008;18(5):1065–70.

33. Oduyebo T, Rauh-Hain AJ, Meserve EE, Seidman MA, Hinchcliff E, George S, et al. The value of re-exploration in patients with inadvertently morcellated uterine sarcoma. Gynecol Oncol. 2014;132(2):360–5.

34. Seidman MA, Oduyebo T, Muto MG, Crum CP, Nucci MR, Quade BJ. Peritoneal dissemination complicating morcellation of uterine mesenchymal neoplasms. PLoS One. 2012;7(11):e50058.

35. Leibsohn S, d'Ablaing G, Mishell DR Jr, Schlaerth JB. Leiomyosarcoma in a series of hysterectomies performed for presumed uterine leiomyomas. Am J Obstet Gynecol. 1990;162(4):968–74; discussion 74–6.

36. Perri T, Korach J, Sadetzki S, Oberman B, Fridman E, Ben-Baruch G. Uterine leiomyosarcoma: does the primary surgical procedure matter? Int J Gynecol Cancer. 2009;19(2):257–60.

37. Van Dinh T, Woodruff JD. Leiomyosarcoma of the uterus. Am J Obstet Gynecol. 1982;144(7):817–23.

38. Bogani G, Cliby WA, Aletti GD. Impact of morcellation on survival outcomes of patients with unexpected uterine leiomyosarcoma: a systematic review and meta-analysis. Gynecol Oncol. 2015;137(1):167–72.

39. Park JY, Kim DY, Kim JH, Kim YM, Kim YT, Nam JH. The impact of tumor morcellation during surgery on the outcomes of patients with apparently early low-grade endometrial stromal sarcoma of the uterus. Ann Surg Oncol. 2011;18(12):3453–61.

40. Park JY, Park SK, Kim DY, Kim JH, Kim YM, Kim YT, et al. The impact of tumor morcellation during surgery on the prognosis of patients with apparently early uterine leiomyosarcoma. Gynecol Oncol. 2011;122(2):255–9.

41. George S, Barysauskas C, Serrano C, Oduyebo T, Rauh-Hain JA, Del Carmen MG, et al. Retrospective cohort study evaluating the impact of intraperitoneal morcellation on outcomes of localized uterine leiomyosarcoma. Cancer. 2014;120(20):3154–8.

42. Wright JD, Tergas AI, Burke WM, Cui RR, Ananth CV, Chen L, et al. Uterine pathology in women undergoing minimally invasive hysterectomy using morcellation. JAMA. 2014;312(12):1253–5.

43. Lurain J, Piver M. Uterine sarcomas: clinical features and management. In: Coppleson M, editor. Gynecologic oncology: fundamental principles and clinical practice. 2nd ed. Edinburgh, New York: Churchill Livingstone; 1992.

44. Harlow BL, Weiss NS, Lofton S. The epidemiology of sarcomas of the uterus. J Natl Cancer Inst. 1986;76(3):399–402.

45. D'Angelo E, Prat J. Uterine sarcomas: a review. Gynecol Oncol. 2010;116(1):131–9.

46. Howlader N, Noone AM, Krapcho M, Garshell J, Miller D, Altekruse SF, et al. SEER Cancer Statistics Review, 1975–2012. http://seer.cancer.gov/csr/1975_2012/, based on November 2014 SEER data submission, posted to the SEER web site, April 2015. National Cancer Institute, Bethesda, MD; 2015. http://seer.cancer.gov/csr/1975_2012/

47. Lieng M, Berner E, Busund B. Risk of morcellation of uterine leiomyosarcomas in laparoscopic supracervical hysterectomy and laparoscopic myomectomy, a retrospective trial including 4791 women. J Minim Invasive Gynecol. 2015;22(3):410–4.

48. Picerno TM, Wasson MN, Gonzalez Rios AR, Zuber MJ, Taylor NP, Hoffman MK, et al. Morcellation and the incidence of occult uterine malignancy: a dual-institution review. Int J Gynecol Cancer. 2016;26(1):149–55.

49. Bojahr B, De Wilde RL, Tchartchian G. Malignancy rate of 10,731 uteri morcellated during laparoscopic supracervical hysterectomy (LASH). Arch Gynecol Obstet. 2015;292(3):665–72.

50. Wright JD, Tergas AI, Cui R, Burke WM, Hou JY, Ananth CV, et al. Use of electric power morcellation and prevalence of underlying cancer in women who undergo myomectomy. JAMA Oncol. 2015;1(1):69–77.

51. American College of Obstetricians and Gynecologists Committee on Gynecologic Practice. ACOG committee opinion. No. 336: tamoxifen and uterine cancer. Obstet Gynecol. 2006;107(6):1475–8.

52. Stewart EA, Morton CC. The genetics of uterine leiomyomata: what clinicians need to know. Obstet Gynecol. 2006;107(4):917–21.

53. Janus C, White M, Dottino P, Brodman M, Goodman H. Uterine leiomyosarcoma—magnetic resonance imaging. Gynecol Oncol. 1989;32(1):79–81.

54. Takemori M, Nishimura R, Sugimura K. Magnetic resonance imaging of uterine leiomyosarcoma. Arch Gynecol Obstet. 1992;251(4):215–8.

55. Pattani SJ, Kier R, Deal R, Luchansky E. MRI of uterine leiomyosarcoma. Magn Reson Imaging. 1995;13(2):331–3.

56. Melia P, Maestro C, Bruneton JN, Gasperoni A, Peyrottes I, Teissier E, et al. [MRI of uterine leiomyosarcoma. Apropos of 2 cases]. J Radiol. 1995;76(1):69–72.

57. Aviram R, Ochshorn Y, Markovitch O, Fishman A, Cohen I, Altaras MM, et al. Uterine sarcomas versus leiomyomas: gray-scale and Doppler sonographic findings. J Clin Ultrasound. 2005;33(1):10–3.

58. Fukunishi H, Funaki K, Ikuma K, Kaji Y, Sugimura K, Kitazawa R, et al. Unsuspected uterine leiomyosarcoma: magnetic resonance imaging findings before and after focused ultrasound surgery. Int J Gynecol Cancer. 2007;17(3):724–8.

59. Exacoustos C, Romanini ME, Amadio A, Amoroso C, Szabolcs B, Zupi E, et al. Can gray-scale and color Doppler sonography differentiate between uterine leiomyosarcoma and leiomyoma? J Clin Ultrasound. 2007;35(8):449–57.

60. Oduyebo T, Hinchcliff E, Meserve EE, Seidman MA, Quade BJ, Rauh-Hain JA, et al. Risk factors for occult uterine sarcoma among women undergoing minimally invasive gynecologic surgery. J Minim Invasive Gynecol. 2016;23(1):34–9.

61. Parker WH, Fu YS, Berek JS. Uterine sarcoma in patients operated on for presumed leiomyoma and rapidly growing leiomyoma. Obstet Gynecol. 1994;83(3):414–8.

62. Milman D, Zalel Y, Biran H, Open M, Caspi B, Hagay Z, et al. Unsuspected uterine leiomyosarcoma discovered during treatment with a gonadotropin-releasing hormone analogue: a case report and literature review. Eur J Obstet Gynecol Reprod Biol. 1998;76(2):237–40.

63. Schwartz LB, Diamond MP, Schwartz PE. Leiomyosarcomas: clinical presentation. Am J Obstet Gynecol. 1993;168(1 Pt 1):180–3.

64. Hata K, Hata T, Makihara K, Aoki S, Takamiya O, Kitao M, et al. Sonographic findings of uterine leiomyosarcoma. Gynecol Obstet Invest. 1990;30(4):242–5.

65. Amant F, Coosemans A, Debiec-Rychter M, Timmerman D, Vergote I. Clinical management of uterine sarcomas. Lancet Oncol. 2009;10(12):1188–98.

66. Schwartz LB, Zawin M, Carcangiu ML, Lange R, McCarthy S. Does pelvic magnetic resonance imaging differentiate among the histologic subtypes of uterine leiomyomata? Fertil Steril. 1998;70(3):580–7.

67. Tanaka YO, Nishida M, Tsunoda H, Okamoto Y, Yoshikawa H. Smooth muscle tumors of uncertain malignant potential and leiomyosarcomas of the uterus: MR findings. J Magn Reson Imaging. 2004;20(6):998–1007.

68. Goto A, Takeuchi S, Sugimura K, Maruo T. Usefulness of Gd-DTPA contrast-enhanced dynamic MRI and serum determination of LDH and its isozymes in the differential diagnosis of leiomyosarcoma from degenerated leiomyoma of the uterus. Int J Gynecol Cancer. 2002;12(4):354–61.

69. Rha SE, Byun JY, Jung SE, Lee SL, Cho SM, Hwang SS, et al. CT and MRI of uterine sarcomas and their mimickers. AJR Am J Roentgenol. 2003;181(5):1369–74.

70. Umesaki N, Tanaka T, Miyama M, Kawamura N, Ogita S, Kawabe J, et al. Positron emission tomography with (18)F-fluorodeoxyglucose of uterine sarcoma: a comparison with magnetic resonance imaging and power Doppler imaging. Gynecol Oncol. 2001;80(3):372–7.

71. Zhang HJ, Zhan FH, Li YJ, Sun HR, Bai RJ, Gao S. Fluorodeoxyglucose positron emission tomography/computed tomography and magnetic resonance imaging of uterine leiomyosarcomas: 2 cases report. Chin Med J (Engl). 2011;124(14):2237–40.

72. Kitajima K, Murakami K, Kaji Y, Sugimura K. Spectrum of FDG PET/CT findings of uterine tumors. AJR Am J Roentgenol. 2010;195(3):737–43.

73. Yoshida Y, Kiyono Y, Tsujikawa T, Kurokawa T, Okazawa H, Kotsuji F. Additional value of 16alpha-[18F]fluoro-17beta-oestradiol PET for differential diagnosis between uterine sarcoma and lciomyoma in patients with positive or equivocal findings on [18F]fluorodeoxyglucose PET. Eur J Nucl Med Mol Imaging. 2011;38(10):1824–31.

74. Wallach EE, Vlahos NF. Uterine myomas: an overview of development, clinical features, and management. Obstet Gynecol. 2004;104(2):393–406.

75. Vellanki VS, Rao M, Sunkavalli CB, Chinamotu RN, Kaja S. A rare case of uterine leiomyosarcoma: a case report. J Med Case Rep. 2010;4:222.

76. Juang CM, Yen MS, Horng HC, Twu NF, Yu HC, Hsu WL. Potential role of preoperative serum CA125 for the differential diagnosis between uterine leiomyoma and uterine leiomyosarcoma. Eur J Gynaecol Oncol. 2006;27(4):370–4.

77. Bansal N, Herzog TJ, Burke W, Cohen CJ, Wright JD. The utility of preoperative endometrial sampling for the detection of uterine sarcomas. Gynecol Oncol. 2008;110(1):43–8.

78. Giuntoli RL 2nd, Gostout BS, DiMarco CS, Metzinger DS, Keeney GL. Diagnostic criteria for uterine smooth muscle tumors: leiomyoma variants associated with malignant behavior. J Reprod Med. 2007;52(11):1001–10.

79. Bell SW, Kempson RL, Hendrickson MR. Problematic uterine smooth muscle neoplasms. A clinicopathologic study of 213 cases. Am J Surg Pathol. 1994;18(6):535–58.

80. Kawamura N, Ichimura T, Ito F, Shibata S, Takahashi K, Tsujimura A, et al. Transcervical needle biopsy for the differential diagnosis between uterine sarcoma and leiomyoma. Cancer. 2002;94(6):1713–20.

81. Milad MP, Sokol E. Laparoscopic morcellator-related injuries. J Am Assoc Gynecol Laparosc. 2003;10(3):383–5.

82. McKenna JB, Kanade T, Choi S, Tsai BP, Rosen DM, Cario GM, et al. The Sydney contained in bag morcellation technique. J Minim Invasive Gynecol. 2014;21(6):984–5.

83. Kanade TT, McKenna JB, Choi S, Tsai BP, Rosen DM, Cario GM, et al. Sydney contained in bag morcellation for laparoscopic myomectomy. J Minim Invasive Gynecol. 2014;21(6):981.

84. Vargas MV, Cohen SL, Fuchs-Weizman N, Wang KC, Manoucheri E, Vitonis AF, et al. Open power morcellation versus contained power morcellation within an insufflated isolation bag: comparison of perioperative outcomes. J Minim Invasive Gynecol. 2015;22(3):433–8.

85. Cohen SL, Einarsson JI, Wang KC, Brown D, Boruta D, Scheib SA, et al. Contained power morcellation within an insufflated isolation bag. Obstet Gynecol. 2014;124(3):491–7.

86. Cohen SL, Greenberg JA, Wang KC, Srouji SS, Gargiulo AR, Pozner CN, et al. Risk of leakage and tissue dissemination with various contained tissue extraction (CTE) techniques: an in vitro pilot study. J Minim Invasive Gynecol. 2014;21(5):935–9.

87. Montella F, Riboni F, Cosma S, Dealberti D, Prigione S, Pisani C, et al. A safe method of vaginal longitudinal morcellation of bulky uterus with endometrial cancer in a bag at laparoscopy. Surg Endosc. 2014;28(6):1949–53.

88. Favero G, Anton C, Silva e Silva A, Ribeiro A, Araujo MP, Miglino G, et al. Vaginal morcellation: a new strategy for large gynecological malignant tumor extraction: a pilot study. Gynecol Oncol. 2012;126(3):443–7.

89. Wu SD, Lesani OA, Zhao LC, Johnston WK, Wolf JS Jr, Clayman RV, et al. A multi-institutional study on the safety and efficacy of specimen morcellation after laparoscopic radical nephrectomy for clinical stage T1 or T2 renal cell carcinoma. J Endourol. 2009;23(9):1513–8.

90. Barrett PH, Fentie DD, Taranger LA. Laparoscopic radical nephrectomy with morcellation for renal cell carcinoma: the Saskatoon experience. Urology. 1998;52(1):23–8.

91. Cohen SL, Morris SN, Brown DN, Greenberg JA, Walsh BW, Gargiulo AR, et al. Contained tissue extraction using power morcellation: prospective evaluation of leakage parameters. Am J Obstet Gynecol. 2016;214(2):257.e1–6.

92. Committee opinion no. 464: patient safety in the surgical environment. Obstet Gynecol. 2010;116(3):786–90.

93. American College of Obstetricians and Gynecologists, Women's Health Care Physicians, American College of Obstetricians and Gynecologists, Committee on Patient Safety and Quality Improvement. Quality and safety in women's health care. 2nd ed. Washington, DC: American College of Obstetricians and Gynecologists; 2010. vii, 112 p.

94. Harris JA, Swenson CW, Uppal S, Kamdar N, Mahnert N, As-Sanie S, et al. Practice patterns and postoperative complications before and after US Food and Drug Administration safety communication on power morcellation. Am J Obstet Gynecol. 2016;214(1):98.e1–e13.

95. Siedhoff MT, Wheeler SB, Rutstein SE, Geller EJ, Doll KM, Wu JM, et al. Laparoscopic hysterectomy with morcellation vs abdominal hysterectomy for presumed fibroid tumors in premenopausal women: a decision analysis. Am J Obstet Gynecol. 2015;212(5):591.e1–8.

96. Bortoletto P, Einerson BD, Miller ES, Milad MP. Cost-effectiveness analysis of morcellation hysterectomy for myomas. J Minim Invasive Gynecol. 2015;22(5):820–6.

97. Wright JD, Cui RR, Wang A, Chen L, Tergas AI, Burke WM, et al. Economic and survival implications of use of electric power morcellation for hysterectomy for presumed benign gynecologic disease. J Natl Cancer Inst. 2015;107(11).

98. Clark Donat L, Clark M, Tower AM, Menderes G, Parkash V, Silasi DA, et al. Transvaginal morcellation. JSLS. 2015;19(2).

99. Joyce A, Hessami S, Heller D. Leiomyosarcoma after uterine artery embolization. A case report. J Reprod Med. 2001;46(3):278–80.

100. Common AA, Mocarski EJ, Kolin A, Pron G, Soucie J. Therapeutic failure of uterine fibroid embolization caused by underlying leiomyosarcoma. J Vasc Interv Radiol. 2001;12(12):1449–52.

101. D'Angelo A, Amso NN, Wood A. Uterine leiomyosarcoma discovered after uterine artery embolisation. J Obstet Gynaecol. 2003;23(6):686–7.

102. Papadia A, Salom EM, Fulcheri E, Ragni N. Uterine sarcoma occurring in a premenopausal patient after uterine artery embolization: a case report and review of the literature. Gynecol Oncol. 2007;104(1):260–3.

Sacrohysteropexy

Bilal Chughtai and Dominique Thomas

Introduction

Pelvic organ prolapse (POP) affects an increasing number of women over the age of 50 as the aging population grows in size [1, 2]. An estimated 300,000 procedures to correct this condition are performed annually in the US alone [3]. Over the last several years, interest in uterine-preservation has been on the rise due to a woman's desire to maintain her sense of self, prolong her childbearing potential, and preserve sexual function [4, 5].

The appropriate surgical approach for patients with POP depends on a number of different factors including the degree of prolapse, the patient's general health status, her current physical activity level, desire for sexual function, and the surgeon's experience and skill with the procedure. Vaginal hysterectomy with apical suspension has been the most common approach of correcting POP [6]; however, a hysterectomy does have significant long-term sequelae that some women with POP are not willing to accept.

Reasons to Utilize a Uterine-Sparing Approach

An increasing number of women are opting for uterine-sparing surgery at the time of POP surgery for a multitude of reasons, including their desire to prolong their childbearing years and maintain a sense of self [6, 7]. In a study of 213 women in which surgical outcomes were similar across different procedure types, 36% preferred uterine-preservation, 20% chose hysterectomy, and 44% had no preference. If uterine-preservation was perceived as being superior, then 46% preferred this method compared to 11% for hysterectomy. Interestingly, even when hysterectomy had a higher success profile, uterine-preservation still remained a popular choice at 21%. Importantly, women who believed the uterus was important to their sense of self had increased odds for preserving their uterus (OR = 28.2; 95% CI, 5.00–158.7) [4].

Hysterectomy has been perceived to also have significant effects on a woman's personality and femininity, as well as her postoperative sexual function [8]. Different factors such as nerve damage and shortening of the vagina following a hysterectomy can all lead to a negative impact on a woman's self-esteem and sexual function. Thus, the utilization of uterine-preserving procedures can help to boost a women's body image, her overall self-esteem, and her sexual femininity [9]. It is important to counsel women that a supracervical

B. Chughtai, M.D. (✉) • D. Thomas, B.S.
Department of Urology, Weill Cornell Medicine/
New-York Presbyterian, 425 East 61st Street,
12th Floor, New York, NY 10065, USA
e-mail: bic9008@med.cornell.edu

© Springer International Publishing AG 2018
J.T. Anger, K.S. Eilber (eds.), *The Use of Robotic Technology in Female Pelvic Floor Reconstruction*, DOI 10.1007/978-3-319-59611-2_9

hysterectomy should not impact either sexual function or hormonal status, as this is a common misconception among women. One disadvantage of preserving the uterus is that women who opt for these procedures are at continued risk for cervical and endometrial cancer [10].

However, because a woman's pelvic anatomy is not altered during uterine-sparing surgery, there are fewer complications such as shorter length of hospital stay, less intraoperative bleeding, and decreased operating times. Studies demonstrating the benefits of uterine-preservation have given momentum to the healthcare field to develop better procedures for POP surgery. The known benefits are faster healing times, less invasive surgery, and a reduction in postoperative risks. In a study by Dietz et al., women were randomized to either undergo a vaginal hysterectomy or sacrospinous hysteropexy [11]. They evaluated recovery time, anatomical outcomes, functional outcomes, and quality of life [11]. Women who did not have their uterus removed took less time to return to work (43 days vs. 66 days, $p = 0.02$) [11]. Both the vaginal hysterectomy and sacrohysteropexy were comparable in terms of functional outcomes and quality of life. However, women who underwent vaginal hysterectomy had a lower incidence of stage 2 uterine descent (3%) when compared to sacrohysteropexy (27%).

Sacrohysteropexy, a uterine-preserving surgical technique, can be achieved via many different surgical approaches including open abdominal, traditional laparoscopy, and robotic-assisted laparoscopy. Despite this, there is no real data explicitly stating which method is superior [9, 10, 12]. When choosing an appropriate technique for a surgical candidate, many factors bear importance such as the surgeon's experience and the patient's general health status.

Abdominal Sacrohysteropexy

The abdominal sacrohysteropexy (ASH) may require both transvaginal and transabdominal access [13, 14]. Patients are placed in a low lithotomy position, and a midline infraumbilical

or Pfannenstiel incision is made to enter the peritoneal cavity [15]. As described by Barranger et al., "... a transverse incision was made through the peritoneum between the uterus and the bladder...Polyester fiber mesh, roughly 3–4 cm wide, was then attached to the anterior [vaginal] wall, with four or five stitches of interrupted nonabsorbable suture, which were then passed through the right and left broad ligaments and then attached to the posterior cervix" [15]. Another mesh is attached to the posterior vaginal wall in similar fashion. In the posterior peritoneum, an incision is made over the sacral promontory, and the anterior and posterior meshes are then attached to the ligament overlying the sacral promontory with two nonabsorbable sutures to elevate the vagina and uterus. The original peritoneal incision can then be closed to cover the mesh using a continuous suture. Care should be taken to avoid the mesocolon and the right ureter [15].

Barranger et al. evaluated the long-term efficacy of ASH in women with prolapse. A total of 30 women with an average age of 35.7 years who underwent the uterine-preserving technique were included in the study between 1987 and 1999 [15]. All women simultaneously underwent a Burch procedure and posterior colporrhaphy. Intraoperative and postoperative complications were relatively low in this cohort, at 6.6% and 13.3%, respectively. Mean follow-up was 94.6 months. Two cases (6.6%) presented with recurrent prolapse at the last physical examination, and one of these patients required surgical retreatment because of symptomatic prolapse, specifically the anterior compartment. No other patients presented with recurrent prolapse, nor did they need surgical re-intervention. In conclusion, ASH was demonstrated to be a safe and effective treatment for women with uterine-prolapse who are of childbearing age.

Costantini et al. evaluated the use of sacrohysteropexy for POP, aiming to report on extended follow-up in 55 patients who underwent the uterine-preserving method [14]. All the participants in the study were followed on an annual basis. Voiding and storage symptoms resolved postoperatively in 42 (93.4%) and 30 (83.3%)

patients, respectively. All patients retained sexual activity [14]. De novo stress urinary incontinence was exhibited in four patients. In summary, this procedure was effective in treating not only POP, but it was also effective in preserving postoperative sexual function.

In another series, Leron and colleagues reported on sacrohysteropexy in 13 women [16]. The mean age of the cohort was 38 years. In total, 12 women had second-degree prolapse and one patient presented with third-degree prolapse. There were no reported intraoperative or postoperative complications. Mean follow-up was 16 months, and at this time period, only one woman had first-degree prolapse [16]. Preoperatively, four women (30.8%) reported constipation, and this number increased to seven (53.8%) women postoperatively [16].

An additional study evaluating abdominal sacrohysteropexy reported on the results of 20 women with uterine-prolapse [17]. The mean age of the participants was not mentioned, but mean follow-up was 25 months. Postoperatively, 19 patients expressed that their sexual function had improved, while three of these patients reported dyspareunia [17]. Postoperative quality of life (QOL) and symptom inventory scores were significantly lower (improved) compared to those taken at baseline, indicating that this cohort had a high rate of satisfaction and no symptoms related to prolapse following the procedure.

Although ASH has acceptable reported outcomes, potential complications of abdominal sacrohysteropexy include bowel injury, small bowel obstruction, wound-site infection, and recurrent prolapse [15, 17]. Dietz et al. reported recurrent prolapse in 22% of women [18].

Laparoscopic Sacrohysteropexy

The two main laparoscopic sacrohysteropexy techniques include laparoscopic suture sacrohysteropexy (LSH) and laparoscopic mesh sacrohysteropexy (LMH) [12]. Either laparoscopic technique is very difficult compared to the open abdominal approach. The surgeon has to not only be well-versed in laparoscopy, but also needs to be very sound with their knowledge of the pelvic as well as the retroperitoneal anatomy.

The advantages of laparoscopic sacrohysteropexy over an open approach are shorter recovery, significantly less blood loss, and more readily visible anatomy. Postoperatively, women experience less pain, length of stay (LOS) in the hospital is much shorter, aesthetically the incision is much smaller and less visible, while maintaining sexual function and vaginal anatomy. Furthermore, the number of intraoperative adhesions is relatively low, which can prevent infertility in the future. This procedure is performed similarly to the open sacrohysteropexy described above [15].

Suture Sacrohysteropexy

Suture sacrohysteropexy is a safe and reliable method for women who need an effective treatment for the management of uterine POP, but wish to avoid the use of mesh. This procedure is unique in that the uterosacral ligaments are attached to the cervix following the closure of the pouch of Douglas. Krause et al. describes the procedure by first introducing a 10-mm laparoscope using the Hasson technique. A total of three ports are inserted: one at each iliac fossa and one suprapubically at the midline. The supravaginal portion of the posterior cervix is suspended from the sacral promontory using suture material that is monofilamentous and nonabsorbable. Exact suture type was not described. Another set of sutures are placed at the posterior end of the cervix and at the insertions of the uterosacral ligaments attached to the promontory, where a stitch is employed back towards the cervix [19].

A study by Maher et al. evaluated laparoscopic suture hysteropexy in 43 women [20]. Mean follow-up was 12 ± 7 months and mean operative time was 42 ± 15 min. The mean blood loss was less than 50 mL. During the follow-up period, it was found that 35 (81%) patients had no symptoms of prolapse. Furthermore, 34 (79%) had no evidence of prolapse on exam. Interestingly, two women subsequently sustained pregnancies without prolapse. Both women underwent elective Cesarean delivery. This procedure is very effective in correcting the prolapse without rendering the cervix incompetent for successful pregnancy.

Krause et al. initiated a prospective study of women who underwent laparoscopic suture hysteropexy [19]. Over the course of 2 years, 81 women underwent this procedure for prolapse. During the follow-up period, a total of 65 (87.8%) women had no symptoms of prolapse. Sixty-four women (82.4%) had a Visual Analog Patient Satisfaction Score (VAS) ≥ 80% (VAS: 0–100, 0 = complete failure, 100 = complete success), indicating an overall satisfaction with surgery.

Mesh Sacrohysteropexy

Laparoscopic mesh sacrohysteropexy (LMH) differs from laparoscopic suture sacrohysteropexy (LSH) in that it uses a nonabsorbable mesh to suspend the uterus as opposed to suturing the uterosacral ligaments [5]. This procedure proves to be effective in correcting the prolapse, maintaining normal vaginal axis and sexual function [10]. When contemplating a uterine-preserving procedure for POP, the LMH is usually the preferred method of choice. Often times, this has to do with the surgeon's skill set as well as experience with performing the surgery.

The surgeon introduces four laparoscopic ports, which include two 5-mm lateral ports, one 11-mm suprapubic ports, and one 11-mm umbilical ports [12]. The uterus is then suspended from the sacral promontory using bifurcated polypropylene mesh.

Price et al. investigated the outcomes of LMH using bifurcated polypropylene mesh [12]. A total of 51 women were included in the study, all of whom had uterine-prolapse that was evaluated in two ways: (1) objectively using the Baden-Walker halfway system via vaginal examination as well as pelvic organ prolapse quantification (POP-Q) scale, and (2) subjectively using the International Consultation on Incontinence Questionnaire of vaginal symptoms (ICIQ-VS). The mean age of the patients was 52.5 years. All of the women in this cohort were sexually active, with some expressing a desire to bear children in the future. The procedure was successful for all but one of the patients. This patient had a

symptomatic, persistent grade-2 uterine-prolapse. This patient had to undergo a repeat laparoscopy and mesh was tightened further (shortened) by mesh plication with Ethibond sutures. This helped to reduce the uterine-prolapse significantly. During the follow-up time period, there was significant improvement in the patients' QoL, sexual well-being, and prolapse symptoms. This study demonstrated the feasibility of this procedure in correcting prolapse with overall favorable outcomes.

In a retrospective case series, Rosenblatt et al. investigated the clinical outcomes of laparoscopic sacrocervicopexy [21]. A total of 40 women underwent the procedure using synthetic mesh. Preoperatively, the mean C value of the Pelvic Organ Prolapse Quantification (POP-Q) staging system was −1.13, and at 6 weeks postoperatively, the mean C was −5.28. At 6 months postoperatively, the mean C value was −5.26, and at 1 year, it was −4.84. The authors determined this was an effective treatment for women desiring uterine-preservation.

A benefit of both LSH and LMH is that the complication rates are very low. The most common complications reported are prolapse recurrence, mesh erosion, and large bowel injury (2%) [5]. Generally, the mesh is attached to the posterior surface of the cervix and upper vagina, then sutured distal to the sacral promontory. An issue arises using this approach when the surgeon is faced with a patient who also has anterior wall prolapse because there may be inadequate support of the anterior vaginal wall with LMH. In fact, any anterior defects should be addressed transvaginally at the time of hysteropexy using a posterior-only strip of mesh, as the anterior vaginal wall support is inferior to that of a sacrocolpopexy with both anterior and posterior mesh strips. In this case, there have been reports of bringing the mesh to the anterior cervix and vagina through the broad ligament, similar to that described for open ASH. One concern with this procedure is that it may inhibit uterine expansion during pregnancy in the future due to potential constriction of the uterine vasculature. Vree et al. described a 50 year old multiparous patient who had mesh placed medial to the uterine vessels during LMH using blunt needles to capture the mesh arms [22]. Whether this is safe in women desiring later pregnancy is unknown.

In summary, laparoscopic sacrohysteropexy is a reliable and effective method for patients with POP who wish to preserve their uteri.

Robotic-Assisted Laparoscopic Sacrohysteropexy

An alternative to traditional laparoscopic sacrohysteropexy for women wishing to undergo a uterine-preserving surgery is robotic-assisted laparoscopic sacrohysteropexy (RALS). Surgeons opting for this method have a three-dimensional view of the pelvic anatomy, which allows for more precise suturing and dissection capabilities [23]. Furthermore, the overall maneuvering capacity is greatly increased. Similar to traditional laparoscopic sacrohysteropexy, RALS also results in shorter LOS in the hospital, less morbidity, and decreased postoperative pain compared with open approaches.

The technique is performed by first positioning the patient similar to that for robotic-assisted sacrocolpopexy as described in previous chapters in this textbook. A total of five incisions are placed in a W-configuration as follows: two 8-mm trocars for the robotic arms, one 12-mm trocar for an assist port, and one 12-mm trocar for the camera above the umbilicus [24]. The uterovesical junction is dissected as well as the peritoneum of the posterior uterus. This is to create tunneling at the broad ligament opening. The surgeon then makes an incision in the peritoneum over the sacral promontory in order to expose the anterior longitudinal ligament. From the promontory, a tunnel is created through the peritoneum until the sacro-uterine ligament region is reached. The posterior vaginal wall and posterior fornix is pushed up by a vaginal retractor. The bladder and the anterior vaginal plane are dissected via the anterior fornix. A nonabsorbable polypropylene monofilament mesh is placed between the vagina and the rectum and a second between the vagina and bladder. Next, the broad ligament is opened on the right side with the anterior mesh taken through this opening. "The anterior and posterior meshes are then combined and drawn through the peritoneal tunnel. The distal ends of these meshes are then fixed on the anterior longitudinal ligament of the sacrum with one or two nonabsorbable sutures. The peritoneum is then re-approximated over the mesh and closed with absorbable sutures" [24].

Mourik et al. evaluated the use of RALS as a uterine-preserving technique by assessing the outcomes on the quality of life [24]. This prospective study involved 50 women with uterine-prolapse. The quality of life for this cohort was assessed using the Urogenital Distress Inventory (UDI) and Incontinence Impact Questionnaire (IIQ) self-questionnaires designed for Dutch speaking persons [24]. The questionnaires were administered pre- and postoperatively. Follow-up assessments were collected up to 29 months. Preoperatively, overall well-being for the patients was approximately 67.7%, and postoperatively, this improved to 82.1% ($p = 0.03\%$). Furthermore, patients reported that their overall feelings of nervousness, embarrassment, and frustration had significantly reduced following the procedure. The overall satisfaction following the procedure was 95.2%. The mean operating time was 223 min, but with more experience the overall operating time decreased. Mean blood loss was less than 50 mL and the average LOS in the hospital was 2 days.

Geller and colleagues assessed the short-term outcomes of robotic sacrocolpopexy in comparison to ASH. The primary outcome was POP-Q score at 6 weeks [23]. Secondary outcomes included blood loss, length of stay (LOS), bowel obstruction, wound infection, and urinary retention. Seventy-three patients underwent the robotic procedure and 105 patients had ASH [23]. The mean C point for the POP-Q system was slightly better for those who had robotic surgery compared to ASH (−9 vs. −8, $p = .008$). Furthermore, mean blood loss was also significantly lower (103 ± 96 mL vs. 255 ± 155 mL, $p < .001$) for the robotic approach.

Pregnancy After Uterine-Sparing Surgery

The current information available on pregnancy following uterine-preserving surgery POP is sparse. Furthermore, there is a paucity of data detailing how women of childbearing age who undergo POP surgery are informed about the possible effects of pregnancy and eventual delivery on the reconstruction. A Cochrane review by Maher et al. found that, of 257 women who had received corrective POP surgery, 9.4% [24] had become pregnant following the procedure [1]. Ten of these women delivered vaginally, six by Cesarean delivery, while eight of the pregnancies were terminated for unknown reasons.

Lewis et al. reported a case of a 35-year old woman who had been treated with a laparoscopic sacrohysteropexy [25]. Following the procedure, the woman was able to successfully conceive 6 months later, delivering via Cesarean section. There were no signs of prolapse 12 months postpartum; however, at the 2-year follow-up she had recurrent apical prolapse. Her recurrent prolapse was treated by robotic-assisted laparoscopic supracervical hysterectomy, sacrocolpopexy, and perineorrhaphy. Two years following this procedure, there were no symptoms of prolapse.

Outcomes of Uterine-Sparing Surgery

A major factor when considering this procedure is understanding the recurrence rate postprocedure. Many studies have been conducted in order to understand this phenomenon in comparison to methods that do not spare the uterus, such as hysterectomy. A study by Hefni et al. found no differences in the recurrence rate between women who opted for the uterine-preserving method compared to hysterectomy [26]. Another study by van Brummen et al. found similar results when comparing sacrospinous hysteropexy and vaginal hysterectomy [27]. Despite this, patients undergoing hysterectomy for POP had a higher risk of "urge incontinence and overactive bladder symptoms compared to sacrospinous hysteropexy; a uterine-preserving procedure" [27].

Conclusions

Sacrohysteropexy has been shown to be safe and effective in women who wish to preserve the uterus, and it allows women to maintain normal sexual activity and potentially bear children in the future [4]. In addition, there is less blood loss, shorter LOS in the hospital, and overall decreased operating times compared to procedures in which the uterus is removed. Furthermore, women undergoing sacrohysteropexy report higher surgery satisfaction, better QOL scores, and overall high self-esteem. Although sacrohysteropexy can be performed in a variety of methods, the robotic-assisted laparoscopic approach has the most literature to support its use. In summary, women with POP who wish to have uterine-preserving surgery can consider sacrohysteropexy a safe and viable option.

References

1. Maher C, Baessler K, Glazener CM, Adams EJ, Hagen S. Surgical management of pelvic organ prolapse in women: a short version Cochrane review. Neurourol Urodyn. 2008;27(1):3–12.
2. Olsen AL, Smith VJ, Bergstrom JO, Colling JC, Clark AL. Epidemiology of surgically managed pelvic organ prolapse and urinary incontinence. Obstet Gynecol. 1997;89(4):501–6.
3. Barber MD, Brubaker L, Burgio KL, Richter HE, Nygaard I, Weidner AC, et al. Comparison of 2 transvaginal surgical approaches and perioperative behavioral therapy for apical vaginal prolapse: the OPTIMAL randomized trial. JAMA. 2014;311(10):1023–34.
4. Korbly NB, Kassis NC, Good MM, Richardson ML, Book NM, Yip S, et al. Patient preferences for uterine preservation and hysterectomy in women with pelvic organ prolapse. Am J Obstet Gynecol. 2013;209(5):470.e1–6.
5. Faraj R, Broome J. Laparoscopic sacrohysteropexy and myomectomy for uterine prolapse: a case report and review of the literature. J Med Case Rep. 2009;3:99.

6. Thakar R, Stanton S. Management of genital prolapse. BMJ. 2002;324(7348):1258–62.
7. Rahmanou P, Price N, Jackson SR. Laparoscopic hysteropexy versus vaginal hysterectomy for the treatment of uterovaginal prolapse: a prospective randomized pilot study. Int Urogynecol J. 2015;26(11):1687–94.
8. Good MM, Korbly N, Kassis NC, Richardson ML, Book NM, Yip S, et al. Prolapse-related knowledge and attitudes toward the uterus in women with pelvic organ prolapse symptoms. Am J Obstet Gynecol. 2013;209(5):481.e1–6.
9. Zucchi A, Lazzeri M, Porena M, Mearini L, Costantini E. Uterus preservation in pelvic organ prolapse surgery. Nat Rev Urol. 2010;7(11):626–33.
10. Costantini E, Mearini L, Bini V, Zucchi A, Mearini E, Porena M. Uterus preservation in surgical correction of urogenital prolapse. Eur Urol. 2005;48(4):642–9.
11. Dietz V, van der Vaart CH, van der Graaf Y, Heintz P, Schraffordt Koops SE. One-year follow-up after sacrospinous hysteropexy and vaginal hysterectomy for uterine descent: a randomized study. Int Urogynecol J. 2010;21:209–16.
12. Price N, Slack A, Jackson SR. Laparoscopic hysteropexy: the initial results of a uterine suspension procedure for uterovaginal prolapse. BJOG. 2010;117(1):62–8.
13. Elliott DS, Krambeck AE, Chow GK. Long-term results of robotic assisted laparoscopic sacrocolpopexy for the treatment of high grade vaginal vault prolapse. J Urol. 2006;176(2):655–9.
14. Costantini E, Lazzeri M, Zucchi A, Bini V, Mearini L, Porena M. Five-year outcome of uterus sparing surgery for pelvic organ prolapse repair: a single-center experience. Int Urogynecol J. 2011;22(3):287–92.
15. Barranger E, Fritel X, Pigne A. Abdominal sacrohysteropexy in young women with uterovaginal prolapse: long-term follow-up. Am J Obstet Gynecol. 2003;189(5):1245–50.
16. Leron E, Stanton SL. Sacrohysteropexy with synthetic mesh for the management of uterovaginal prolapse. BJOG. 2001;108(6):629–33.
17. Demirci F, Ozdemir I, Somunkiran A, Doyran GD, Alhan A, Gul B. Abdominal sacrohysteropexy in young women with uterovaginal prolapse: results of 20 cases. J Reprod Med. 2006;51(7):539–43.
18. Dietz V, Huisman M, de Jong JM, Heintz PM, van der Vaart CH. Functional outcome after sacrospinous hysteropexy for uterine descensus. Int Urogynecol J Pelvic Floor Dysfunct. 2008;19(6):747–52.
19. Krause HG, Goh JT, Sloane K, Higgs P, Carey MP. Laparoscopic sacral suture hysteropexy for uterine prolapse. Int Urogynecol J Pelvic Floor Dysfunct. 2006;17(4):378–81.
20. Maher CF, Carey MP, Murray CJ. Laparoscopic suture hysteropexy for uterine prolapse. Obstet Gynecol. 2001;97(6):1010–4.
21. Rosenblatt PL, Chelmow D, Ferzandi TR. Laparoscopic sacrocervicopexy for the treatment of uterine prolapse: a retrospective case series report. J Minim Invasive Gynecol. 2008;15(3):268–72.
22. Vree FE, Cohen SL, Kohli N, Einarsson JI. Case report: a novel method for uterine-sparing hysteropexy. Female Pelvic Med Reconstr Surg. 2012;18(4):247–8.
23. Geller EJ, Siddiqui NY, Wu JM, Visco AG. Short-term outcomes of robotic sacrocolpopexy compared with abdominal sacrocolpopexy. Obstet Gynecol. 2008;112(6):1201–6.
24. Mourik SL, Martens JE, Aktas M. Uterine preservation in pelvic organ prolapse using robot assisted laparoscopic sacrohysteropexy: quality of life and technique. Eur J Obstet Gynecol Reprod Biol. 2012;165(1):122–7.
25. Lewis CM, Culligan P. Sacrohysteropexy followed by successful pregnancy and eventual reoperation for prolapse. Int Urogynecol J. 2012;23(7):957–9.
26. Hefni M, El-Toukhy T, Bhaumik J, Katsimanis E. Sacrospinous cervicocolpopexy with uterine conservation for uterovaginal prolapse in elderly women: an evolving concept. Am J Obstet Gynecol. 2003;188(3):645–50.
27. van Brummen HJ, van de Pol G, Aalders CI, Heintz AP, van der Vaart CH. Sacrospinous hysteropexy compared to vaginal hysterectomy as primary surgical treatment for a descensus uteri: effects on urinary symptoms. Int Urogynecol J Pelvic Floor Dysfunct. 2003;14(5):350–5; discussion 5.

Additional Gynecologic Indications for Robotic-Assisted Surgery

M. Jonathon Solnik and Lea Luketic

Introduction

The introduction of contemporary, minimally invasive procedures designed for the female reproductive system dates back to 1898 [1], when early forms of intrauterine evaluation, currently termed hysteroscopy, were first described by Duplay and Clado. Gynecologic surgeons began to investigate the role of diagnostic laparoscopy in the late 1960s [2], but they did not begin to tackle more complex procedures, such as hysterectomy, until the first case was described in 1988 by Dr. Harry Reich [3]. Several decades later, innovative technologies such as the Zeus robotic surgical system (Computer Motion, Goleta, CA) were devised to facilitate more intricate procedures and enable surgeons to operate in difficult to reach locations. Despite its technology, this particular device was not widely adopted by

M. Jonathon Solnik, M.D., F.A.C.O.G., F.A.C.S. (✉)
University of Toronto Faculty of Medicine, Mount Sinai Hospital, 700 University Avenue, Room 8-813, Toronto, ON, Canada, M5G 1Z5
e-mail: jsolnik@mtsinai.on.ca

L. Luketic, M.Sc., M.D.
Department of Obstetrics and Gynecology, Mount Sinai Hospital, 700 University Avenue, Room 8-813, Toronto, ON, Canada, M5G1Z5
e-mail: lea.luketic@medportal.ca

gynecologists and was discontinued in 2003, only two years after being cleared by the US Food and Drug Administration (FDA), likely because of low volume of procedures.

The next robotic surgical system that was introduced to the market was the da Vinci platform (Intuitive Surgical, Sunnyvale, CA), which, unlike Zeus, rapidly gained popularity and received FDA approval for gynecologic procedures in 2005. Since that time, the da Vinci surgical system has been used by gynecologic surgeons for myomectomy, hysterectomy, microscopic tubal reanastomosis (MTR), sacrocolpopexy, excision of endometriosis, extirpative surgery for reproductive cancers, and adnexal surgery.

The introduction of robotic-assisted surgery (RAS) has not been without controversy or debate. This, in part, is borne from financial and competitive pressures at the institutional and physician levels. The relative saturation documented in both urologic and certain gynecologic procedures represents a strong indicator of these pressures to change and how best to provide surgical care. The combination of the almost "too-quick" implementation of a complex device into the healthcare setting represents a potential quagmire of large-scale safety concerns, but also limits our capacity to evaluate these tools in a systematic fashion. This dilemma is further heightened by the related challenge of how we should implement multi-disciplinary educational programs. The lack of consistent outcomes reporting further restricts our ability to establish treatment paradigms specific to RAS, especially when proven, non-robotic minimally approaches already exist.

The objective of this chapter is to provide the reader with a current and evidence-based review to facilitate a thoughtful approach to the surgical care for women. Please see Table 10.1 for a summative comparison of the below disease states and how they compare based on surgical approach.

Disease States

Uterine Myoma

One of the most perplexing findings when evaluating women with a variety of pelvic complaints is the presence of uterine myomas, frequently called fibroids. These benign tumors of the reproductive tract are so common that in population studies they can be detected by ultrasound in 40–60% of women by age 35 and 70–80% by age 50, with a higher prevalence among those of African ancestry [4]. The clinician is then faced with the task of linking the findings with the symptoms, rather than simply treating something which could otherwise be coined an unrelated bystander, given the high prevalence in women. Uterine myomas can cause pelvic pressure, urinary frequency, constipation, and abnormal uterine bleeding. In specific circumstances, depending on location and size, they can be linked with reduced fertility in couples trying to conceive. Surgical management of uterine myoma, the focus of this segment, represents only one of many options for women who are symptomatic. Figure 10.1 demonstrates location of myoma and their potential for abnormal uterine bleeding or pressure-related symptoms.

Myomectomy

The original uterus-sparing surgical concept is actually a group of procedures collectively called myomectomy, whereby the myoma is enucleated and the muscular defect reconstructed with suture in a layered fashion. This repair is critical to the integrity and contractile function of this smooth muscle during pregnancy. The open approach was first reported by Atlee in 1845 [5] and is considered the gold standard for women wishing to conceive.

The most appropriate myomectomy approach and technique depends upon a number of factors including the patient's desire for future fertility as well as the size, number, location, and relationship of the deepest aspect of the myoma(s) to the uterine serosa. An abdominal approach [open, laparoscopic (LM) or robotic-assisted laparoscopic myomectomy (RALM)] is most appropriate for transmural lesions, when the myoma extends from a submucosal location to the serosa.

The principle potential advantages of LM and RALM, compared to the open approach, include reduced morbidity, shorter hospitalization, improved cosmesis, and faster return to normal activity (Table 1) [6]. Notwithstanding these benefits, an open approach remains a commonplace procedure due to the complexity of the laparoscopic approach, primarily due to the skillset needed to identify the myoma(s) of interest with less tactile feedback and to place multiple sutures laparoscopically, which are often in deep and difficult-to-access spaces.

The da Vinci robotic surgical system was designed to overcome these dynamic surgical obstacles. The first case series of RALM was reported by Advincula more than a decade ago [7]. Although the average procedural time was 230 min, the perioperative outcomes were promising. As a result, the robotic platform seemed to represent an enabling device for an otherwise complex procedure. Early adopters believed that the instrument articulation, which allowed the surgeon to enucleate anatomically challenging myomas and effectively reconstruct large surgical defects, may be the defining feature of the device when it comes to myomectomy. Evidence-based guidelines for surgical candidacy of either LM or RALM have yet to be defined. Experts typically refer to 15 cm as a relative maximum size limit for an isolated myoma when considering a laparoscopic or robotic-assisted approach, but location, number of myomas, and volume of

Table 10.1 Comparison of outcomes based on surgical approach

	RAS vs. laparotomy	RAS vs. laparoscopy
Myomectomy		
OR time	Longer	Same (slightly longer)
EBL	Less	Less
LOS	Shorter	Same
Recovery	Faster	Same
Complications	Fewer	Same
Clinical outcome	Same	RAS: more complex cases
Hysterectomy		
OR time	Longer	Longer
EBL	Less	Same
LOS	Shorter	Same
Recovery	Faster	Same
Complications	Fewer	Same
Clinical outcome	Same	Same
Endometriosis		
OR time	Longer	Longer
EBL	Less	Same
LOS	Shorter	Same
Recovery	Faster	Same
Complications	–	Same
Clinical outcome	–	Same
Fallopian tube surgery		
OR time	Longer	Longer
EBL	Same	Greater
LOS	Same	Same
Recovery	Faster	Same
Complications	–	–
Clinical outcome	Similar pregnancy rate	Similar pregnancy rate
Adnexal surgery		
OR time	Longer	Same (slightly longer)
EBL	Less	Same
LOS	Shorter	Same
Recovery	Faster	–
Complications	–	Higher
Clinical outcome	–	–
Endometrial CA		
OR time	Longer	Same (slightly shorter)
EBL	Less	Less
LOS	Shorter	Shorter
Recovery	Fewer	Same
Complications	Shorter	–
Clinical outcome	More nodes	More nodes; obese women
Cervix CA		
OR time	Same	Similar
EBL	Less	Less
LOS	Shorter	Similar
Complications	Same	Similar
Recovery	–	–
Clinical outcome	–	Similar nodes

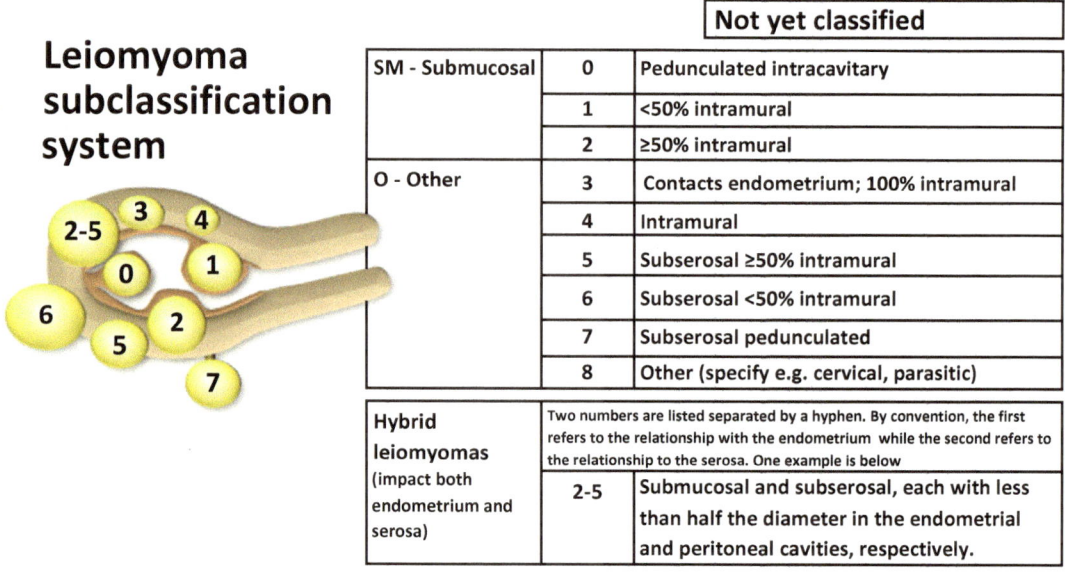

Fig. 10.1 Leiomyoma subclassification system

disease represent equally critical variables when considering this approach.

With clear benefits of a minimally invasive approach to myomectomy, both LM and RALM, specific questions remain as to which represents the ideal approach for the individual patient. The leiomyoma recurrence rates and likelihood of severe complications appear to be similar in women undergoing myomectomy by either approach [8], but it would appear that when performed by a skilled operator, RALM may allow for a minimally invasive completion of more complex cases. The data currently available on fertility outcomes indicate that the two approaches are also similar, with about 50–60% conception rates in the follow-up period with resulting pregnancy outcomes, as well comparable risk of spontaneous abortion, preterm delivery, and uterine rupture [9].

Gargiulo and colleagues evaluated the perioperative outcomes of similar groups of women undergoing either LM or RALM, both by high-volume surgeons who had a preference for surgical approach. Both the laparoscopic and robotic surgeons had reached the perceived learning curves for the respective technique. In this observational study, the authors documented similar

findings in each group with two exceptions: a longer operating time (absolute difference of 77 min) and a higher estimated blood loss (absolute difference 24 mL) for the robotic group. A major confounder was the introduction of barbed suture, only utilized by the laparoscopic group. This suture type allowed for faster uterine reconstruction with the potential for decreased blood loss because of its ability to close the defects more efficiently and by creating an internal tourniquet within the myometrium [9]. Barakat and colleagues evaluated the outcome of 575 women undergoing myomectomy performed at a single institution, comparing all three approaches [10]. The majority of cases (68.3%) were performed by laparotomy with the remaining evenly distributed between LM and RALM. Consistent with other study findings, patients undergoing the open approach experienced a shorter procedure compared to LM (absolute difference 29 min), whereas those undergoing RALM experienced the longest operating time (absolute difference of 55 min vs. 26 min for open and LM, respectively). Patients who underwent open myomectomy had more blood loss compared to both LM or RALM, as well as a longer hospital stay. Mean myoma size and weight of those in the RALM were closer to that of those undergoing open myomectomy, suggesting an increased capacity to address larger myomas. Reproductive outcomes were not assessed in this retrospective trial. The authors concluded that RALM may allow surgeons to perform more difficult cases laparoscopically and prevent conversion to laparotomy.

One critical surgical tenet for performing RALM is that the surgeon utilizes the same technique(s) described for the abdominal counterpart. Surgical planning with appropriate imaging and knowledge of where the myomas sit within the uterus allows for better efficiency in the operating room. Specifically, this allows the surgeon to decide which myomas to address and in what particular order, allowing for streamlined removal and repair. Maintaining proper surgical planes between the myoma itself and overlying myometrium will minimize bleeding and subsequent hematoma formation which impedes muscular repair. Gentle tissue handling and appropriate use of electrosurgery will further aid in tissue repair and minimize adhesion formation.

Robotic instruments commonly used are monopolar Metzenbaum scissors or hook, using a low voltage setting, a Maryland dissector that can aid in enucleation of the myoma from its bed, and a single tooth tenaculum or claw grasper that can be used to place traction on the myoma. Many surgeons typically use a dilute form of vasopressin (example: 20 units vasopressin diluted in 50 mL normal saline) to minimize bleeding as the overlying serosa and myometrium are incised. Bleeding during this portion is expected since these muscular tissues have abundant blood supply, and so a combination of vasoactive agents and electrosurgery will help to keep the surgical field clear. An incision is created to allow for adequate exposure, but smaller serosal injuries will minimize subsequent adhesion formation.

Enucation is the process by which the myoma is removed from its bed. Typically, there is a relatively avascular cleavage plane between the myoma surface and myometrium. Excessive bleeding during this portion of the procedure may indicate dissection within an incorrect plane. Once removed, the defect must be repaired in layers with absorbable suture of the surgeon's

choosing. The advent of barbed suture resulted in a similar phenomenon as did the robotic platform, allowing for a more efficient and hemostatic myometrial reconstruction and enabling surgeons not as skilled in laparoscopic suturing to offer this procedure.

Upon completion of the myomectomy, the myomas must be extracted from the peritoneal cavity. With the current and limited use of mechanical morcellators, many surgeons are removing uterine myomas with a scalpel and some form of a containment system. Adhesion prevention with use of a barrier remains a separate discussion, but it is the opinion of this author that surgical technique and use of a minimally invasive approach are key to reducing this potentially morbid phenomenon.

Hysterectomy

Notwithstanding an arsenal of options currently available for women with uterine myoma, hysterectomy remains one of the most commonly performed procedures in North America, with over 400,000 cases performed on an inpatient basis [11]. Common indications for hysterectomy include both benign and malignant disorders, with myoma being the most common. Substantive literature exists in support of vaginal hysterectomy as the route of choice when feasible, given the excellent outcomes and shorter convalescence when compared to abdominal hysterectomy (AH) [12]. Nevertheless, the utilization of this approach seems to have stalled at approximately 20% of all cases performed in the U.S. [12]. Laparoscopic approach to hysterectomy (LH) confers similar outcomes, but at a higher overall direct cost, primarily due to longer operating times and use of disposable instruments such as trocars and electrosurgical devices.

Early publications addressing the role of robotic assistance in hysterectomy focused on patients who had undergone multiple prior Cesarean deliveries and developed significant anterior cul de sac adhesions [13]. Although only six patients were described in this retrospective review, the authors believed the tool could enable surgeons to undertake more challenging cases. Since then, two randomized trials were published evaluating perioperative outcomes of robotic-assisted laparoscopic hysterectomy (RALH) and LH for benign disorders, representing more typical clinical scenarios. Both studies, of similar design, documented significantly longer total operating times (31–72 min) in the robotic arms for a comparable group of patients with uterine weights of approximately 250 g. Other variables related to the procedure, including postoperative complications, were similar in both arms of both studies. In an attempt to minimize the impact of surgical experience, both groups enlisted surgeons skilled in conventional laparoscopy and who had completed at least 20 robotic procedures. Other reasons that could account for differences in operative time include setup and the complexity of the device, both of which require a well-versed team in the operating room and electrosurgical instrumentation. It could be argued, however, that the robotic surgeons were still in the early phase of their learning curve. At the time of publication, it was felt that only 20 cases were needed for the average surgeon. However, for effective team functionality, the flattening of the learning curve more likely occurs upward of 50 cases [14].

In 2007, less than 1% of all hysterectomies in the U.S. were performed with robotic assistance [11]. An astonishing uptake of procedures was noted nationwide, such that by 2010, the number of cases increased to 9.5%. Early adopters were seeing rates as high as 22% only 3 years after implementing this service within their institutions (Fig. 10.2). Prior to the introduction of the robot, the rates of all minimally invasive hysterectomies remained relatively static in prior years. It was felt that this disruptive technology could represent the next phase in surgical management for women with reproductive disorders. A robust database review of sample cases from 2007 to 2010 documented similar findings from earlier work with regard to clinical outcomes and cost, with a typical RALH resulting in a direct cost increase of over $2000. Perhaps limited by errors in misclassification and missing variables, this population-based analysis provided data consistent with other prospective trials and highlighted the need to strategically implement robotic services.

Using the same database, reviewing outcomes from 2005 to 2010, a separate group of authors demonstrated slightly different findings [15]. They found that more surgeons performing RALH were able to perform hysterectomy on larger uteri (>250 g) compared to those using conventional laparoscopy (7.4% vs. 5.5%), while operating on women with more comorbidities (21.6% vs. 15.2%) and experiencing fewer conversions to laparotomy (2.5% vs. 7.2%). An interesting and unexpected finding, in contrast to other studies, was that the overall complication rate was significantly lower in the robotic group, even when compared to women who underwent any other approach to hysterectomy including open, laparoscopic, and vaginal hysterectomy. Women undergoing open hysterectomy had a mortality rate ten times higher compared to any other approach; however, the rate of this event was low at ≤0.2% in all groups. Selection bias may have also contributed to worse outcomes in the open group.

Endometriosis

Endometriosis is defined as the existence of endometrial glands and stroma external to the endometrial cavity and myometrium. It is a common condition that occurs in approximately 15% of reproductive aged women, but has been documented in all stages of life [16, 17]. The prevailing theory of pathogenesis of endometriosis, postulated over 90 years ago by Sampson, is one of reimplantation of endometrial glands and stroma that gain access to the peritoneal cavity via retrograde menstruation. It has been suggested that, in women with endometriosis, there is a deficient cell-mediated immune response and therefore a resultant failure of the peritoneal mechanisms designed to clear the menstrual effluent. Separately, the peritoneum may demonstrate altered physiology and response to foreign stimuli resulting in increased levels of inflammatory markers in women with endometriosis, resulting in adherence and perpetuation of endometrial glands and stroma [18].

Endometriosis is frequently asymptomatic, and its presence in a patient with pain may not

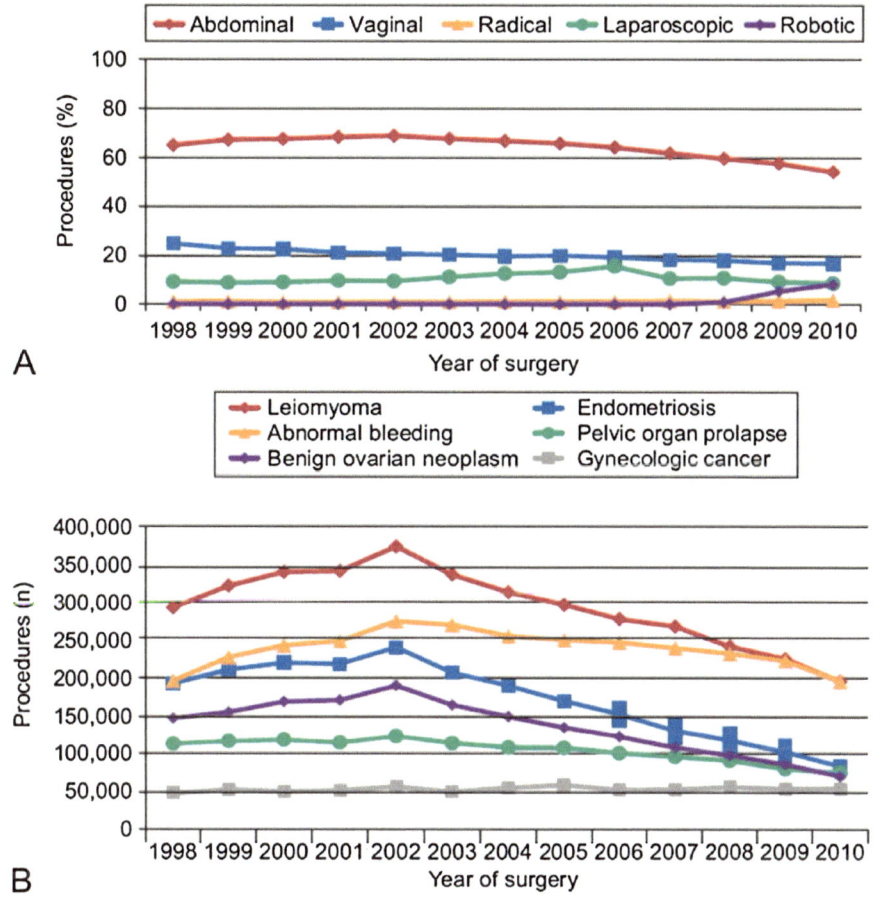

Fig. 10.2 (**a**) Hysterectomies (%) performed via each surgical route by year of procedure. (**b**) Procedures (*n*) performed each year stratified by indication for surgery. From [11]; with permission

always be the actual cause of the pain. In fact, endometriosis is commonly encountered in women with pelvic pain of other etiologies. However, in many instances, endometriosis is clearly the cause of any one or combination of dyspareunia (pain with sexual intercourse), dyschezia (pain with bowel movements during menstrual period), dysmenorrhea (cyclic menstrual pain), and other types of pelvic pain. Although neither the stage of endometriosis nor the site of implantation necessarily correlates with the degree of pain experienced, the depth of infiltration beneath the peritoneal or mesothelial surface does [19]. Furthermore, it appears that noncyclical pain is more common in women with deep infiltrating endometriosis. Women with endometriosis may also experience subfertility, even in the absence of pain.

Although a host of nonsurgical treatment paradigms exist, women with deep infiltrating endometriosis are more likely to represent a group of women recalcitrant to medical therapy. Radical excisional procedures are often required to improve chronic pain, and the infiltrative process of this category of endometriosis represents a known surgical challenge, even in the most experienced of hands. Significant alteration in normal anatomic relationships not only predisposes to inadequate resection, but also predisposes the patient to surgical complications. Historically, surgical options were managed by laparotomy, followed by the advent of modern day laparoscopy. The role of robotic surgery for deep infiltrating endometriosis remains to be defined, as outcomes data have been limited to retrospective analyses. Nezhat and colleagues published one of the larger initial series, describing 30-day perioperative outcomes in 86 women. In this single surgeon review, the majority of patients (>75%) had more advanced stages of endometriosis, yet outcomes were similar in both robotic and conventional laparoscopic groups [20]. The main difference between the groups was operative time, with the robotic group requiring an additional 77 min (mean difference) (longer operative time in the robotic group). The use of hysterectomy as part of the treatment plan and rate of surgical complications were also similar.

In 2015, Magrina and colleagues published data on 493 women, all of whom had advanced stages of disease [21]. A large team was involved in their care and surgeons were adept in both traditional and robotic-assisted surgical techniques. Although surgeon preference influenced which patient was treated with which modality, perioperative outcomes were not drastically different among the groups, with the exception of two key patient characteristics: those who were managed with RAS were more likely to have undergone more procedures and more radical procedures specific to endometriosis-related surgery during the incident. This finding likely accounted for the difference in operating time of 26 min. In the absence of a randomized trial, which is currently underway, the role of RAS for patients for deep infiltrating endometriosis remains controversial. At this point in time and for this indication, surgeon preference remains the driving force for perioperative decision making.

Fallopian Tube Surgery

Microsurgical tubal anastomosis allows for reconstruction of the fallopian tube after interruptive procedures designed for permanent sterilization. A small percentage of these women will reinvest in their desire to conceive, and this option, if successful, represents their ongoing ability to conceive in the future and avoid costly cycles of in vitro fertilization (IVF). Further, the success rates are quite high, making this an attractive option for some couples. This procedure requires delicate tissue handling, and the reanastomosis is dependent on the use of

extremely fine suture. Historically performed by laparotomy under microscopic guidance, the procedure has more recently been performed by conventional laparoscopy. Falcone described the first robotic technique in 2007, having performed his first case in 2001, and all studies since have been retrospective in design [22]. Similar to other procedures within gynecology, operative times have been consistently longer when compared to laparoscopy or mini-laparotomy, at greater cost and with similar reproductive outcomes (tubal patency and subsequent rate of pregnancy) [23]. Robotic assistance represents yet another option for surgeons who offer this procedure.

Adnexal Surgery

Surgical management of benign adnexal masses involves either adnexectomy (removal of the ovary and tube) or cystectomy (removal of the cystic portion while preserving the ovary and/or tube) and can be managed either by laparotomy or conventional laparoscopy. In an attempt to define the role of RAS for managing adnexal masses, Wright and colleagues evaluated surgical outcomes from 87,514 women who underwent either conventional laparoscopic surgery or robotic-assisted surgery for this indication [24]. They found that the rate of intraoperative complications was significantly higher in women who underwent both robotic adnexectomy and cystectomy, although the absolute difference was small (3.4% vs. 2.1%, OR = 1.60; 95% CI, (1.21–2.13) and (2.0% vs. 0.9%, OR = 2.40; 95% CI, (1.31–4.38), respectively. Based on these findings, it would be difficult to justify use of the device for this indication as a standalone procedure. However, when performed at the time of robotic sacrocolpopexy, the additional cost of oophorectomy is little more than operative time and pathological processing.

The above data specifically refers to adnexal pathology as the primary surgical indication. Offering women salpingoophorectomy (removal of the ovary and tube) as a concomitant procedure during hysterectomy or sacrocolpopexy depends on the age and desire of the patient, as well as incidental abnormal findings encountered during surgery. Emerging data regarding women's heart health has changed the historical paradigm of removing ovaries prematurely [25]. Mathematical models that reference population-based studies suggest women should strongly consider preserving their ovaries if younger than 50 years if no increased genetic predisposition exists. Since many women undergoing sacrocolpopexy are well into menopause, offering salpingoophorectomy is quite reasonable. Adnexal structures are not always imaged in anticipation of pelvic reconstructive surgery, so awareness of some abnormality may not always be known beforehand. If an abnormal appearing ovary is encountered in a younger patient who might otherwise preserve her ovaries, intraoperative consultation with a gynecologist may help to guide urologists with the decision to leave the ovary in place or to recommend removal.

Reproductive Cancers

Reproductive cancers were readily targeted as disease states amenable to robotic-assisted surgery, and prior to the introduction into mainstream surgery, the majority of women with such cancers were treated by laparotomy. A recent survey published in 2015 of the Society of Gynecologic Oncology members showed a remarkable increase in the overall use of robotic surgery among members compared to the previous survey in 2007 [26]. This survey demonstrated that 97% of respondents performed robotic surgery compared to 27% who responded in the previous survey less than a decade prior [26]. Similar to trends in urologic oncology, robotic-assisted laparoscopic hysterectomy with lymphadenectomy for endometrial and cervical cancers were procedures identified by gynecologic oncologists as almost more appropriate or commonly performed than by conventional laparoscopic approach.

Endometrial Cancer

In the developed world, endometrial cancer is the most common cancer of the female genital tract with an estimated 60,050 new cases in the most recent cancer statistics report [27]. Obesity represents an established risk factor, and as the rates of obesity increase in North America, epidemiologists predict a continued increase in the rates of endometrial cancer. Fortunately, most patients present with early stage disease and treatment are focused on surgical staging followed by adjuvant treatment for more advanced stages of disease and with more aggressive cell types. Hysterectomy and bilateral salpingoophorectomy, with or without nodal assessment, is the mainstay of surgical management. For grade 1 endometrioid adenocarcinoma, the most commonly diagnosed variant, no further treatment is needed. RAS has been performed for endometrial cancer since 2005.

Studies have consistently demonstrated the feasibility of RAS for surgical staging of endometrial cancers and report significantly reduced surgical morbidity while maintaining similar survival curves when compared to laparotomy [28]. Perioperative measures such as estimated blood loss, length of stay, and cancer-specific markers including lymph node yield are enhanced with RAS [29]. When evaluating outcomes of this approach to surgery based on age, an independent risk factor for postoperative morbidity, RAS had an improved safety profile in women over the age of 65 years when compared to a similarly aged group undergoing laparotomy [30]. Although most of the trials to date are nonrandomized, comparative, or observational, even larger scale multi-centered trials evaluating women with higher grade disease demonstrate similar safety and outcome profiles of minimally invasive approaches compared to laparotomy [31]. A 2010 meta-analysis reported findings from trials comparing robotic to conventional laparoscopic approach and found that women who underwent RAS experienced less blood loss and a lower rate of complications, although not statistically significant [8]. What remains difficult to assess from these studies is the experience of the operator and bias towards using one approach over the other, especially as the trend in the US has been shifted towards robotic surgery in recent years. Nevertheless, consistent with literature focusing on benign disease, longer operative times were seen with robotic surgery compared to laparotomy [29].

Of real clinical significance, however, is the demonstration by several studies of the safety of robotic surgery in the obese and super obese populations [Body Mass Index (BMI) greater than 40 and 50, respectively] [32, 33]. Women with significant BMI represent surgical challenges not only to the surgeon, but also to the anesthesiologist, and are at greater risk for perioperative morbidity. When the robotic platform was used in these populations of women, no differences were seen when comparing outcomes to women with lower BMI with respect to length of stay, blood loss, complication rates, number of nodes retrieved, recurrence, and ultimate survival [32]. Not surprisingly, there was a correlation between increasing BMI and conversion to an open procedure [33].

Cervical Cancer

Cervical cancer is the third most common malignancy found in women worldwide [26]. Fortunately, due to good screening programs, the majority of patients in North America are diagnosed in early stages of disease and survival rates are relatively high. Radical hysterectomy is the standard surgical procedure for the treatment of early stage disease. As with endometrial cancer, laparotomy represents the historical benchmark for surgical management. The first case series of robotic radical hysterectomy for cervix cancer was published in 2008 [34]. Since that time, numerous studies have further evaluated the role of the robotic platform. A recent systematic review and meta-analysis comparing intraoperative and short-term postoperative outcomes of robotic radical hysterectomy to laparoscopic and open approaches for early stage cancer has been conducted [35]. The study found that robotic-assisted radical hysterectomy may be superior to open approaches, with lower blood loss, shorter hospital stays, less febrile morbidity, and fewer wound-related complications [35]. When compared to conventional laparoscopy, robotic radical hysterectomy resulted in comparable outcomes.

While radical hysterectomy is the standard surgical procedure for the treatment of early stage cervical cancer, another option that exists for women who desire to preserve fertility and have a tumor size of less than 2 cm is radical trachelectomy. During the trachelectomy procedure, a cervical cerclage is typically placed to assist with future pregnancies and decreased risk of preterm birth. The first robotic-assisted trachelectomy was performed in 2007 [36]. In 2012, a study examined the accuracy and reproducibility of robot-assisted trachelectomy in women with early stage cervical cancer and demonstrated no differences between this approach and vaginal radical trachelectomy, in terms of remaining cervical length, a marker for future pregnancy outcomes [36]. The placement of the cerclage, however, was more precise with the robotic-assisted surgery [36]. This procedure remains a viable option for select women.

Ovarian Cancer

While ovarian cancer is a relatively uncommon tumor of the female reproductive tract [27], it is the most common cause of cancer death from a gynecologic tumor in the developed world, accounting for 5% of all cancer deaths. Because early ovarian cancer causes minimal, nonspecific symptoms or no symptoms at all, the majority of cases are diagnosed in the advanced stage, with only 15–20% of cancers diagnosed in early stages. The traditional surgical approach consisted of a midline laparotomy incision to perform staging and debulking. While robotic surgery has become widely accepted for treatment of endometrial and cervical cancer, its role in managing ovarian cancer remains controversial. Data to support the role of robotic-assisted surgery in ovarian cancer is currently limited to case reports and case series [37, 38] for staging procedures for those with early disease and surgical debulking in patients with advanced and recurrent disease [39].

Conclusions

Technological advances and innovation play an integral role in how gynecologists provide surgical care for women, but few have had such a dramatic and rapid impact as the da Vinci surgical platform. The mechanical advantages enable surgeons trained in minimally invasive techniques to offer patients nontraditional surgical options and add clinical value to patients with more complex disease states. From an epidemiological viewpoint, this technology has transformed surgical practice more than any other device in such a short period of time. Whether this trajectory continues on the same path remains uncertain. Nevertheless, as surgical performance becomes more of a transparent measure and the dollars for healthcare more restricted, surgeons must be strategic about new modalities until well-designed studies demonstrate consistent and true benefit.

References

1. Russell JB. History and development of hysteroscopy. Obstet Gynecol Clin North Am. 1988;15(1):1–11. [Cited 2 Jun 2016].
2. Palmer R. [Gynecological celioscopy; its possibilities and present indications]. La Sem des hôpitaux organe fondé par l'Association d'enseignement médical des hôpitaux Paris [Internet]. 1954;30(79):4440–3. [Cited 2 Jun 2016].
3. Reich H, McGlynn F, Wilkie W. Laparoscopic management of stage I ovarian cancer. A case report. J Reprod Med [Internet]. 1990;35(6):601–4; discussion 604–5. [Cited 2 Jun 2016].
4. Baird DD, Dunson DB, Hill MC, Cousins D, Schectman JM. High cumulative incidence of uterine leiomyoma in black and white women: ultrasound evidence. Am J Obstet Gynecol [Internet]. 2003;188(1):100–7. [Cited 17 May 2016].
5. Atlee W. Case of successful extirpation of a fibrous tumor of the peritoneal surface of the uterus by the large peritoneal section. Am J Med Sci. 1845;9:309–35.
6. Seracchioli R, Rossi S, Govoni F, Rossi E, Venturoli S, Bulletti C, et al. Fertility and obstetric outcome after laparoscopic myomectomy of large myomata: a randomized comparison with abdominal myomectomy. Hum Reprod. 2000;15(12):2663–8.
7. Advincula AP, Xu X, Goudeau S IV, Ransom SB. Robot-assisted laparoscopic myomectomy versus abdominal myomectomy: a comparison of short-term surgical outcomes and immediate costs. J Minim Invasive Gynecol. 2007;14(6):698–705.
8. Reza M, Maeso S, Blasco JA, Andradas E. Meta-analysis of observational studies on the safety and effectiveness of robotic gynaecological surgery. Br J Surg. 2010;97(12):1772–83.
9. Gargiulo AR, Srouji SS, Missmer SA, Correia KF, Vellinga T, Einarsson JI. Robot-assisted laparoscopic myomectomy compared with standard laparoscopic myomectomy. Obstet Gynecol. 2012;120(2 Pt 1):284–91.
10. Barakat EE, Bedaiwy MA, Zimberg S, Nutter B, Nosseir M, Falcone T. Robotic-assisted, laparoscopic, and abdominal myomectomy: a comparison of surgical outcomes. Obstet Gynecol [Internet]. 2011;117(2 Pt 1):256–65.
11. Wright JD, Herzog TJ, Tsui J, Ananth CV, Lewin SN, Lu Y-S, et al. Nationwide trends in the performance of inpatient hysterectomy in the United States. Obstet Gynecol [Internet]. 2013;122(2 Pt 1):233–41. [Cited 2 Jun 2016].
12. Aarts JWM, Nieboer TE, Johnson N, Tavender E, Garry R, Mol BWJ, et al. Surgical approach to hysterectomy for benign gynaecological disease. Cochrane Database Syst Rev. 2015;8:CD003677. doi:10.1002/14651858.CD003677.pub5.
13. Advincula AP, Reynolds RK. The use of robot-assisted laparoscopic hysterectomy in the patient with a scarred or obliterated anterior cul-de-sac. JSLS. 2005;9(3):287–91.
14. Woelk JL, Casiano ER, Weaver AL, Gostout BS, Trabuco EC, Gebhart JB. The learning curve of robotic hysterectomy. Obstet Gynecol [Internet]. 2013;121(1):87–95. [Cited 5 Jun 2016]. http://www.ncbi.nlm.nih.gov/pubmed/23262932
15. Luciano AA, Luciano DE, Gabbert J, Seshadri-Kreaden U. The impact of robotics on the mode of benign hysterectomy and clinical outcomes. Int J Med Robot [Internet]. 2016;12(1):114–24. [Cited 5 Jun 2016]. http://www.ncbi.nlm.nih.gov/pubmed/25753111
16. Giudice LC. Endometriosis. N Engl J Med [Internet]. 2010;362(25):2389–98. [Cited 11 Mar 2015]. http://www.pubmedcentral.nih.gov/articlerender.fcgi?artid=3108065&tool=pmcentrez&rendertype=abstract
17. Moen MH. Endometriosis in women at interval sterilization. Acta Obstet Gynecol Scand [Internet]. 1987;66(5):451–4. [Cited 5 Jun 2016]. http://www.ncbi.nlm.nih.gov/pubmed/3425247
18. Young VJ, Brown JK, Saunders PTK, Horne AW. The role of the peritoneum in the pathogenesis of endometriosis. Hum Reprod Update [Internet]. 2013;19(5):558–69. [Cited 5 Jun 2016]. http://www.ncbi.nlm.nih.gov/pubmed/23720497
19. Fauconnier A, Chapron C, Dubuisson J-B, Vieira M, Dousset B, Bréart G. Relation between pain symptoms and the anatomic location of deep infiltrating endometriosis. Fertil Steril [Internet]. 2002;78(4):719–26. [Cited 5 Jun 2016]. http://www.ncbi.nlm.nih.gov/pubmed/12372446
20. Nezhat FR, Sirota I. Perioperative outcomes of robotic assisted laparoscopic surgery versus conventional laparoscopy surgery for advanced-stage endometriosis. JSLS J Soc Laparoendosc Surg [Internet]. 2014;18(4):e2014.00094. http://www.ncbi.nlm.nih.gov/pmc/articles/PMC4254472/

21. Magrina JF, Espada M, Kho RM, Cetta R, Chang YHH, Magtibay PM. Surgical excision of advanced endometriosis: perioperative outcomes and impacting factors. J Minim Invasive Gynecol [Internet]. 2015;22(6):944–50. http://dx.doi.org/10.1016/j.jmig.2015.04.016. Elsevier Ltd.

22. Rodgers AK, Goldberg JM, Hammel JP, Falcone T. Tubal anastomosis by robotic compared with outpatient minilaparotomy. Obstet Gynecol [Internet]. 2007;109(6):1375–80. http://www.ncbi.nlm.nih.gov/entrez/query.fcgi?cmd=Retrieve&db=PubMed&dopt=Citation&list_uids=17540810

23. Goldberg JM, Falcone T. Laparoscopic microsurgical tubal anastomosis with and without robotic assistance. Hum Reprod. 2003;18(1):145–7.

24. Wright JD, Kostolias A, Ananth CV, Burke WM, Tergas AI, Prendergast E, et al. Comparative effectiveness of robotically assisted compared with laparoscopic adnexal surgery for benign gynecologic disease. Obstet Gynecol. 2014;124(5):886–96.

25. Parker WH, Feskanish D, Broder MS, et al. Long-term mortality associated with oophorectomy compared with ovarian conservation in the nurses' health study. Obstet Gynecol. 2013;121(4):709–16.

26. Conrad LB, Ramirez PT, Burke W, Naumann RW, Ring KL, Munsell MF, et al. Role of minimally invasive surgery in gynecologic oncology: an updated survey of members of the Society of Gynecologic Oncology. Int J Gynecol Cancer. 2015;25(6):1121–7. http://www.ncbi.nlm.nih.gov/pubmed/25860841

27. Siegel RL, Miller KD, Jemal A. Cancer statistics. CA Cancer J Clin. 2016;66(1):7–30.

28. Park HK, Helenowski IB, Berry E, Lurain JR, Neubauer NL. A comparison of survival and recurrence outcomes in patients with endometrial cancer undergoing robotic versus open surgery. J Minim Invasive Gynecol. 2015;22(6):961–7. http://dx.doi.org/10.1016/j.jmig.2015.04.018. Elsevier Ltd.

29. Boggess JF, Gehrig PA, Cantrell L, Shafer A, Ridgway M, Skinner EN, et al. A comparative study of 3 surgical methods for hysterectomy with staging for endometrial cancer: robotic assistance, laparoscopy, laparotomy. Am J Obstet Gynecol. 2008;199(4):360.e1–9.

30. Guy MS, Sheeder J, Behbakht K, Wright JD, Guntupalli SR. Comparative outcomes in older and younger women undergoing laparotomy or robotic surgical staging for endometrial cancer. Presented at

the Annual Clinical Congress in the Surgical Forum of the American College of Surgeons, San Francisco, CA, 26–30 Oct 2014. Am J Obstet Gynecol. 2016;214(3):350.e1–350.e10. Elsevier Inc.

31. Fader AN, Seamon LG, Escobar PF, Frasure HE, Havrilesky LA, Zanotti KM, et al. Minimally invasive surgery versus laparotomy in women with high grade endometrial cancer: a multi-site study performed at high volume cancer centers. Gynecol Oncol [Internet]. 2012;126(2):180–5. [Cited 6 Jun 2016].

32. Pavelka JC, Ben-Shachar I, Fowler JM, Ramirez NC, Copeland LJ, Eaton LA, et al. Morbid obesity and endometrial cancer: surgical, clinical, and pathologic outcomes in surgically managed patients. Gynecol Oncol. 2004;95(3):588–92.

33. Stephan JM, Goodheart MJ, McDonald M, Hansen J, Reyes HD, Button A, et al. Robotic surgery in supermorbidly obese patients with endometrial cancer. Am J Obstet Gynecol [Internet]. 2015;213(1):49.e1–8. Elsevier Inc.

34. Fanning J, Hojat R, Johnson J, Fenton B. Robotic radical hysterectomy. Minerva Ginecol. 2009;61(1):53–5.

35. Shazly SAM, Murad MH, Dowdy SC, Gostout BS, Famuyide AO. Robotic radical hysterectomy in early stage cervical cancer: a systematic review and meta-analysis. Gynecol Oncol. 2015;138(2):457–71. Elsevier Inc.

36. Persson J, Kannisto P, Bossmar T. Robot-assisted abdominal laparoscopic radical trachelectomy. Gynecol Oncol [Internet]. 2008;111(3):564–7. Elsevier Inc.

37. Brown JV, Mendivil AA, Abaid LN, Rettenmaier MA, Micha JP, Wabe MA, et al. The safety and feasibility of robotic-assisted lymph node staging in early-stage ovarian cancer. Int J Gynecol Cancer. 2014;24(8):1493–8.

38. Magrina JF, Zanagnolo V, Noble BN, Kho RM, Magtibay P. Robotic approach for ovarian cancer: perioperative and survival results and comparison with laparoscopy and laparotomy. Gynecol Oncol. 2011;121(1):100–5. Elsevier B.V.

39. Escobar PF, Levinson KL, Magrina J, Martino MA, Barakat RR, Fader AN, et al. Feasibility and perioperative outcomes of robotic-assisted surgery in the management of recurrent ovarian cancer: a multi-institutional study. Gynecol Oncol [Internet]. 2014;134(2):253–6. Elsevier Inc.

Robotic Surgical Management of Combined Vaginal and Rectal Prolapse

Emily Siegel, Beth A. Moore, and David P. Magner

Introduction

Rectal prolapse is a dynamic disorder caused by damage to the pelvic support structures, which has been attributed to the shearing forces of vaginal childbirth, connective tissue disorders, neuropathy, congenital defects, chronic constipation, or pelvic surgery [1]. This pelvic floor weakness often affects the entire pelvic floor muscular diaphragm resulting in the descent of one or more of the pelvic organs (i.e., uterus, vagina, bladder, rectum). It is estimated that up to 50% of parous females will experience partial or complete prolapse of one or more organs in their lifetime

E. Siegel, M.D.
Department of Surgery, Division of Colorectal
Surgery, Cedars Sinai Medical Center,
8700 Beverly Blvd, #8215, Los Angeles,
CA 90048, USA
e-mail: Siegel@cshs.org

B.A. Moore, M.D., F.A.C.S., F.A.S.C.R.S. (✉)
Department of Surgery, Division of Colorectal
Surgery, Cedars-Sinai Medical Center,
8737 Beverly Boulevard, Suite 402, Los Angeles,
CA 90048, USA
e-mail: mooreb@cshs.org

D.P. Magner, M.D., F.A.C.S.
Department of Surgery, Division of Colorectal
Surgery, Cedars-Sinai Medical Center,
8700 Beverly Blvd., #402, Los Angeles,
CA 90048, USA
e-mail: david.magner@cshs.org

[2, 3]. Pelvic organ prolapse is becoming a significant concern in the aging population, and the prevalence in the United States is expected to increase by 46% to 4.9 million cases by the year 2050 [4].

Traditionally, the medical and surgical management of pelvic organ dysfunction was confined to each specialty. Urologists and gynecologists would repair pelvic organ prolapse of the anterior and middle (apical) compartments, while separate treatment would be performed by a colorectal surgeon for posterior compartment (rectal) prolapse. Addressing the combined pathology in a piecemeal approach likely alters the physical stressors of the non-treated compartments. This compartmentalized approach resulted in higher prolapse recurrence, worsening prolapse of a different compartment, and worsening bowel symptoms. In addition, it results in additional surgeries for the patient. Virtanen and colleagues found that isolated treatment of middle compartment prolapse by sacrocolpopexy resulted in 26% of patients developing constipation, 22% developing difficulty with evacuation, and 26% developing pain and pressure during defecation (this can be from the prolapse and possibly enterocele) [5]. In fact, concomitant pelvic floor disorders such as cystocele, enterocele, and rectocele are present in 15–30% of patients with rectal prolapse [6, 7]. A multidisciplinary approach combining the expertise of colorectal surgeons, gynecologists, and urologists is

© Springer International Publishing AG 2018
J.T. Anger, K.S. Eilber (eds.), *The Use of Robotic Technology in Female Pelvic Floor Reconstruction*, DOI 10.1007/978-3-319-59611-2_11

essential for the treatment of women suffering from multi-compartment prolapse in order to optimize surgical outcomes aiming for the lowest recurrence, improved bowel function, and better quality of life.

Patient Evaluation

Every woman being evaluated for pelvic floor dysfunction should be routinely questioned regarding the presence or absence of symptoms within all three pelvic compartments: anterior (bladder), apical (vault/uterus), and posterior (rectum). Specific questioning for symptoms associated with pelvic floor disorders such as urinary incontinence, fecal incontinence, or organ prolapse needs to be performed. Many women suffering from these disorders are too embarrassed to inform their doctor or have the perception that these symptoms are a normal part of aging and, therefore, untreatable. Patients with pelvic organ prolapse can present with a myriad of symptoms (Table 11.1). Important questions to ask patients regarding rectal prolapse include:

1. Do you have a protrusion from the rectum?
2. How often does the protrusion occur? With each bowel movement? Does it occur with standing or coughing?
3. Do you need to push the prolapse in or does it spontaneously reduce?
4. How long have you had the prolapse?
5. Do you have a history of constipation and straining?
6. Do you suffer from fecal incontinence? If so, to what extent?

Table 11.1 Symptoms of pelvic organ dysfunction

Pelvic pressure or heaviness
Urinary incontinence or retention
Fecal incontinence
Constipation
Protrusion or bulge from vagina and/or rectum
Pain
Rectal bleeding or mucous discharge

A thorough physical examination evaluating all the pelvic floor compartments is essential for determining what surgical treatment to recommend. It is important to note that complete rectal prolapse (rectal procidentia) is a full-thickness protrusion of the rectum through the anus (Fig. 11.1), while incomplete rectal prolapse (partial rectal procidentia) consists of internal rectal prolapse to, but not through, the anal canal. Both represent degrees of severity along the continuum of pelvic floor prolapse and should be appropriately diagnosed and treated.

The simplest method of diagnosing complete rectal prolapse is to visualize this in the office by having the patient reproduce the prolapse while straining in the left lateral position or while sitting on a commode. Sometimes it can be difficult to reproduce, and we have found it helpful for patients to take a photograph at home. In addition, rectal examination should focus on evaluation of sphincter tone and function, as well as the presence of a patulous anus, rectocele, solitary rectal ulcer, and/or rectal mass. How do we know who should be referred for more than a

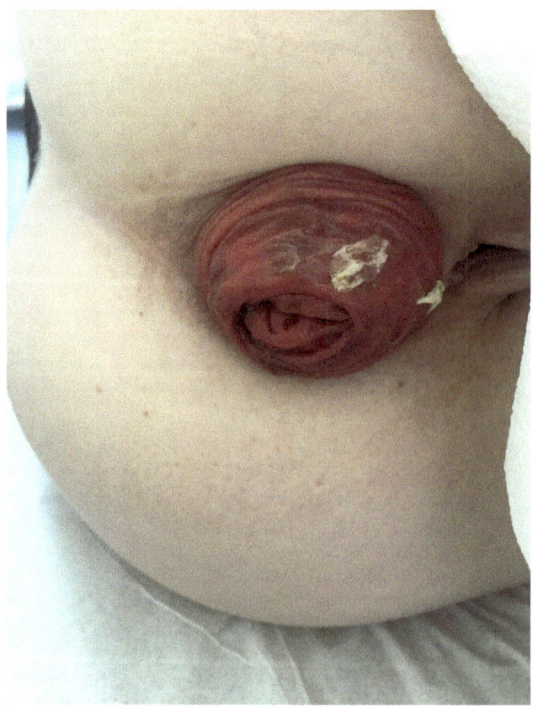

Fig. 11.1 Complete rectal prolapse (rectal procidentia)

sacrocolpopexy? If patients deny having a protrusion or defecation problems, we do not think any further work up is necessary. But, the right questions need to be asked. Many patients will not openly tell you unless you ask. In addition, many patients either think it is their hemorrhoids or are afraid it may be something worse such as cancer and so they don't inform anyone.

While vaginal and rectal prolapse are diagnosed by physical examination, the presence and extent of associated pelvic floor dysfunction requires dedicated imaging studies. Fluoroscopic defecography (Fig. 11.2) or dynamic magnetic resonance imaging (MRI) (Fig. 11.3) prove

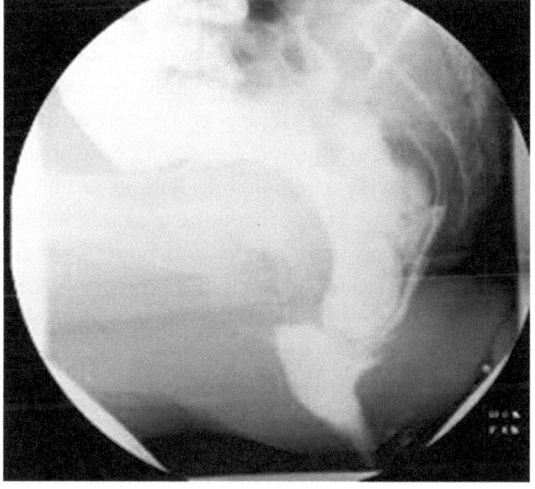

Fig. 11.2   Example of flouroscopic defecography

critical in identifying the various anatomic defects present and ensuring the involvement of appropriate specialties in an attempt to improve surgical outcomes and decrease recurrence. There is consensus that most types of vaginal prolapse can be staged and surgery planned without imaging. In fact, most "enteroceles" that occur in the setting of high stage vaginal vault prolapse are without symptoms and are addressed by a sacrocolpopexy without formal enterocele repair. However, rectal prolapse is often caused by severe straining caused by an enterocele that protrudes between the posterior vaginal wall and the anterior rectum (usually in the setting of good apical vaginal support). In the setting of rectal prolapse, it is very important to obtain if the patient has an enterocele. A common mistake is to correct the prolapse without repairing the enterocele. This results in a very high recurrence rate. Additional preoperative studies may be warranted based on the patient's clinical evaluation which are beyond the scope of this chapter (Table 11.2).

Surgical Treatment of Multi-visceral Organ Prolapse

Although much progress has been made regarding the preoperative assessment and necessity for a combined surgical repair when addressing multi-visceral organ prolapse, the optimal

Fig. 11.3   Dynamic magnetic resonance imaging of rectal prolapse. Note the enterocele, which results in severe straining and likely exacerbated her rectal prolapse symptoms

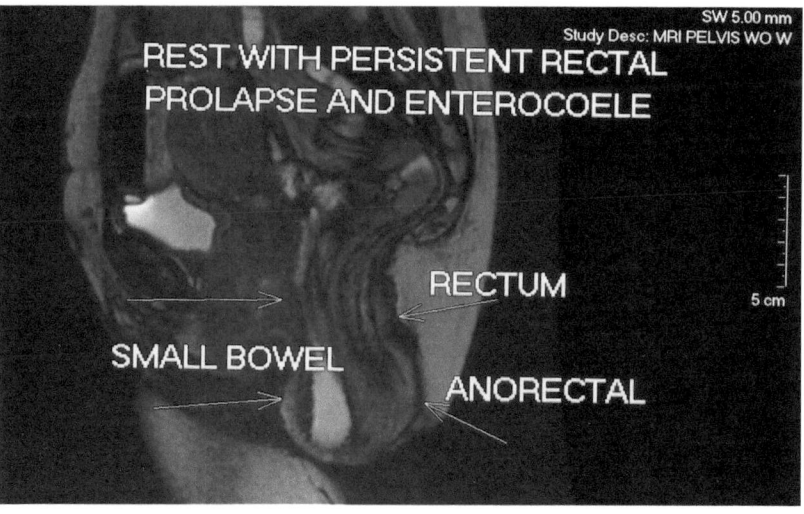

Table 11.2 Ancillary preoperative studies and imaging

Colonoscopy
Anal manometry
Urodynamics
Cystoscopy
Colonic Transit Marker Study

procedure for treatment of this disorder is still not defined. In our practice, we approach all pelvic reconstruction surgery through a multidisciplinary approach with colorectal surgeons, urologists, and gynecologists discussing the pathology, patient selection, and approach. In our opinion, this offers the best chance for curative intervention with the aim of improving symptoms and quality of life.

Abdominal sacrocolpopexy is considered the gold standard procedure for the surgical correction of vaginal vault prolapse. Sacrohysteropexy is an option for women who wish to preserve their uterus (*see* Chap. 9). Simultaneous repair of rectal prolapse includes anterior or posterior rectopexy, with or without placement of mesh, and with or without sigmoid resection. Watadani and colleagues studied open sacrocolpopexy and rectopexy for combined middle and posterior compartment prolapse, demonstrating that it is a safe procedure with low risk of recurrence, improved bowel function, and improved quality of life scores [8]. Many surgeons have transitioned to performing this procedure through a minimally invasive approach, initially with laparoscopic instrumentation and, more recently, with robotic technology. This evolution of approach is born from the enhanced capabilities of robotic instrumentation for operating in the deep pelvis as compared to rigid laparoscopic instruments. For years, surgeons operating in the pelvis have had to adapt to the limitations of laparoscopic instrumentation, which include operating at an oblique angle in the cone-shaped pelvis utilizing static instrumentation. However, robotic surgery mimics the surgeon's maneuvers and is more consistent with open surgical techniques. The da Vinci surgical system has several advantages including three-dimensional visualization, wristed instrumentation that restores seven degrees of freedom, zoom magnification,

and a third working arm. The end result is finer dissection with improved exposure, visualization, and suturing (particularly anteriorly and deep to the sacral promontory). Previously, deep pelvic dissection and the required pelvic suturing proved challenging and was limited to expert laparoscopic surgeons. The learning curve for robotic surgery, especially in the pelvis, does not appear as steep as for traditional laparoscopic surgery [9].

Combined Robotic Sacrocolpopexy and Posterior Rectopexy: Techniques and Surgical Options

Rectopexy vs. sigmoid resection. There is no consensus among colorectal surgeons about the best approach for repair of rectal prolapse. Traditionally, if a patient has severe constipation associated with a redundant sigmoid colon and rectal prolapse, she is recommended to have sigmoid resection and rectopexy. If there is no evidence of a redundant sigmoid colon, then a rectopexy alone is advised. This continues to evolve as new techniques emerge such as the ventral mesh rectopexy that will be discussed later in this chapter.

Step 1. Intubation

The patient is placed directly on a thick foam pad on the operating table in order to prevent sliding with Trendelenberg position during the operation. After general endotracheal anesthesia is administered, the patient is placed in low lithotomy position in Allen stirrups. The patient's arms are padded with foam and tucked at the sides. A urinary catheter is then placed in a sterile field.

Step 2. Port Placement

Once the abdomen and perineum are prepped and draped, a 12 mm curvilinear incision is made in the periumbilical position. A Veress needle or a Hassan technique is used to achieve trocar placement, followed by insufflation to 12–15 mmHg

Fig. 11.4 Port placement

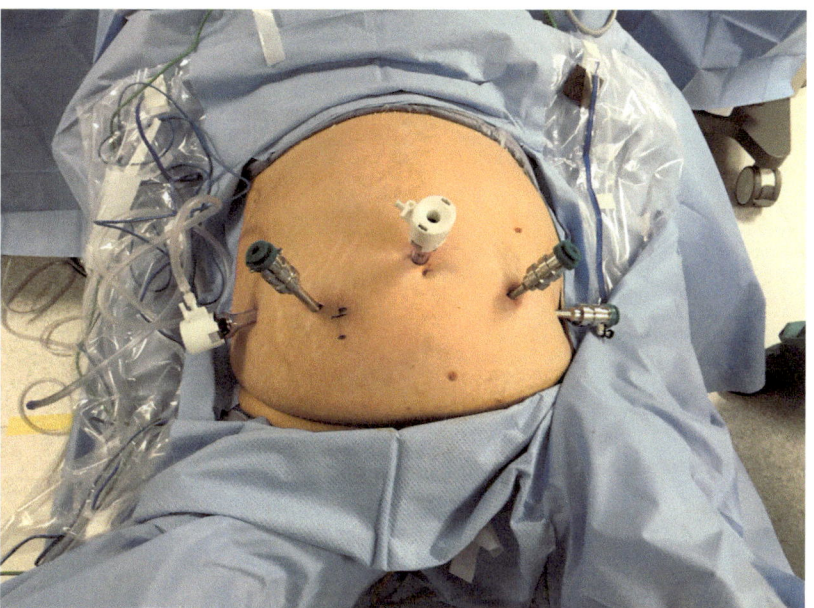

CO_2 pneumoperitoneum. The da Vinci camera (Intuitive Surgical, Sunnyvale, CA) is introduced and a general inspection is performed. A 0° or 30° down camera can be used, based on surgeon preference. We prefer the 30° down scope because we can visualize over the sacral promontory better in the presacral space.

Under direct visualization, two 8-mm trocars are placed on each side along the mid-clavicular line just below the umbilicus. A third 8-mm trocar is placed in the left lower abdomen along the mid-axillary line. Finally, a 1-mm trocar is placed at the right lower abdomen along the mid-axillary line as an assistant port approximately 4 cm above the anterior superior iliac spine. The Si robot arms should be placed a minimum of 10 cm apart in order to avoid arm collisions; however, the robotic arms can be placed closer with the Xi robot (Fig. 11.4).

Step 3. Docking

The patient is placed in steep Trendelenberg position with slight left side up. The da Vinci bedside cart is side-docked in order to maintain access to the vagina and rectum during the course of the procedure (Fig. 11.5). The small bowel is retracted out of the pelvis and the relevant pelvic landmarks are identified.

Step 4. Instrumentation

Once the robot is docked, monopolar shears are placed in the number 4 (right lower quadrant) port. A bipolar grasper is placed in the number 3 (left mid-clavicular) port, and either a Prograsp forceps or Cadiere forceps is placed in the number 1 (left mid-clavicular) port with the camera at the supraumbilical port. For the left-handed surgeon, the instruments in ports 1 and 3 are reversed. The Cadiere forceps is less traumatic for retracting the sigmoid mesentery, while the Prograsp forceps improves traction for manipulation of the more sturdy pelvic structures. We would recommend starting with the Cadiere forceps and only switch to the Prograsp forceps if the Cadiere is unable to properly retract the tissues such as the mesentery.

Step 5. Mobilization of the Sigmoid Colon and Rectum

The sigmoid colon is mobilized out of the pelvis. The sigmoid mesentery is retracted up and towards the left to identify the superior hemorrhoidal vessels and sacral promontory. Using the monopolar shears, the peritoneal reflection is opened starting approximately 2 cm above and just to the right of the sacral promontory and

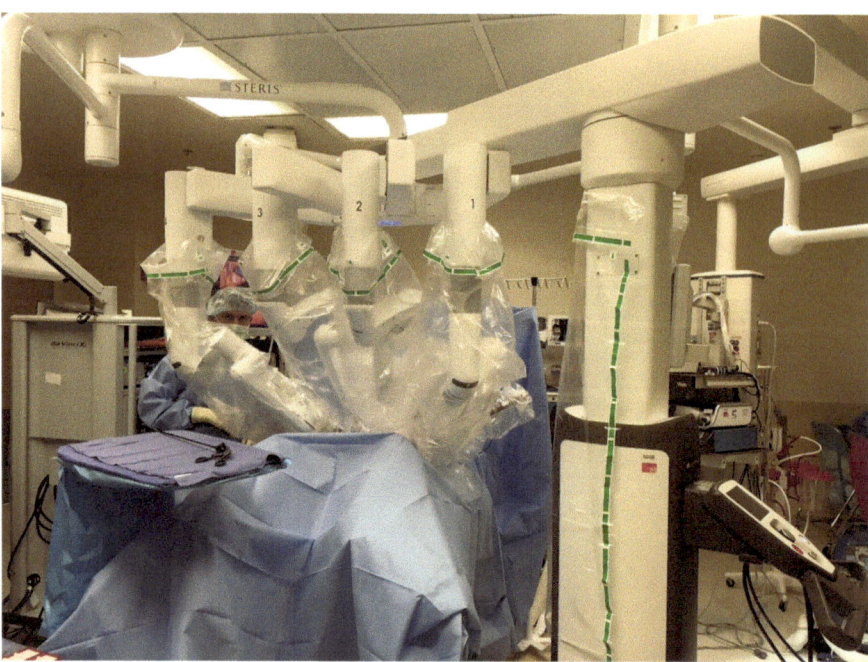

Fig. 11.5 DaVinci Xi Robot system docked in place using a side-docking technique

extending down to the rectovaginal septum. Care is taken to identify and preserve the right ureter. Using careful dissection, the superior hemorrhoidal vessels are elevated off the retroperitoneum and the left ureter is identified through the length of the dissection. Once all anatomic structures are properly identified, the rectum and mesorectum are mobilized using monopolar shears to complete the dissection as far inferiorly as the pelvic floor musculature. The hypogastric nerves are identified posteriorly and carefully preserved during this dissection. This portion of the dissection is usually performed by the colorectal surgeon.

Step 6. Sacrocolpopexy

Once the rectum is mobilized, the sacrocolpopexy is performed by the urologist, urogynecologist, or gynecologist as described by several authors [10, 11]. The presacral dissection is facilitated by the sigmoid mobilization already performed, though often Female Pelvic Medicine and Reconstructive Surgery (FMPRS) surgeons

perform additional dissection until the anterior longitudinal ligament is fully exposed. The vaginal peritoneum is incised and the vagina is dissected free from the bladder and prerectal fat. A Y-shaped piece of mesh or graft (or two separate pieces, based on surgeon preference) is sutured to the vaginal apex and anterior and posterior vaginal walls with permanent suture. The tail end of the mesh is attached to the anterior longitudinal ligament at the sacral promontory as described elsewhere in this book.

Step 7. Posterior Rectopexy

The colorectal surgeon returns to the console to perform the rectopexy. The rectum is elevated cephalad and the cuff of the mesorectum is sutured to the sacrocolpopexy mesh or just above it with permanent suture. We prefer to use 2-0 Gortex or 2-0 Ethibond suture. We place two to three figure-of-eight sutures on the right side of the mesorectum. The peritoneum is closed over the mesh with absorbable sutures of 2-0 Vicryl.

Surgical Options

Redundant Sigmoid Colon

In patients with a redundant sigmoid colon diagnosed by either colonoscopy, barium enema or dynamic MRI, and constipation symptoms, a concomitant sigmoid colon resection may be warranted. In this situation, the sigmoid colon and rectum are mobilized as previously described. The distal transection is performed at the top of the rectum, identified as the individual taenia coli splay out to cover the rectum circumferentially. The mesentery is ligated with either with a vessel sealer or a vascular-loaded stapler. The rectum is transected with the robotic stapler (usually with a green load stapler that have larger size staples). The proximal resection point is selected by identifying an area of healthy colon that will allow for a tension-free anastomosis with removal of the redundant portion of colon and also allow for the remaining colon to cradle without tension along the left lateral side wall. Once this is completed, the robot is temporarily undocked and a small Pfannenstiel incision is made. The redundant colon is removed and the proximal bowel is transected. A circular anvil is placed in the colotomy. A purse-string suture is created using 2-0 Prolene at the end colotomy. A circular anvil is placed through the colotomy and secured in place with the purse-string suture. The colon is then returned to the abdomen and the fascia is closed. The abdomen is re-insufflated, an endoanal circular stapler is introduced transanally, and the anastomosis is performed in the traditional manner with straight laparoscopic instruments. Once insufflation is re-established, the proximal colon is aligned properly along the left lateral side wall. The mesentery should be facing medially to avoid a rotation of the colon. Following a rectal examination, the endoanal circular stapler is introduced in the rectum and carefully advanced to the staple line. Under direct visualization, the spike is brought out adjacent to the staple line in the middle of the end rectum. The anvil on the proximal bowel is grasped and secured to the spike. Prior to closing the instrument, all areas are carefully inspected to make sure the bowel is aligned properly again as well as to assure there is no incorporation of any surrounding tissues. The circular stapler is closed, fired, and removed. The anastomosis is evaluated both with an air leak test and flexible sigmoidoscopy. After normal saline is placed in the pelvis, the proximal bowel is gently occluded with a grasper. A sigmoidoscopy is performed to check for any evidence of an air leak at the anastomosis and to visually inspect the anastomosis. Upon completion of the anastomosis, the robot is returned to the field and the remaining portion of the surgery is continued.

When the sigmoid resection and sacrocolpexy are combined, there are unique considerations to consider surgically. First, based on surgeon preference, we often use acellular human dermis allograft instead of mesh (Flex HD® allograft, extra thick) in the event of a colon leak. Second, we take a "tag team" approach. After the sigmoid resection, the presacral and vaginal dissections are performed (± hysterectomy). Based on surgeon preference, the vaginal mesh/graft attachments can be performed prior to the sigmoid resection, so that as much surgery is completed before the bowel anastomosis is done. Then, the vaginal mesh/graft is attached to the sacral promontory with two, 2-0 Gore-Tex sutures. At this time, the rectopexy is performed by tacking the sigmoid directly to the sacrocolpopexy graft/mesh (our preferred approach), or by tacking it to the promontory directly. Any concomitant vaginal procedures are performed at the end of the case, often at the time of port closure.

Ventral Mesh Rectopexy

Anterior placement of mesh to the rectum and a ventral rectopexy has gained popularity. This technique allows for anterior mobilization of the rectum with the mesh secured between the ventral aspect of the rectum and posterior aspect of the vagina and then attached at the sacral promontory [12]. This avoids dissecting in proximity to the pelvic nerves and sacral venous plexus as required with the posterior approach. Ventral mesh rectopexy has become an established procedure for the treatment of both internal and external rectal prolapse [13]. This technique has been performed in Europe for a number of years and is currently establishing footsteps in the United States. A combined sacrocolpopexy can readily be performed with this technique. The general consensus in the United States is to use biologic mesh for the ventral rectopexy. Biologic or synthetic mesh can be used for the sacrocolpopexy.

Robotic Sacrohysteropexy

In women who desire a uterine-sparing procedure, robotic sacrohysteropexy is an option, as described by Rosenblum [9]. Laparoscopic or robotic approaches have been shown to have less operative bleeding, shorter operative times, and fewer post-operative symptoms as compared to an open approach for sacrohysteropexy [14].

In a study reviewing their experience with laparoscopic sacrohysteropexy, Rosenblum et al. documented zero intraoperative complications (0/15) and that uterine prolapse improved in all patients undergoing this procedure. However, the same study noted that only 12 (80%) women appreciated symptomatic improvement [15]. On the contrary, a larger European trial reported overall patient satisfaction to be above 95% after undergoing this procedure [16]. Robotic sacrohysteropexy is described in more detail in Chapter 9, but deserves mention here since we see young women with symptomatic rectal prolapse who are found to have significant uterine prolapse by exam or by history. Many of these women are of childbearing age and wish to preserve fertility. In these cases, we have had success with a posterior strip sacrocolpopexy with acellular human dermis (Flex HD® allograft, extra thick), often in combination with an anterior repair performed vaginally at the end of the case. It should be mentioned that numbers are small, follow-up is short, and data is lacking on outcomes of delivery after sacrohysteropexy. Nonetheless, with proper patient counseling, this is a safe option for women at a uniquely high risk of vaginal and rectal prolapse recurrence.

Mesh: Biologic Versus Synthetic

With the increased public awareness of the FDA safety communications regarding synthetic mesh and vaginal prolapse repair, the use of mesh versus biologic graft, especially in the setting of concomitant sigmoid resection, remains a very highly debated issue. Some studies have compared native tissues (cadaveric fasica lata) to mesh-based sacrocolpopexy and have showed poor long-term results with fascia lata (93% success at 1 year in mesh group vs. 62% in fascia lata group [17]). This increase in anatomic success comes with the cost of significant mesh extrusion rates (up to 19%). In our hospital's experience of 78 women randomized to robotic versus laparoscopic ASC, however, mesh-related complications were acceptably low. Covering the mesh with peritoneum and performing supracervical (vs. total) hysterectomy for uterine prolapse are important steps in reducing mesh-related complications. When biologic graft is preferred, it is likely that newer biologic materials, specifically acellular cadaveric dermis, hold more promise than cadaveric fascia lata. No difference has been uncovered in terms of dyspareunia or sexual function between mesh and non-mesh repairs [18].

Given the concern for erosion and other postoperative complications with the use of synthetic mesh (most commonly polypropylene), many have investigated the use of biologic mesh as a substitute. This material is much more costly, but comes with easier handling properties and is less prone to infection. Thus, when performing sigmoid colectomy in addition to vaginal floor repair as described above, biologic mesh may be considered. In addition, the biologic meshes confer a lesser degree of adhesiogenesis and may decrease the rate of post-operative bowel obstructions. They also allow us to forego the step of covering the mesh with peritoneum, which saves time. While the final outcome on the biologic versus synthetic mesh debate remains unknown, a small study has compared synthetic and biologic mesh in ventral mesh rectopexy. In this study, there was no difference in recurrence or mesh complications (3.7 vs. 4.0% and 0.7 vs. 0.0%) [12].

Outcomes

As discussed previously, a combined multidisciplinary approach is essential for the best possible surgical outcomes. When looking at combined sacrocolpopexy and rectopexy, there are significant improvements in the pelvic floor distress inventory (PFDI) and patients with mixed symptoms significantly improved in terms of their colorectal distress [8, 19].

Mesh can be safely inserted, but further data is needed to clarify the biologic versus synthetic debate. In addition, sacrocolpopexy can be performed in an open manner, but can also be done with a minimally invasive technique. While there is a paucity of data comparing the efficacy of a laparoscopic versus robotic technique [20], some small studies have shown that urinary and gastrointestinal symptom improvement is better with robotic procedures [21].

Conclusions

Pelvic organ prolapse remains an important clinical problem for many women with the expectation of an increased incidence in the future. Surgical management with a multidisciplinary approach remains the procedure of choice for cure. Both laparoscopic and robotic approaches are viable and likely represent an improvement over open techniques.

The use of mesh has been shown to decrease recurrence, although this comes with the addition of the risk for mesh extrusion and mesh infection (in the setting of bowel injury or an anastomotic leak). Both synthetic and biologic grafts have been used safely, and the choice should be determined by the concomitant procedures (i.e., bowel resection), graft availability, and the results of future, well-designed studies.

References

1. Womack NR, Morrison JF, Williams NS. The role of pelvic floor denervation in the aetiology of idiopathic fecal incontinence. Br J Surg. 1984;73:404–7.
2. Olsen AL, Smith VJ, Bergstrom JD, Colling DC, Clark AL. Epidemiology of surgically managed pelvic organ prolapsed and urinary incontinence. Obstet Gynecol. 1997;89:501–6.
3. Nygaard I, Barber MD, Burgio KL, et al. Prevalence of symptomatic pelvic floor disorders in US women. JAMA. 2008;300:1311–6.
4. Wu JM, Hundley AF, Fulton RG, Myers ER. Forecasting the prevalence of pelvic floor disorders in U.S. women: 2010 to 2050. Obstet Gynecol. 2009;114:1278–83.
5. Virtanen HS, Mäkinen JI. Retrospective analysis of 711 patients operated on for pelvic relaxation in 1983-1989. Int J Gynaecol Obstet. 1993;42(2):109–15.
6. Gonzalez-Argenté FX, Jain A, Nogueras JJ, Davila GW, Weiss EG, Wexner SD. Prevalence and severity of incontinence and pelvic genital prolapsed in females with anal incontinence or rectal prolapsed. Dis Colon Rectum. 2001;44:920–6.
7. Pomerri F, Zuliani M, Mazza C, et al. Defecographic measurements of rectal intussusceptions and prolapsed in patients and in asymptomatic subjects. Am J Roentgenol. 2001;176:641–5.
8. Watadani Y, Vogler SA, Warshaw JS, Sueda T, Lowry AC, Madoff RD, Mellgren A. Sacrocolpopexy with rectopexy for pelvic floor prolapsed improves bowel function and quality of life. Dis Colon Rectum. 2013;56:1415–22.
9. Rosenblum N. Robotic approaches to prolapse surgery. Curr Opin Urol. 2012;22:292–6.
10. White WM, Pickens RB, Elder RF, Firoozi F. Robotic-assisted sacrocolpopexy for pelvic organ prolapse. Urol Clin N Am. 2014;41(4):549–57.
11. Pollard ME, Eilber KS, Anger JT. Abdominal approaches to pelvic prolapsed repairs. Curr Opin Urol. 2013;23:306–11.
12. Smart NJ, Pathak S, Boorman P, Daniels IR. Synthetic or biological mesh use in laparoscopic ventral mesh rectopexy—a systematic review. Color Dis. 2013;15(6):650–4.
13. Samaranayake CB, Luo C, Plank AW, Merrie AE, Plank LD, Bissett IP. Systematic review on ventral rectopexy for rectal prolapse and intussusception. Color Dis. 2010;12(6):504–12.
14. Paek J, Lee M, Kim BW, Kwon Y. Robotic or laparoscopic sacrohysteropexy versus open sacrohysteropexy for uterus preservation in pelvic organ prolapse. Int Urogynecol J. 2016;27(4):593–9.
15. Lee T, Rosenblum N, Nitti V, Brucker BM. Uterine sparing robotic-assisted laparoscopic sacrohysteropexy for pelvic organ prolapse: safety and feasibility. J Endourol. 2013;27(9):1131–6.
16. Mourik SL, Martens JE, Aktas M. Uterine preservation in pelvic organ prolapse using robot assisted laparoscopic sacrohysteropexy: quality of life and technique. Eur J Obstet Gynecol Reprod Biol. 2012;165(1):122–7.
17. Tate SB, Blackwell L, Lorenz DJ, Steptoe MM, Culligan PJ. Randomized trial of fascia lata and

propylene mesh for abdominal sacrocolpopexy: 5-year follow-up. Int Urogynecol J. 2011;22:137–43.

18. Nieminen K, Hiltunen R, Takala T, Heiskanen E, Merikari M, Niemi K, Heinonen PK. Outcomes after anterior vaginal wall repair with mesh: a randomized, controlled trial with a 3-year follow-up. Am J Obstet Gynecol. 2010;203(3):235.

19. Lim M, Sagar PM, Gonsalves S, Thekkinkattil D, Landon C. Surgical management of pelvic organ prolapse in females: functional outcome of mesh sacrocolpopexy and rectopexy as a combined procedure. Dis Colon Rectum. 2007;50(9):1412–21.

20. Anger JT, Mueller ER, Tarnay C, Smith B, Stroupe K, Rosenman A, Brubaker L, Bresee C, Kenton K. Robotic compared with laparoscopy sacrocolpopexy: a randomized controlled trial. Obstet Gynecol. 2014;123:5–12. Erratum in: Obstet Gynecol 2014;124:165.

21. Mehmood RK, Parker J, Bhuvimanian L, Qasem E, Mohammed AA, Zeeshan M, Grugel K, Carter P, Ahmed S. Short-term outcome of laparoscopic versus robotic ventral mesh rectopexy for full-thickness rectal prolapse. Is robotic superior? Int J Color Dis. 2014;29(9):1113–8.

Enterocele

David P. Magner, Adam Truong,
and Beth A. Moore

Prevalence

Unlike cystocele and rectocele, considered to be pseudo-hernias, an enterocele is a true herniation of the small bowel through the rectovaginal septum. Initially considered a rare entity, enterocele was first described as a condition chiefly affecting elderly, multiparous females and thought to occur secondary to pelvic floor atrophy and aging [1]. As interest in pelvic floor pathology grew, it became clear that the prevalence of symptomatic enterocele proves much more common and affects a wider age range than previously believed. In radiologic studies of healthy female volunteers, approximately two-thirds of women with enterocele had previously undergone hysterectomy (18%), leaving a significant number (10%) who had spontaneously developed an enterocele [2]. A prospectively maintained defecography database of 912 patients revealed 104 enteroceles (11% incidence) with a mean age of 63 years (range, 21–86 years), with the vast majority occurring in females (18 males, 0.02%). Only 25 patients had an isolated enterocele (defined as reaching within 3 cm of the anorectal angle), with the majority (76%) displaying additional pelvic floor organ prolapse, rectocele, or perineal descent [3]. These numbers correlate well with those regarding the expected accompaniment of vaginal vault prolapse with other pelvic floor pathology, such as cystocele, rectocele, and enterocele found in 72% of patients [4]. Clearly, enterocele is not as rare as once believed, and an effort must be made to identify this entity in all patients presenting with symptomatic pelvic floor prolapse.

D.P. Magner, M.D., F.A.C.S. (✉)
Department of Surgery, Division of Colorectal Surgery, Cedars-Sinai Medical Center, 8700 Beverly Blvd., Los Angeles, CA 90048, USA
e-mail: david.magner@cshs.org

A. Truong, M.D.
Department of Surgery, Division of Colorectal Surgery, Cedars-Sinai Medical Center, Los Angeles, CA, USA

B.A. Moore, M.D., F.A.C.S., F.A.S.C.R.S.
Department of Surgery, Division of Colorectal Surgery, Cedars-Sinai Medical Center, 8737 Beverly Boulevard, Suite 402, Los Angeles, CA 90048, USA
e-mail: mooreb@cshs.org

Anatomic and Physiologic Considerations

An enterocele defect is not a pathology of a given pelvic floor compartment per se, but rather a defect of the support structures attaching and defining these compartments. There is some controversy over the etiology of these defects. The traditional theory is that of gradual stretching and weakening of the pelvic fascia that allows for the potential spaces between pelvic organs to widen, deepen, and eventually allow symptomatic organ prolapse

© Springer International Publishing AG 2018
J.T. Anger, K.S. Eilber (eds.), *The Use of Robotic Technology in Female Pelvic Floor Reconstruction*, DOI 10.1007/978-3-319-59611-2_12

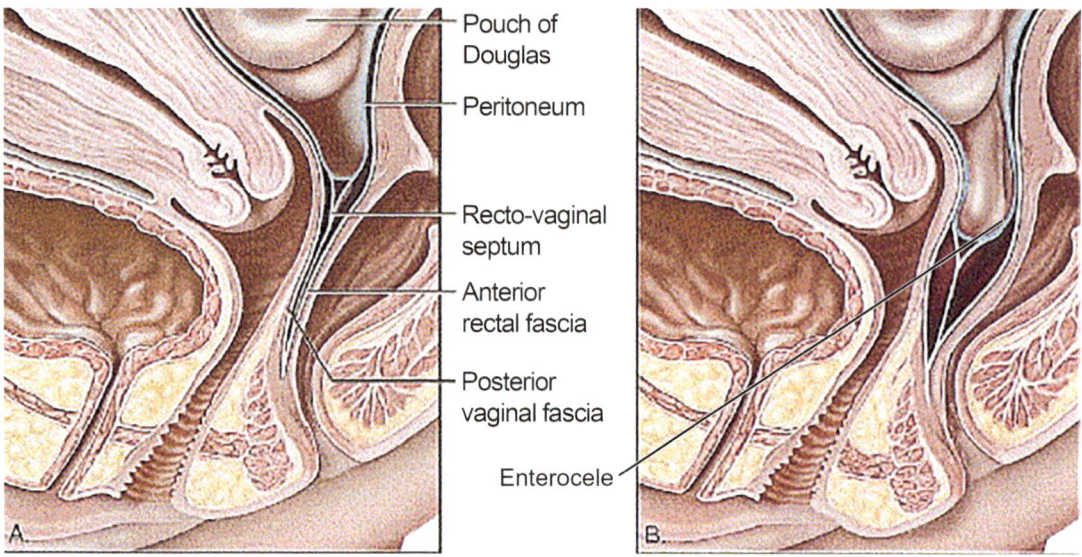

Pouch of
Douglas

Peritoneum

Recto-vaginal
septum

Anterior
rectal fascia

Posterior
vaginal fascia

Enterocele

Fig. 12.1 A natural increase in intraabdominal pressure during the sensation to defecate exacerbates the enterocele intrusion through the Pouch of Douglas (Reprinted from American Journal of Obstetrics and Gynecology, 180(4), Cruikshank SH, Kovac SR, Randomized comparison of three surgical methods used at the time of vaginal hysterectomy to prevent posterior enterocele, 859–65., Copyright (1999), with permission from Elsevier)

Fig. 12.2 Small bowel herniating through the vaginal apex forming an apical enterocele (Reprinted from American Journal of Obstetrics and Gynecology, 179(6 Pt 1), Miklos JR, Kohli N, Lucente V, Saye WB, Site-specific fascial defects in the diagnosis and surgical management of enterocele, 1418–22, Copyright (1998), with permission from Elsevier)

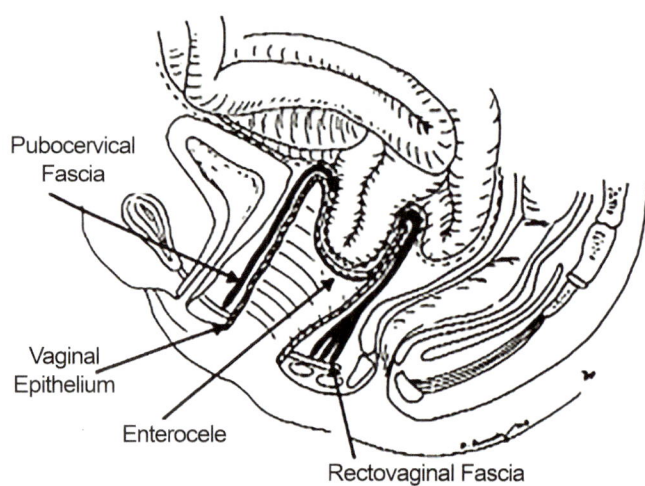

Pubocervical
Fascia

Vaginal
Epithelium

Enterocele

Rectovaginal Fascia

and/or herniation [5] (Fig. 12.1). Other researchers suggest that the pathophysiology of enterocele lies in specific defects and detachments of the pubocervical fascia or rectovaginal septum [6, 7]. The "site specific" theory of enterocele development is supported by the creation of an apical enterocele which occurs after failure to close the resulting endopelvic fascial defect overlying the vaginal cuff (which is created during hysterectomy) (Fig. 12.2). The recognition of the defective supporting structure(s) leading to a given enterocele is key in achieving successful repair.

A brief review of the key supporting structures and potential spaces within the pelvis is important in understanding enterocele defects and in serving as a guide to the appropriate repair. By viewing the pelvis as three compartments: anterior (bladder, urethra), middle (vagina, cervix, uterus), and posterior (anal canal, rectum), we are able to conceptualize pelvic organ prolapse in an organized way. However, it is important not to lose sight of the pathology causative of pelvic organ prolapse. The organ structures are bystanders in the process, though often blamed as the perpetrators. Defects in the pubocervical, endopelvic, and rectovaginal fasciae are the root cause of organ prolapse. Study of the anterior, middle, and posterior compartments will reveal the specific defects present and guide repair.

In the structurally sound pelvis, the vagina is anchored anteriorly to the bladder by the pubocervical fascia and posteriorly to the rectum by the rectovaginal fascia. A natural hiatus is present for the cervix and uterine fundus. The upper quarter of the vagina is suspended by the cardinal-uterosacral ligaments, the middle half by lateral attachments, and lower quarter by the urogenital diaphragm/perineal body fusion plane [8]. These levels correspond to De Lancey's levels 1, 2, and 3, respectively (see Chap. 3). Failure of any, or a combination, of these levels will cause vaginal vault prolapse and allow the small bowel to occupy the potential space between the vagina and rectum, producing a posterior enterocele. The distinct apical enterocele will occur when the endopelvic fascia overlying the vaginal cuff is disrupted and/or thinned, typically during hysterectomy. The small bowel is then afforded direct contact with the uncovered vaginal epithelium and an apical enterocele occurs [6].

The sensation to defecate is likely created, or contributed to, by the sensation of pressure and stretch of the levator ani musculature. Patients with enterocele experience the herniated small intestine pressing upon the pelvic musculature and anterior rectal wall. This produces the misinterpreted urge to defecate. Subsequent straining at unproductive defecation increases the intraabdominal pressure, intensifying this sensation as the small intestine is pushed more strongly against these receptors. This leads to further attenuation of Denonvillier's fascia, widening of the Pouch of Douglas, and deepening of the enterocele as symptoms continue to worsen [19]. A simple test is useful in identifying this process. Explain this process to the patient and, at the next occurrence, have the patient leave the toilet and position themselves with hips well above shoulders (i.e., hips elevated on cushions). Relief of the sensation to defecate suggests that gravity has assisted the small intestine in falling out of Pouch of Douglas and predicts success after surgical repair of the enterocele.

Presenting Symptoms

The symptoms of enterocele can be classified into two categories: (1) pelvic discomfort and (2) altered bowel function. Symptoms of pelvic discomfort from an enterocele can include pelvic pain, pressure, a sensation of prolapse/protrusion, and dyspareunia. Symptoms of obstructed defecation are the most common symptoms of enterocele. Patients describe a sensation of a ball in the rectum, which leads them to making several unsuccessful visits to the toilet in an attempt to relieve this sensation. Others will complain of the sensation of incomplete emptying, straining, infrequent bowel movements, or episodes of fecal incontinence. A history of chronic straining and constipation is often present; however, there is some question as to the role of enterocele in causing the symptoms of obstructed defecation and concomitant partial or complete rectal prolapse may be the true cause of the symptoms. This highlights the need for complete pelvic floor evaluation prior to embarking on repair [9]. One study of 310 women with pelvic organ prolapse found no difference in bowel function among those with and without enterocele [10]. Often, the patient will detail a history of chronic constipation that has been present for years, but has more recently become associated with additional pelvic complaints. This supports the notion that functional symptoms are likely due to multiple factors which are gradually worsening and eventually come to the clinician's attention once they have passed an individual's pain and bowel function threshold of complaint. By this time, multiple pathologies are likely to be present and the identification and correction of each pelvic compartment is paramount. The history must seek out the symptoms typical of enterocele cited above, as well as other possible contributing factors. Questions regarding urinary incontinence, the presence of a vaginal bulge, difficulty evacuating bowel movements, and rectal prolapse should all be routine. The development of symptoms occurring after hysterectomy should alert the clinician to the possibility of an apical enterocele as the causative agent. Lastly, patients with enterocele and associated obstructed defecation often develop symptomatic anorectal disorders such as hemorrhoids or fissuring and pelvic floor pathology may prove to be the unifying diagnosis.

Diagnostic Evaluation

Physical Examination

A thorough, focused pelvic exam with the intent of uncovering pathology in all compartments is paramount. The pelvic exam should evaluate the anterior and posterior vaginal walls, cervix, urethra, rectum, anus, and perineum. This is usually achieved in the lithotomy position; however, subsequent bimanual exam for enterocele may be better achieved in standing position. After static exam is performed, the patient should be asked to strain and each component evaluated with attention to cervical descent, cystocele, perineal descent, rectal prolapse, rectocele, and presence of a patulous anus. During bimanual exam, the examiner should attempt to palpate bowel interposed between the vagina and rectum. Again, this is often better demonstrated with the patient standing.

In advanced cases, enterocele with complete loss of fascial attachments will herniate through the vaginal orifice. Rarely will the diagnosis be so obvious. The majority of patients will have a lesser degree of enterocele, remaining a hidden diagnosis contributing to, rather than solely responsible for, a litany of complaints generally focused around pelvic discomfort, sensation of prolapse, and the act of defecation. Even in cases where the diagnosis is clearly evident, it is important to fully evaluate the pelvic floor for synchronous pathology. This allows one to address all surgical aspects of pelvic floor dysfunction during a single intervention, while, at the same time, increasing the probability of a successful outcome.

Imaging

The vast majority of enteroceles are not detected on physical exam and require designated imaging to detect their presence [11]. Dynamic imaging of the pelvic floor is the key component to identify and address all aspects of pelvic floor pathology.

Traditionally, this has been obtained with X-ray defecography studies. More recently, magnetic resonance imaging (MRI) defecography is supplanting classic defecography. Some suggest this is due less to improved images and detection, but more to reluctance on the part of both patient and radiologist to pursue classic defecography. We, however, believe that dynamic MRI with rectal contrast (MRI defecography) provides superior anatomic and physiologic detail of all three compartments in both static and functional states. The limitation of MRI defecography stems from the inability to truly document the patient's anatomy during the act of defecation—as we are generally instructing patients to "push as if you are passing stool," rather than having them defecate out contrast material as with a flouroscopic defecography study.

Evacuation proctography was initially limited to a fluoroscopic technique. This requires the patient's rectum to be filled by a thick, radiopaque paste via rectal tube, followed by defecation while undergoing fluoroscopic imaging seated on a radiolucent commode (Fig. 12.3). This often produces consternation on the patient's part, in addition to significant radiation exposure. It does provide excellent images and a true physiologic evaluation of defecation. It is important that the small bowel has also been opacified with oral contrast prior to imaging to enhance identification of the small intestine.

The advent of MRI defecography allows for excellent images of all three compartments and obviates the need for additional studies if the bladder, uterus, or other pelvic organs require imaging. Patients find the procedure much more agreeable, as they do not need to actually defecate during the process. In addition, they are spared exposure to ionizing radiation. MRI in the seated position is best suited for this exam, but it is not readily available at many institutions. Regardless, we have been very satisfied with images obtained with standard, supine MRI. The addition of an evacuation phase, rather than simple instruction to bear down, is considered mandatory by some [12]. Gousse et al. compared physical examination, MRI, and intraoperative findings and found the sensitivity, specificity, and positive predictive value of MRI in identifying

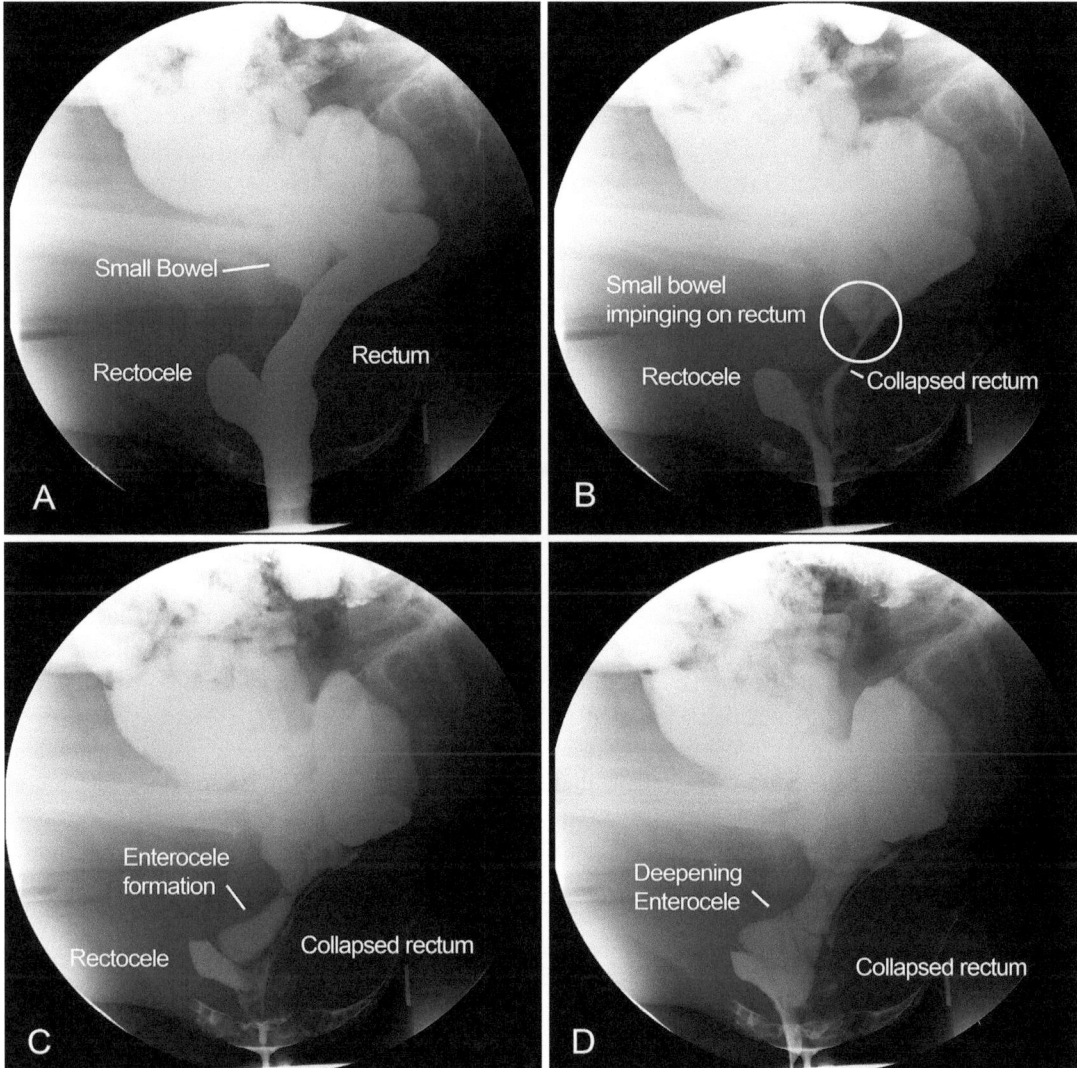

Fig. 12.3 X-ray defacography. (**a**) Resting. The patient has an incidental rectocele. (**b**) Patient initiates bear-down, collapsing the rectum. (**c**) Enterocele forming as patient continues to bear-down. (**d**) Enterocele deepens as intra-abdominal pressure increases

enterocele to be 87%, 80%, and 91%, respectively [13]. In a systematic review of dynamic MRI imaging for pelvic organ prolapse, Broikhuis et al. confirmed that dynamic MRI proves useful within the subset of identifying the presence of enteroceles as a component of pelvic floor prolapse [14]. For those interested, we highly recommend an excellent review of dynamic MRI, available online by searching: Dynamic MR Imaging of the Pelvic Floor: a Pictorial Review [15] (Table 12.1).

Table 12.1 Grading of enterocele as visualized by evacuation proctography

Grade
1. Enterocele descending to the upper one third of the vagina
2. Enterocele descending to the middle one third of the vagina
3. Enterocele descending to the lower one third of the vagina

Additional Studies

Obtaining a history consistent with enterocele, a confirmatory physical exam and appropriate dynamic imaging of the pelvis allow us to correctly identify all components of a given patient's pelvic floor pathology, leading to selection of appropriate interventions. On occasion, certain adjunctive studies are indicated. First and foremost, colonoscopy should be performed to evaluate for significant redundancy of the sigmoid colon or "kinking" of the rectosigmoid junction, which would alter the choice of surgery to include resection of this segment of bowel. Moreover, other possible causes of the patient's symptoms, such as tumor, stricture, and solitary rectal ulcer, must be ruled out.

In the patient with complaints of constipation, functional studies of the bowel are also indicated. In our practice, we routinely order a SITZMARKS® study (Fig. 12.4) to distinguish whether the cause of constipation is due to colonic inertia or obstructed defecation. A capsule is ingested by the patient, which dissolves in the upper GI tract releasing 24 radiopaque rings. The patient then returns for serial abdominal X-rays on certain days over the following week—we typically obtain films on post-ingestion days three, five and seven. This allows for determination of overall colorectal function and aids in determining if constipation is due to colonic motility (i.e., colonic inertia) or defecatory dysfunction (i.e., obstructed defecation). If greater than 80% of the rings have been evacuated in the one-week evaluation period, the test is considered normal. If the test is abnormal (i.e., five or more markers remain), then we focus on where the markers are located. If all have advanced to and clustered in the rectum, this sug-

gests that the patient's colonic motility is normal and the constipation is due to obstructed defecation of either functional or anatomic nature (such as rectal prolapse, enterocele, rectocele, descending perineum syndrome, and paradoxical puborectalis contraction/anismus). If the remaining markers are scattered throughout the colon or have not reached the rectum, then this represents colonic inertia and the pathology lies in the motility of the colon and not in a functional/anatomic issue with defecation.

Patients with anismus (a.k.a. paradoxical puborectalis contraction) experience dysynergistic contraction of pelvic floor musculature. The puborectalis muscle forms a sling around the rectum with both ends of the muscle anchored anteriorly at the pubis. The muscle is usually contracted, creating a kink (anorectal angle) in the rectum which helps maintain continence. During normal defecation, the puborectalis muscle should relax, allowing for straightening of the anorectal angle and passage of stool. Patients who experience paradoxical puborectalis contraction/anismus exhibit a further tightening of this muscle during attempts to defecate. This leads to increased "kinking" of the anorectal angle and an inability to pass stool. We have been satisfied with the ability of dynamic pelvic MRI (MRI defecography) in revealing the non-coordinated muscular activity present in these patients. However, some clinicians will directly measure the anorectal pressures present during defecation by obtaining dedicated anorectal manometry studies on any patient with suspected obstructed defecation. Lastly, a urologic workup should be considered for all patients in order to diagnose occult urinary stress incontinence or other disorder, which may worsen if not addressed at the time of enterocele or vaginal prolapse repair.

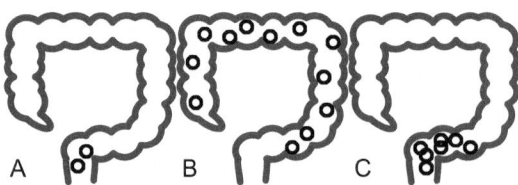

Fig. 12.4 *Sitzmarker* study interpretation. (**a**) Normal colonic motility with <5 residual *Sitzmarkers* at 1 week. (**b**) Residual *Sitzmarkers* throughout the colon due to colonic inertia. (**c**) Residual *Sitzmarkers* are concentrated in the rectum due to obstructed defecation

Robotic-Assisted Enterocele Repair

Multiple options exist for the treatment of enterocele. Both transvaginal and transabdominal surgical approaches are available, but for the purposes of this textbook, we will focus on our preferred approach (robotic-assisted transabdominal) followed by an evaluation of outcomes. The transvaginal approach is not within the scope of this chapter and it appears inferior to abdominal repair (see section "Outcomes"). The key to preventing an apical enterocele is in preventing its formation—we encourage specific attention to prophylactic cul-de-sac obliteration and vaginal support performed at the time of hysterectomy.

Pre-operative Considerations

We prepare all patients as for bowel surgery, even in cases when we do not anticipate a concomitant bowel resection. This includes giving both mechanical and antibiotic bowel preparation the evening before surgery. This includes a mechanical bowel preparation with either an osmotic and/ or stimulant laxative. Please note that sodium phosphate preparations should not be used in patients with decreased renal function, hypercalcemia, or those on ACE inhibitors due to possibility of irreversible renal failure secondary to phosphate deposition. These patients should be given an osmotic-only PEG (polyethylene glycol) solutions. In addition to mechanical bowel preparation, we also perform antibiotic preparation with modified Nichols and Condon protocol the night prior to surgery of 1 g oral neomycin at 2:00 pm, 3:00 pm, and 10:00 pm and 500 mg metronidazole at 3:00 pm and 10:00 pm. This not only ensures proper practice if a bowel resection is required, but also reduces the weight of the colon and provides easier, less traumatic handling. In addition, all patients receive an appropriate pre-operative antibiotic, sequential compression devices and thromboprophylaxis in the pre-operative area. Pre-operative glucose levels are checked and addressed prior to surgery and normothermia is ensured prior to, and throughout, the case. An orogastric tube is placed and the urinary catheter should be prepped into the surgical field.

Positioning/Exposure

As enterocele repair chiefly involves suturing, patients should be positioned according to the primary procedure being performed (i.e., sig-

moidectomy, rectopexy, sacrocolpopexy, etc.). For repair of an isolated enterocele defect, we recommend lithotomy positioning with a minimal amount of Trendelenburg and the patient's left side up, which allows gravity to displace the small intestine out of the pelvis. Proper exposure requires retraction of the uterus, when present, anteriorly. This can be easily achieved with the use of a fan retractor, transvaginal EEA sizer, or by introducing a Keith needle and temporarily tacking the uterus to the anterior abdominal wall.

Docking/Port Placement/Equipment

The bedside cart is docked along the patient's left side, either with right angle "side-docking" or oblique docking at the patient's left hip. Side-docking has the benefit of affording easy access to the perineum during the course of the case.

Port placement is dependent on the platform being employed (da Vinci Si versus Xi). Again, one should place ports based on the primary procedure being performed. For an isolated enterocele repair, the ports can be limited to a camera port at the umbilicus and two working ports 6 cm to either side. The final arm does not need to be docked. An assistant port should also be placed for suctioning, suture passing, and anterior retraction of the uterus (Fig. 12.5).

We preferentially utilize the monopolar shears and either ProGrasp or Cadiere forceps for

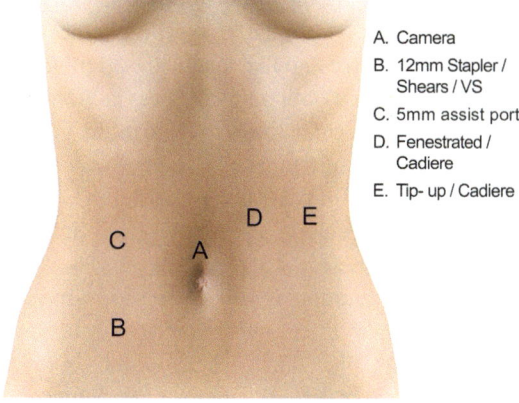

A. Camera
B. 12mm Stapler / Shears / VS
C. 5mm assist port
D. Fenestrated / Cadiere
E. Tip- up / Cadiere

Fig. 12.5 Optimal port placement using the da Vinci Si/ Xi platform

manipulating tissue. Our suture of choice is 2-0 Ethibond for both its strength and superior handling qualities/ease of intra-corporeal suturing.

Surgical Technique

1. After positioning the patient, the small bowel is placed into the upper abdomen providing exposure of the rectosigmoid colon, sacral promontory, uterus, vagina, and bladder. Key landmarks are identified, including the ureters and pelvic vasculature. If present, adhesive bands are taken down to achieve adequate working space/visualization.
2. Any simultaneous procedure is performed per standard robotic/laparoscopic technique. In all instances, the enterocele repair is performed after completion of the concomitant procedure. For instance, in conjunction with a sigmoid resection and rectopexy, the dissection, resection, anastomosis, and rectopexy are all performed prior to repairing the enterocele defect. Likewise, the enterocele defect is closed as the final step in a combined sacrocolpopexy/enterocele repair.
3. Once the primary procedure has been completed, an end-to-end anastomosis (EEA) sizer is placed into the vagina to assist with traction and reveal the extent of the enterocele defect. If present, the uterus is reflected towards the anterior abdominal wall, while the rectosigmoid junction is gently retracted cephalad.
4. The deepest portion of the enterocele is then grasped and multiple, concentric purse-string sutures of 2-0 Ethibond (Ethibond Excell polyester suture) are used at the peritoneal level. Between three and five layers are often needed to completely obliterate the sac. Caution must be paid to avoid damage to the rectum and ureters. The closure must be complete, as any gap ("air knots") in tying down the suture will risk internal herniation of small bowel into the remaining defect [16] (Fig. 12.6).
5. A Halban culdoplasty can be used to buttress this repair after hysterectomy. Additional sutures are placed in a posterior/anterior direction to incorporate the native peritoneum posteriorly, outermost layer of the rectum, vaginal cuff and, finally, the peritoneum of the enterocele repair anteriorly [16] (Fig. 12.7).

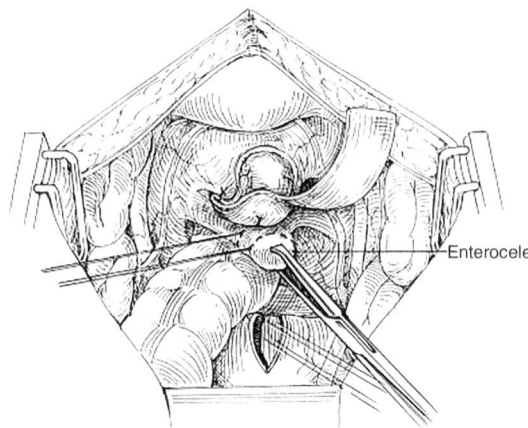

Fig. 12.6 A purse-string suture is placed at the enterocele cul-de-sac [Reprinted from Urology, 56(6 Suppl 1), Winters JC, Cespedes RD, Vanlangendonck R., Abdominal sacral colpopexy and abdominal enterocele repair in the management of vaginal vault prolapse, 55–63, Copyright (2000), with permission from Elsevier]

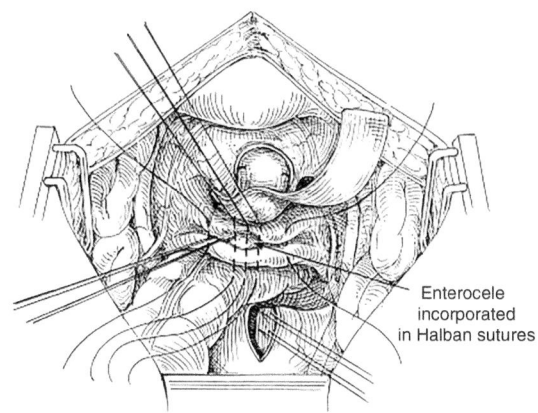

Fig. 12.7 Stitches in the anterior/posterior direction are used to incorporate pelvic structures and buttress the repair [Reprinted from Urology, 56(6 Suppl 1), Winters JC, Cespedes RD, Vanlangendonck R., Abdominal sacral colpopexy and abdominal enterocele repair in the management of vaginal vault prolapse, 55–63, Copyright (2000), with permission from Elsevier]

Notes:

- When a sacrocolpopexy has been performed, it is critical to completely cover any exposed mesh with peritoneum. Closing peritoneum over the mesh after completion of sacrocolpopexy will go a long way in obliterating the enterocele defect. The remaining defect can then be obliterated (see step 2 above).

- In the case of an isolated apical vaginal defect subsequent to hysterectomy, site-specific defect repair is indicated. Several techniques have been described and an excellent review is provided by James Carter [8]. The key is the obliteration of the defect by systematically recreating the pericervical ring at the vaginal apex. This is achieved by identifying the uterosacral ligaments, which are buttressed in an anterior/posterior orientation, followed by obliterating the remaining apical defect as the pubocervical and rectovaginal fascial edges are brought together to recreate coverage of the vaginal apex (this often requires mesh implantation due to tissue attenuation).

Closure

All trocar sites of 10 mm or larger are closed with 0-Vicryl at the fascial level, and if an extraction site was employed (i.e., for simultaneous bowel resection), the fascia is closed with #1-PDS. Skin can be approximated with a subcuticular closure; however, in cases with a concomitant bowel resection, we generally use skin staples.

Outcomes

Surgery for enterocele repair should have three aims: (1) objective repair of the defect, (2) relief of symptoms, and (3) durability. Eradication of the defect is best studied by pre- and post-operative imaging studies. Determining the corresponding resolution of symptoms proves more difficult due to the subjective nature and difficulty in assessing/attributing patient outcomes to a given portion of, an often, multi-component surgery. Finally, the durability of any given repair requires longer term study, which will aid in directing us towards native tissue techniques versus mesh reinforcement as more data becomes available.

Objective evidence of the successful eradication of an enterocele defect is illustrated through a comparison of pre-operative and post-operative defecography studies in patients. Oom et al. revealed that 90% of enteroceles were success-

fully treated by the abdominal approach; however, 25% of patients experienced recurrence of pelvic discomfort and 75% noted persistent obstructed defecation [2, 17]. These findings are echoed by several groups [3, 17].

A second method of assessing the success of an enterocele repair is through comparison of pre-operative and post-operative symptoms of pelvic pressure, abdominal pain, obstructed defecation, and fecal/urinary incontinence. Jean et al. evaluated these metrics in 62 consecutive women undergoing enterocele repair by a single surgeon. Pelvic pressure was less frequent after abdominal colporectosacropexy than prior to surgery ($p < 0.01$), with complete resolution in 41/56 patients and improvement in 10/56 patients at 27 ± 13 months after surgery. Importantly, there were no significant differences found in symptoms of obstructed defecation, lower abdominal pain, or fecal or urinary incontinence after surgery [17]. These findings are also supported by Takahashi et al. who found that the characteristic symptoms of difficulty emptying (61 patients), post-evacuation discomfort (54 patients), and pelvic pain (28 patients) were improved or resolved after surgery. Eleven patients (10 females) underwent enterocele repair. Three of the 11 patients reported complete resolution of pelvic pain. The remaining eight patients experienced reduced symptoms, mainly resolution of pelvic heaviness, but still had difficulty emptying or post-evacuation discomfort. This study supports the notion that the common symptoms of pelvic pain or heaviness respond better to enterocele repair than do either post-evacuation discomfort or difficulty in defecation; they conclude that selected patients with pelvic pain rather than obstructed defecatory symptoms might benefit more from surgical repair.

An important distinction should be made in regard to obstructed defecation in the presence of sigmoidocele. Although less common than enterocele, sigmoidoceles are not rare and these patients have shown significant improvement of constipation symptoms after surgical repair of the support defects [18].

Stephen Cruikshank et al. evaluated three methods of prophylactic enterocele repair at the time of vaginal hysterectomy [19]. One hundred consecutive women undergoing vaginal hysterectomy were randomly assigned to a vaginal Moschcowitz repair, an abdominal McCall-type repair with culdoplasty/plication of uterosacral and cardinal ligaments/elevation of vaginal apex and, finally, a peritoneal-only closure of the pouch of Douglas. The patients were evaluated at six-weeks, three-months, and annually for three years. The first prolapses were detected at one year (11 with stage 1 or 2) and this increased to 16 at two years. The McCall-type procedure proved statistically superior at three years ($p = 0.004$), with only two of 32 patients developing recurrence. The other two procedures carried failure rates of 30% (10 of 33) with vaginal Moschcowitz-type repair and 39% (13 of 33) with peritoneal closure only. This study underscores the importance of including fascial repair and re-establishing the fascial support structures in order to produce a lasting result. This follows suit with other studies evaluating vaginal versus abdominal approaches to pelvic organ prolapse. A randomized study of 80 women (vaginal 42, abdominal 38) with follow-up ranging from one to 5.5 years (mean 2.5 years) was performed by Benson, et al. The groups were similar in age, weight, parity, and estrogen status, and history of previous pelvic surgery (56%). Surgical success was present in 58% of abdominal approaches versus 29% of vaginal approaches. No significant difference existed in morbidity, complications, hemoglobin change, dyspareunia, pain, or hospital stay [20].

Conclusions

Successful treatment of symptomatic enterocele demands a thorough workup to identify any contributing pelvic pathology and an interdisciplinary team approach in the selection and performance of the appropriate procedure. As evidenced above, patient selection is also key and a frank discussion must occur with each patient regarding their specific set of symptoms and whether and to what extent surgery can be expected to rectify them. This may be one area of surgery that goes against the age-old adage of "if you operate for pain, you (the surgeon) get pain," as it appears that pelvic discomfort and pressure complaints fare better than resolution of obstructive defecation. Having decided to embark on repair, we feel strongly that an abdominal approach, with both suspension and closure components, best achieves a durable repair of the enterocele defect. We have migrated to performing this with the da Vinci robot and find several advantages. A single center randomized trial found no difference in operative time, length of hospital stay, or technical success (based on postoperative MRI) between laparoscopic and robotic ventral rectopexy [21]. We have completely transitioned from the laparoscopic to a robotic approach in our practice. We have found that the technical advantages achieved with wristed instruments, 3D visualization, and improved ergonomics greatly simplify pelvic surgery. These attributes combine to make working and suturing in the deep pelvis more precise and enjoyable. By erasing the difficulties of working in the deep pelvis, particularly caudal to the sacral promontory, that are encountered when using straight-line laparoscopic instrumentation, the robotic approach is extremely well-suited for enterocele and pelvic floor surgery and we strongly encourage its use.

References

1. Holley RL. Enterocele: a review. Obstet Gynecol Surv. 1994;49:284–93.
2. Oom DM, Gosselink MP, Schouten WR. Enterocele: diagnosis and treatment. Gastroenterol Clin Biol. 2009;33:135–7.
3. Takahashi T, Yamana T, Sahara R, Iwadare J. Enterocele: what is the clinical implication? Dis Colon Rectum. 2006;49:S75–81.
4. Herbst A, Mishell D, Stenchever M. Disorders of the abdominal wall and pelvic support. In: Comprehensive gynecology. 2nd ed. St. Louis: Mosby; 1992. p. 594–612.
5. Nichols DH. Types of enterocele and principles underlying choice of operation for repair. Obstet Gynecol. 1972;40:257–63.
6. Miklos JR, Kohli N, Lucente V, Saye WB. Site-specific fascial defects in the diagnosis and surgical management of enterocele. Am J Obstet Gynecol. 1998;179:1418–23.

7. Richardson AC, Lyon JB, Williams NL. A new look at pelvic relaxation. Am J Obstet Gynecol. 1976;126:568–73.
8. Carter JE. Enterocele repair and vaginal vault suspension. Curr Opin Obstet Gynecol. 2000;12:321–30.
9. Peters WA III, Smith MR, Drescher CW. Rectal prolapse in woman with other defects of pelvic floor supports. Am J Obstet Gynecol. 2001;184:1488–95.
10. Chou Q, Weber AM, Piedmonte MR. Clinical presentation of enterocele. Obstet Gynecol. 2000;96:599–603.
11. Kelvin FM, Maglinte DD, Benson JT. Evacuation proctography (defecography): an aid to the investigation of pelvic floor disorders. Obstet Gynecol. 1994;83:307–14.
12. Foti PV, Farina R, Riva G, et al. Pelvic floor imaging: comparison between magnetic resonance imaging and conventional defecography in studying outlet obstruction syndrome. Radiol Med. 2013;118:23–39.
13. Gousse AE, Barbaric ZL, Safir MH, Madjar S, Marumoto AK, Raz S. Dynamic half Fourier acquisition, single shot turbo spin-echo magnetic resonance imaging for evaluating the female pelvis. J Urol. 2000;164:1606–13.
14. Broekhuis SR, Fütterer JJ, Barentsz JO, Vierhout ME, Kluivers KB. A systematic review of clinical studies on dynamic magnetic resonance imaging of pelvic organ prolapse: the use of reference lines and anatomical landmarks. Int Urogynecol J. 2009;20:721–9.
15. Colaiacomo MC, Masselli G, Polettini E, Lanciotti S, Casciani E, Bertini L, Gualdi G. Dynamic MR imaging of the pelvic floor: a pictorial review. Radiographics. 2009;29(3):e35.
16. Winters JC, Cespedes RD, Vanlangendonck R. Abdominal sacral colpopexy and abdominal enterocele repair in the management of vaginal vault prolapse. Urology. 2000;56(6 Suppl 1):55–63.
17. Jean F, Tanneau Y, Le Blanc-Louvry I, Leroi AM, Denis P, Michot F. Treatment of enterocele by abdominal colporectosacropexy: efficacy on pelvic pressure. Color Dis. 2002;4(5):321.
18. Fenner DE. Diagnosis and assessment of sigmoidoceles. Am J Obstet Gynecol. 1996;175:1438–42.
19. Cruikshank SH, Kovac SR. Randomized comparison of three surgical methods used at the time of vaginal hysterectomy to prevent posterior enterocele. Am J Obstet Gynecol. 1999;180:859–65.
20. Benson JT, Lucente V, McClellan E. Vaginal versus abdominal reconstructive surgery for the treatment of pelvic support defects: a prospective randomized study with long-term outcome evaluation. Am J Obstet Gynecol. 1996;175:1418–22.
21. Mäkelä-Kaikkonen J, Rautio T, Pääkkö E, Biancari F, Ohtonen P, Mäkelä J. Robot-assisted versus laparoscopic ventral rectopexy for external or internal rectal prolapse and enterocele: a randomized controlled trial. Color Dis. 2016;18:1010–5.

Robotic-Assisted Vesicovaginal Fistula Repair

13

Devin Patel and Jennifer T. Anger

Introduction

The etiology and incidence of urogenital tract fistulas varies geographically. In developing countries, urogenital fistulas are a common complication of obstructed labor during childbirth [1]. In the United States and other developed countries, these fistulas are uncommon and are most often sequelae of gynecologic surgery, and less often as a result of radiation therapy or obstetric injury [2]. Vesicovaginal fistulas (VVF) are the most common type of urogenital fistula, with approximately 5,000 repairs for this condition performed annually in the United States [3].

Successful VVF repair is dependent on the health of the surrounding tissues and surgical technique. As such, the optimal method of repair continues to be debated. Traditionally, repair techniques have been via either a transvaginal or

D. Patel, M.D., M.B.A. (✉)
Department of Surgery, Division of Urology,
Cedars Sinai Medical Center, 8635 West 3rd Street,
#1070-W, Los Angeles, CA 90048, USA
e-mail: devin.patel@cshs.org

J.T. Anger, M.D., M.P.H.
Department of Surgery, Division of Urology,
Cedars-Sinai Medical Center, 99 N La Cienega Blvd.,
Suite 307, Beverly Hills, CA, USA

an abdominal approach. The transvaginal approach is associated with a faster recovery and decreased morbidity, while the abdominal approach allows for easier access to proximal fistulas and affords the opportunity to provide secondary coverage with an omental or peritoneal flap. Over the past 20 years, minimally invasive laparoscopic techniques have been developed and utilized in an effort to replicate the advantages of an abdominal approach while minimizing morbidly and recovery time.

Laparoscopic dissection and intracorporeal suturing are technically challenging. By providing the advantage of improved instrument dexterity, range of motion, motion scaling, and three-dimensional magnified imaging, robotic assistance has helped overcome these difficulties and decreased the learning curve for this procedure [4].

This chapter focuses on techniques and issues surrounding robot-assisted laparoscopic surgical repair of VVF. Literature regarding optimum patient selection, post-surgical follow-up, and outcomes will be discussed. An overview of surgical techniques will also be presented.

Patient Selection

Prior to selecting a candidate for robotic VVF repair, it is important to consider if surgical repair can be done via a transvaginal approach. As a

© Springer International Publishing AG 2018
J.T. Anger, K.S. Eilber (eds.), *The Use of Robotic Technology in Female Pelvic Floor Reconstruction*, DOI 10.1007/978-3-319-59611-2_13

natural orifice, transvaginal approach to VVF repair remains the most minimally invasive form of repair. The procedure can be performed in an outpatient setting with minimal morbidity and blood loss. Multiple layers of closure can be performed with or without flap coverage. Both a peritoneal and Martius flap can be used during transvaginal repair. Efficacy of transvaginal VVF repair is upwards of 90% [5]. Sexual function and continence rates appear to be similar following either transvaginal or abdominal approach [6].

Most pelvic surgeons are trained in vaginal approaches to vesicovaginal fistula repair. When discussing the role of robotic approaches, one may hear a reconstructive surgeon say "all vesicovaginal fistulae can be repaired vaginally. There is no role for the robot here." Although in many cases this is true, there are certain circumstances where robotic technology changes an operation from a trainee-dependent struggle for exposure to an artistic, secure repair, performed in the same amount of time with comparable morbidity.

The decision to perform a robotic VVF primarily depends on the location of the fistula tract as well as the mobility of the vaginal apex, often a function of parity. A more distal VVF might best be addressed vaginally. However, in the case of a VVF that occurs at the time of hysterectomy, the fistula is usually located at the vaginal cuff, the most proximal aspect of the vagina. In a woman with a high apex (such as a woman who has not given birth vaginally), vaginal exposure can be difficult and require the aid of one or more assistant surgeons. Robotic assistance can be quite useful here.

There are other instances when a vaginal surgeon may choose an abdominal approach to fistula repair, regardless of robotic technology. An abdominal approach may be favored in cases of a fistula located in close proximity (<1 cm distance) to the ureter. An abdominal approach should be considered when there is diminished vaginal access, which can be seen following radiationassociated vaginal narrowing. Another is the rare fistula that involves a tract from the bladder to the uterus or, after supracervical hysterectomy, the cervical os. And lastly, an abdominal approach

is preferred for the combined surgical management of a ureteral injury and a VVF. Any time, if such an abdominal approach is planned and the patient is a candidate for laparoscopy, robotic assistance may be considered.

Timing of Repair

In addition to surgical approach, there is debate regarding the optimal timing of VVF repair. With two to three weeks of catheter drainage alone, spontaneous closure of VVF can occur in approximately 7% of cases [7]. This is especially true in cases of small fistulas with catheter drainage initiated prior to tissue epithelialization. If spontaneous closure does not occur, formal repair is required. Traditionally, timing of fistula repair depends on the readiness of the surrounding tissue. Favorable tissue conditions include good vascularity, absence of infection, and reduced inflammation. Most inflammatory granulation tissue will dissipate after six to 12 weeks after gynecologic surgery.

In the robotic VVF literature, four series reported have specified timing of repair [8–11]. In each of these cases, a minimum of three months elapsed prior to repair. The main advantage of expedient VVF repair is minimizing patient distress and concern due to continuous incontinence [12, 13]. While data regarding outcomes following early robotic-assisted VVF repair is lacking, several reports of laparoscopic repairs have illustrated good outcomes following more immediate closure. A series of 16 patients with VVF following abdominal hysterectomy underwent laparoscopic repair at ten to 28 days following inciting event without a trial of conservative management. In this group, the average fistula size was 2 cm at presentation. Outcomes were confirmed by cystogram and no recurrences were reported with follow-up for an average of nearly 6 months [14]. A second series of 13 patients undergoing early laparoscopic repair at two to four weeks found only one failure at an average of 21 months of follow-up [15]. Although experience with early robotic-assisted repair has not been published, based on successful outcomes from previous literature describing laparoscopic repairs, early robotic repairs should be feasible if the surrounding tissue is healthy. Until more data is established in the literature, we consider six weeks to be the minimum time period to wait before repair. One must not be pressured by surgeons involved in the initial surgery (that caused the injury), who wish for immediate problem resolution, to operate sooner than is optimal for the patient.

A final consideration prior to planning robotic VVF repair is the nature of previous repair attempts. Robotic VVF repair has been successfully done following prior transabdominal and transvaginal repairs with success reported at 12 months follow-up [10]. Results of outcomes between open and robotic in repair of recurrent supratrigonal VVF have been compared in one study. Patients undergoing robotic repair had less operative blood loss and shorter hospital stay with equal success rates [16]. Unavailability of omentum, due to adhesions or use in prior repair, may necessitate the use of alternative tissue interpositioning with peritoneal or colonic epiploica flaps. We have also used cadaveric dermis as interposition tissue with good success. Following previous abdominal repairs, adhesiolysis with laparoscopic scissors may be required to allow for placement of additional ports.

Pre-operative Work-up

Evaluation for a urogenital fistula begins with a history and physical. Fistulas between the urinary tract and vagina typically result in painless urinary leakage. Continuous urine leakage is seen with vesicovaginal fistulas. Intermittent, positional leakage is more characteristic of a ureterovaginal fistula. Other causes of vaginal drainage after gynecological surgery as well as overflow urinary incontinence should be excluded. Though normally of a thicker consistentcy, watery discharge can occur from the cervix or the vagina. Transient drainage of a seroma can also produce vaginal leakage

On speculum exam, a recent fistula may appear as an area of granulation tissue. For small

or proximally located fistulas, examination under anesthesia or a dye test may be necessary for visualization. A cystoscopy should be performed in all patients to assess for other bladder injuries, surgical sutures or clips and to determine the number of intravesical fistula orifices. A conventional or computed tomography (CT) cystogram with at least 300 milliliters of contrast can facilitate detection and localization as well.

As approximately 12% of patients with a vesicovaginal fistula will have a concomitant ureterovaginal fistula or ureteral injury, it is important to evaluate for upper tract injury with either CT urogram or retrograde pyelogram [17].

Operative Technique and Considerations

There are important operative considerations and techniques for successful robotic VVF repair. Prior to repair, it is important to consider antibiotic coverage as well as identification of the fistula tract and ureters. Technical aspects unique to robotic surgery include the induction of pneumoperitoneum, port placement, and fistula dissection. Closure technique is also critical. The use of tissue interposition during robotic VVF repair, though not always needed, is a good option in certain cases.

Antibiotic Prophylaxis

Prior to repair, patients should be tested and treated for the presence of bacteruria. While infection prophylaxis is important for outcomes, there is a lack of strong evidence regarding the duration of prophylaxis [17]. A survey of surgeons performing VVF repair found that 30% use a single dose of antibiotics, 15% use for 24 h, and 45% use for more than 24 h [18]. Our preference is to give coverage with parenteral antibiotics starting just prior to the procedure. A first- or second-generation cephalosporin is usually given orally for the first five days after surgery [19]. Oral antibiotic prophylaxis is continued until all catheters and drains are removed.

Cystoscopy and Ureteral Catheterization

During the initial portion of the procedure, the patient should be placed in low lithotomy position to facilitate cystoscopy and vaginal exam. If feasible, the fistula should be identified and catheterized on vaginal exam to allow for later cystoscopic and intra-operative localization. Alternatively, a ureteric catheter can be placed cystoscopically through the fistula and retrieved through the vaginal introitus. Placement of a fistula catheter (such as a Foley catheter or a Fogarty catheter if the fistula is small) can be helpful for subsequent laparoscopic localization. In cases of large fistula, a catheter can be placed transvaginally into the bladder and the balloon inflated to allow bladder distention for cystoscopy. Ureteral localization and protection should be done by placing retrograde ureteral catheters or double J stents over a guided wire. In cases where the fistula is too close to the ureteral opening to allow for retrograde placement, robotic-assisted bilateral ureteral catheterization has been done. However, such a close proximity to the ureteral orifice (<1 cm) more likely warrants a concomitant reimplant. Following cystoscopy, a 20–22 Fr urethral catheter should be placed as well to allow for intra-operative bladder filling. Suprapubic catheters can also be placed intra-operatively for post-operative management, but we usually manage patients with just a large urethral catheter (in addition to a peritoneal drain).

Pneumoperitoneum

While in lithotomy position, the robot should be docked with the patient in the steep Trendelenberg position. The robot is placed between the patient's legs; thus, these should be positioned with maximum separation to facilitate robot docking and manipulation of the vaginal apex by the assistant during the procedure. Pneumoperitoneum is induced using the Veress needle technique at the level of the umbilicus, where the optical trocar is positioned (as in a robotic sacrocolpopexy). Maintenance of pneumoperitoneum can be achieved with traction on the urethral catheter and a petroleum jelly-soaked sponge in the vagina. Alternatively, an occlusion balloon placed over an end-to-end anastomotic (EEA) sizer can be used to allow for position maintenance and manipulation of the vaginal apex while preserving pneumoperitoneum [20]. We have also placed a bulb syringe vaginally to occlude the vagina during cuff closure.

Port Placement

Port placement is similar to that in a sacrocolpopexy. Once the abdomen is insufflated, the upper margin of the pubic bone and the anterior superior iliac spines are identified and marked. A 12 mm camera port is placed in the midline approximately 21 cm from the upper margin of the pubic bone (arm 2 = camera arm). Our preference is to use a direct-vision placement technique to introduce the initial 12 mm trocar. The 8 mm robotic camera (for SI and recent models) is placed through the obturator of a 12 mm clear-tipped trocar, and the trocar is twisted to visualize peritoneal entry. Older models of the robot (such as the S) necessitate the use of a smaller camera (such as a cystosopic lens) to allow for direct vision through the camera port. The remaining trocars are placed under vision as well. Two 8-mm robotic arm ports (arms 1 and 3) are placed lateral to the rectus muscle bilaterally, located 17 cm from the pubic bone. These ports are placed at least 10 cm from the midline port, to prevent outside robotic arm collision. A robotic fourth arm port is placed on the left, just superior to the anterior iliac spine. An assistant port, ranging from 8 mm to 12 mm is placed just superior to the right anterior iliac spine. The fourth arm port and also the assistant port are also placed 10 cm from robotic arms 1 and 3, again to prevent collision.

Initial Dissection

Initial dissection is performed using a combination of blunt and sharp dissection with Maryland fenestrated bipolar forceps and monopolar curved scissors, respectively (Fig. 13.1). A fenestrated bipolar may actually grasp the tissue better than the Maryland, especially when there is significant adherence of the vagina to the bladder. The anterior surface of the vagina and the superior aspect

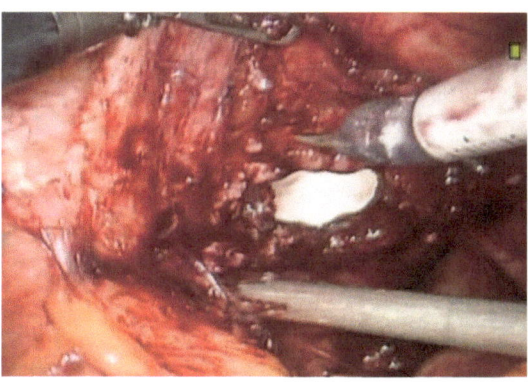

Fig. 13.1 Initial dissection with monopolar scissors. Fenestrated grasper used for tissues handling and retraction

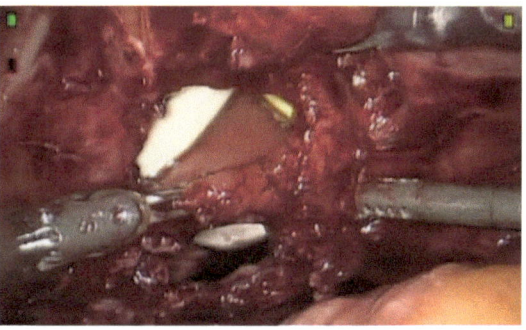

Fig. 13.2 Fistula localization using previously placed fistula catheter (*yellow*) can help minimize cystotomy

of the bladder should be exposed. Intestinal contents are packed superiorly either by the assistant with a laparoscopic retractor or by the surgeon using the fourth robotic arm. Often the steep Trendelenburg obviates the need for additional retraction of the intestines. The dissection is extended until the rectovaginal pouch is completely free of any tissue content.

Fistula Localization: Transvesical vs. Extravesical Technique

Following initial dissection, the next step involves fistula localization and excision (Fig. 13.2). Two techniques have been described in the literature. The traditional transperitoneal approach to VVF repair was popularized by O'Conor and involves a transvesical approach. This technique requires bivalving the bladder to localize the fistula [21]. The advantage of the transvesical O'Conor dissection is the ability to identify the fistula tract and completely dissect it free. Liberal cystostomy can also help identify the ureteric orifices. The transvesical approach was performed via laparotomy until the first laparoscopic case was published in 1994 [22].

However, improved visualization and angled camera offered by the robotic approach has opened up debate as to whether a large opening of the bladder is necessary at all. Long posterior vesical incisions may compromise bladder function and capacity and increase operative time and blood loss. Laparoscopic and robotic VVF repair with extravesical approaches have been performed with good success. Pooled data from laparoscopic and robotic repairs indicate nearly equal representation in the literature of both the transvesical and extravesical approaches, and that both techniques have similar success rates [23]. Three cases of robotic extravesical repair have been reported with recurrence-free results in each [8, 24, 25].

Numerous methods have been described to identify the fistula location in order to perform VVF repair without bivalving the bladder. Transvaginal manipulation of the previously placed fistula catheter can facilitate extravesical fistula localization. Transillumination, via cystoscopy or vaginoscopy, has also been reported. In one series, the authors described the use of concomitant cystoscopy to aid with developing the vesicovaginal plane and localizing the fistula tract [26]. Other authors have described the use of vaginal transillumination via vaginoscopy to facilitate dissection and localization of the fistula [27]. Focusing the light of the cystoscope or vaginoscope on the fistula while switching off the robotic camera light allows for improved intra-abdominal visualization and localization.

The robotic approach to fistula repair provides exceptional magnification, making identification of the fistula much easier than a vaginal approach. Since more fistulas occur at the time of hysterectomy and involve the vaginal cuff, we take the same approach to fistula repair as we do a colpo-pexy and separate the bladder from the anterior vaginal wall. The area that is most adherent is usually the fistula tract. Once it is identified and opened and fluid is seen, it is the urethral cathe-ter. Then the critical component of the dissection is further separating the bladder and vagina distal to the fistula tract, so that the bladder and vagina are no longer adherent.

No randomized or comparative trials exist to compare the results of transvesical and extravesi-cal approach to laparoscopic or robotic VVF repair. It is likely that adherence to the proper techniques of fistula surgery is likely more impor-tant than the approach. Regardless of technique, it is important to have clear and wide exposure of the fistula tract to allow for closure of the fistula edges (and, based on surgeon preference, exci-sion of the fistula tract), while preserving both ureteric orifices.

Fistula Excision and Bladder Mobilization

Once the fistula tract is identified and the poste-rior wall of the bladder is dissected off the ante-rior vaginal wall, the fistula tract can excised using monopolar scissors. The excised portion is sent for pathological examination. Bladder mobi-lization allows for a tension-free closure. Blunt and wide dissection should be limited to avoid injury to the trigone and ureteral orifices. Bleeding in the region of the fistula is best con-trolled with bipolar cautery in order to minimize excessive tissue necrosis from monopolar energy.

Bladder Closure and Conclusion

The bladder should be closed in vertical fashion to minimize the contact between the planned hor-izontally closed vaginal suture line. The bladder is closed in two layers using absorbable suture (2-0 Vicryl). Following bladder closure, the integrity of the repair should be tested. Data pooled from 44 studies of laparoscopic and robotic VVF showed that success rates were 6% higher in cases where a bladder fill test was per-formed [23]. The bladder should be filled with 180–200 mL of saline through the urethral cath-

eter to assess for the absence of extravasation. Any defects should be closed with interrupted, absorbable suture.

Vaginal Closure

Once the bladder is closed, reapproximation of the vagina begins (Fig. 13.3). A horizontal clo-sure with absorbable suture (2-0 Vicryl) in a run-ning, locking fashion is usually used (re-creating a new vaginal cuff). However, if the bladder repair was performed horizontally, the vaginal closure should be vertical such that the suture lines do not overlap. The integrity of the vaginal closure can be tested by removing the vaginal sponge or sizer and assessing for the preservation of pneumoperitoneum.

Tissue Interposition

Following vaginal closure in a non-radiated patient, mobilization and placement of tissue interposition is usually not necessary (Fig. 13.4). The need for flap interposition for VVF repair has been evaluated during time of open transab-dominal VVF repair. Several retrospective series have shown success rates ranging from 63 to 97.5% for fistulas less than 10 mm repaired with-out interposition flaps [28, 29]. Laparoscopic repair of VVF without tissue interposition has been reported with good success, though num-bers are limited. Two separate series of five and two VVFs, each less than 10 mm, repaired lapa-roscopically without interposition showed 100% success at one-year follow-up [13, 30]. As noted

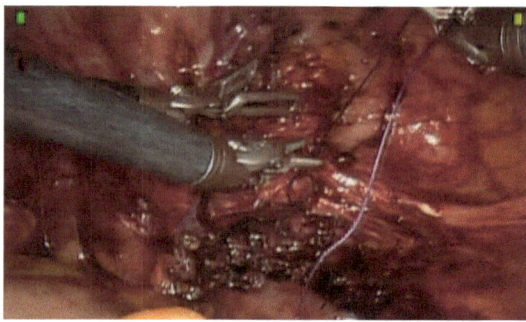

Fig. 13.3 Horizontal vaginal closure with absorbable suture in a running locking fashion

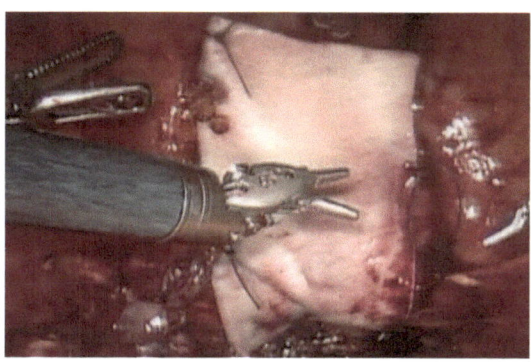

Fig. 13.4 Tissue interposition with Alloderm sutured in place

by Miklos et al., flap coverage is not a substitute for careful dissection and closure. However, omental or peritoneal interposition in the vesicovaginal space takes limited time and morbidity to perform and provides an additional layer to prevent recurrence.

The advantage of a transperitoneal approach is the ability to use a vascularized pedicle for flap coverage between the bladder and vagina. If one is planning to use omentum, it is wise to suture the omentum to the abdominal wall (to be used for the later interposition) before placing the patient in steep Trendelenburg. Often the omentum retracts entirely and is difficult to find robotically. One disadvantage of the robotic approach is the relative lack of flexibility when preparation of the omentum would be necessary. As such, several authors have described the use of regional flaps and other techniques of interposition during robotic VVF repair. A commonly reported technique is a peritoneal flap interposition, which avoids the need for omental preparation or colon mobilization [10, 11]. Other authors have described success with interposition using the epiploic appendices of the sigmoid colon [8, 10]. Fibrin glue was used as interpositioning material in the first reported case of robotic VVF repair [31]. A cadaveric amniotic graft has also been used for robotic-assisted VVF following radiation-induced damage [32].

An omental interposition can also be done robotically by taking the patient out of Trendelenberg position, but this requires undocking and repeat docking. If omentum is unavailable or cannot be adequately mobilized, the epiploic appendices of the sigmoid colon or a peritoneal flap from a nearby location (usually the peritoneum overlying the bladder) can be used as tissue for interposition. The interpositioned tissue should be fixed using absorbable suture on the distal and lateral vaginal walls. The fixation sutures should be adequately distanced from the suture line of the vaginal closure. Importantly, the graft needs to be located such that it prevents the suture lines from re-establishing the fistula tract. When interposition tissue is not available, as in the case of a fistula with surrounding inflammation or large fistula, we have used acellular cadaveric dermis as interposition tissue with good success.

Following satisfactory fistula closure, a drain is left in the rectovaginal pouch. At conclusion, the robotic and assistant trocars are removed under optical guidance. The fascia of the 12-mm trocars is closed with monofilament non-absorbable, number one running suture.

Patient Follow-up, Outcomes, and Complications

Bladder drainage following repair is important for successful outcomes. Most authors have foregone the use of suprapubic drainage, especially in cases where the bladder is not bivalved. If hemostasis is a concern, a suprapubic catheter should be placed. In the absence of injury or extensive peri-ureteral dissection, the ureteral catheters can usually be removed at the conclusion of the procedure. The surgical drain can be removed once output has minimized. The reported duration of urethral catheter drainage following robotic VVF repair ranges from 10 to 21 days. Most authors perform imaging with either retrograde cystogram or voiding cystourethrogram (VCUG) at the time of catheter removal.

Ten reports of robotic VVF repair in 31 patients have been reported. Follow-up ranged from three to 24 months with no recurrences reported (Table 13.1). Reported cases of robotic

Table 13.1 Robotic-assisted VVF repair: results

Study	Patients, *n*	Etiology	Prior repairs	Approach	Interposition	Mean OR time	Duration of catheter (days)	Imaging at time of catheter removal	LOS (days)	Follow-up (months)
Melamud et al. (2008)	1	Vaginal hysterectomy	None	Transvesical	Fibrin sealant	280	14	None	3	4
Sundaram et al. (2006)	5	Abdominal hysterectomy (4), myomectomy (1)	None	Transvesical	Omentum	233	10	VCUG	4–7	6
Schmipf (2007)	1	Abdominal hysterectomy	None	Extravesical	Colonic epiploica	270	21	Cystogram	2	3
Sears (2007)	1	None	None	Transvesical	Omentum	n/a	n/a	None	n/a	n/a
Hemal (2008)	7	Hysterectomy (3), caesarian section (2), obstetric injury (2)	Transabdominal and transvesical	Transvesical	Omentum, colonic epiploica, peritoneum	141	14	VCUG	3	12
Kurz (2012)	3	Abdominal hysterectomy	None	Transvesical	Peritoneal	240	14	Cystogram	5	4
Rogers (2012)	2	Hysterectomy	None	Extravesical	Omentum	n/a	12	Cystogram	3	12
Dutto (2013)		Abdominal hysterectomy	None	Extravesical	Perisigmoid fat	n/a	10	Cystogram	2	6
Agrawal (2016)	10	Abdominal hysterectomy (7), vaginal hysterectomy (3)	None	Transvesical	Peritoneal (2), bladder adventitua (3), peritoneal fat (1), colonic epiploica (3), fibrin sealant (1)	214	9–6 days	Cystogram	1–5	24
Price (2015)	1	Abdominal hysterectomy +radiation for cervical cancer	None	Transvesical	Amniotic allograft patch	305	21	Cystogram	1	5

VVF have shown a mean operative time ranging from 141 to 305 min. The length of stay ranged from one to seven days with the majority of patients having a post-operative stay less than 3 days. The largest systematic review of laparoscopic and robotic VVF repair found a 2% rate of conversion to laparotomy. The rates of urinary tract infection, wound infection, and enterotomy were all less than 1% [23].

Conclusion

Robotic-assisted VVF repair is a safe and feasible option. Outcomes appear comparable to vaginal, abdominal, and laparoscopic repair. In cases where vaginal repair is not ideal, robotic assistance offers a minimally invasive technique that is technically feasible. Compared to traditional open abdominal repair, robotic repair appears to have decreased morbidity with shorter hospital length of stay.

References

1. Wall LL, et al. The obstetric vesicovaginal fistula: characteristics of 899 patients from Jos, Nigeria. Am J Obstet Gynecol. 2004;190(4):1011–9.
2. Tancer ML. Observations on prevention and management of vesicovaginal fistula after total hysterectomy. Surg Gynecol Obstet. 1992;175(6):501–6.
3. Hall MJ, et al. National Hospital discharge survey: 2007 summary. Natl Health Stat Rep. 2010;(29):1-20-24.
4. Cassily R, et al. Optimizing motion scaling and magnification in robotic surgery. Surgery. 2004;136(2):291–4.
5. Eilber KS, et al. Ten-year experience with transvaginal vesicovaginal fistula repair using tissue interposition. J Urol. 2003;169(3):1033–6.
6. Mohr S, et al. Sexual function after vaginal and abdominal fistula repair. Am J Obstet Gynecol. 2014;211(1):74.e1–6.
7. Singh O, Gupta SS, Mathur RK. Urogenital fistulas in women: 5-year experience at a single center. Urol J. 2010;7(1):35–9.
8. Schimpf MO, et al. Vesicovaginal fistula repair without intentional cystotomy using the laparoscopic robotic approach: a case report. JSLS. 2007;11(3):378–80.
9. Sundaram BM, Kalidasan G, Hemal AK. Robotic repair of vesicovaginal fistula: case series of five patients. Urology. 2006;67(5):970–3.
10. Hemal AK, Kolla SB, Wadhwa P. Robotic reconstruction for recurrent supratrigonal vesicovaginal fistulas. J Urol. 2008;180(3):981–5.
11. Kurz M, Horstmann M, John H. Robot-assisted laparoscopic repair of high vesicovaginal fistulae with peritoneal flap inlay. Eur Urol. 2012;61(1):229–30.
12. Wang Y, Hadley HR. Nondelayed transvaginal repair of high lying vesicovaginal fistula. J Urol. 1990;144(1):34–6.
13. Lee JH, et al. Immediate laparoscopic nontransvesical repair without omental interposition for vesicovaginal fistula developing after total abdominal hysterectomy. JSLS. 2010;14(2):187–91.
14. Zhang Q, et al. Laparoscopic transabdominal transvesical repair of supratrigonal vesicovaginal fistula. Int Urogynecol J. 2013;24(2):337–42.
15. Nagraj HK, Kishore TA, Nagalaksmi S. Early laparoscopic repair for supratrigonal vesicovaginal fistula. Int Urogynecol J Pelvic Floor Dysfunct. 2007;18(7):759–62.
16. Gupta NP, et al. Comparative analysis of outcome between open and robotic surgical repair of recurrent supra-trigonal vesico-vaginal fistula. J Endourol. 2010;24(11):1779–82.
17. Muleta M, Tafesse B, Aytenfisu HG. Antibiotic use in obstetric fistula repair: single blinded randomized clinical trial. Ethiop Med J. 2010;48(3):211–7.
18. Arrowsmith SD, Ruminjo J, Landry EG. Current practices in treatment of female genital fistula: a cross sectional study. BMC Pregnancy Childbirth. 2010;10:73.
19. Wolf JS Jr, et al. Best practice policy statement on urologic surgery antimicrobial prophylaxis. J Urol. 2008;179(4):1379–90.
20. Sears CL, Schenkman N, Lockrow EG. Use of end-to-end anastomotic sizer with occlusion balloon to prevent loss of pneumoperitoneum in robotic vesicovaginal fistula repair. Urology. 2007;70(3):581–2.
21. O'Conor VJ Jr, et al. Suprapubic closure of vesicovaginal fistula. J Urol. 1973;109(1):51–4.
22. Nezhat CH, et al. Laparoscopic repair of a vesicovaginal fistula: a case report. Obstet Gynecol. 1994;83(5 Pt 2):899–901.
23. Miklos JR, Moore RD, Chinthakanan O. Laparoscopic and robotic-assisted vesicovaginal fistula repair: a systematic review of the literature. J Minim Invasive Gynecol. 2015;22(5):727–36.
24. Rogers AE, et al. Robotic assisted laparoscopic repair of vesico-vaginal fistula: the extravesical approach. Can J Urol. 2012;19(5):6474–6.

25. Dutto L, O'Reilly B. Robotic repair of vesico-vaginal fistula with perisigmoid fat flap interposition: state of the art for a challenging case? Int Urogynecol J. 2013;24(12):2029–30.

26. Sotelo R, et al. Laparoscopic repair of vesicovaginal fistula. J Urol. 2005;173(5):1615–8.

27. Garcia-Segui A. Laparoscopic repair of vesicovaginal fistula without intentional cystotomy and guided by vaginal transillumination. Actas Urol Esp. 2012;36(4):252–8.

28. Pshak T, et al. Is tissue interposition always necessary in transvaginal repair of benign, recurrent vesicovaginal fistulae? Urology. 2013;82(3):707–12.

29. Evans DH, et al. Interposition flaps in transabdominal vesicovaginal fistula repairs: are they really necessary? Urology. 2001;57(4):670–4.

30. Miklos JR, Moore RD. Vesicovaginal fistula failing multiple surgical attempts salvaged laparoscopically without an interposition omental flap. J Minim Invasive Gynecol. 2012;19(6):794–7.

31. Melamud O, et al. Laparoscopic vesicovaginal fistula repair with robotic reconstruction. Urology. 2005;65(1):163–6.

32. Price DT, Price TC. Robotic repair of a vesicovaginal fistula in an irradiated field using a dehydrated amniotic allograft as an interposition patch. J Robot Surg. 2016;10(1):77–80.

Christopher J. Dru and Hyung L. Kim

Introduction

Background

Ureteral reimplantation, also referred to as a ureteroneocystostomy, is the general term used to
describe the surgical re-anastomosis of the ureter
to the bladder and is typically performed for ureteral injury or inadequate drainage of the kidney
due to a ureteral defect. It can be performed using
an open, laparoscopic, or robotic-assisted laparoscopic technique.

Embryology and Anatomy of the Ureter

The ureter begins to develop in utero at approximately the fourth to fifth weeks of life when the
ureteric bud arises as an outpouching from the
mesonephric duct. The ureteric bud grows later-

C.J. Dru, M.D. (✉)
Department of Surgery, Division of Urology,
Cedars-Sinai Medical Center, Los Angeles, CA, USA
e-mail: CHRISTODRU@GMAIL.COM

H.L. Kim, M.D.
Department of Surgery, Division of Urology,
Cedars-Sinai Medical Center, Los Angeles, CA, USA

ally and fuses with the developing metanephros,
which eventually develops into the fetal kidney.
At this point, the ureter is patent, although no
urine is produced by the metanephros. As the
metanephros ascends, the ureteric bud continues
to branch and forms the renal pelvis. The ureter
temporarily loses its lumen, but regains its
patency at approximately 40 days. Patency of the
ureter is maintained when the metanephros
begins to produce urine at nine weeks of development [1, 2].

The mature ureter has three areas of natural
relative narrowing: (1) the ureteropelvic junction,
(2) crossing of the iliac vessels, and (3) the ure-
terovesical junction. The blood supply to the ureter is drawn from multiple overlapping and
redundant vessels; however, none of the tributar-
ies are named given their small size and high
degree of variability. The proximal (upper third)
ureter receives its blood supply from the renal
artery. The middle third of the ureter receives its
blood supply from branches of the common iliac
arteries, abdominal aorta, and the gonadal arteries (testicular artery in males; ovarian artery in
females). The distal (lower third) ureter receives
its blood supply from branches of the internal
iliac artery, superior vesical artery, and middle
rectal artery. In females, the ureter receives additional blood supply from the uterine artery and
vaginal arteries. In males, the ureter receives
additional blood supply from the inferior vesical
artery. Each ureter is encased in a relatively thick

© Springer International Publishing AG 2018
J.T. Anger, K.S. Eilber (eds.), *The Use of Robotic Technology in Female
Pelvic Floor Reconstruction*, DOI 10.1007/978-3-319-59611-2_14

adventitial layer where these vessels form vast and extensive anastamotic networks. Due to this diffuse arterial network, devascularization of the ureter is rare [3, 4].

Etiology and Diagnosis of Ureteral Injury

Ureteral injury is most commonly caused by laparoscopic or open surgical dissection adjacent to the ureter using monopolar cautery. In laparoscopic hysterectomy, the incidence of thermal injury to the ureter requiring intervention is approximately 1–2% [5–7]. A similar injury can also be seen during colon and rectal surgery, pelvic lymphadenectomy, tubal ligation, and thermal ablation of endometriosis [8–10]. Ureteral injury is less common with vaginal hysterectomy compared with open and laparoscopic hysterectomy [11]. Additional iatrogenic causes of ureteral injury include partial or complete division, application of vascular clips to control bleeding that inadvertently ligate the ureter, and blunt dissection next to the ureter causing devascularization of a ureteral segment. Non-iatrogenic causes of ureteral occlusion that may require ureteral reimplantation include malignancy (internal filling defects or mass effect from external ureteral compression), urolithiasis, infection, or trauma.

Identification of a subtle intraoperative ureteral injury can be difficult and is often missed during surgery. Accumulation of small areas of amber, clear fluid can easily be confused with peritoneal fluid, lymphatic fluid, or irrigant. As most ureteral injuries are due to thermal injury and do not violate the ureteral lumen, the surgeon cannot rely upon the presence of hematuria or pneumaturia to aid in the diagnosis, as in the case of bladder perforation.

The vast majority of operative ureteral injuries are identified several days after surgery. Patients present with signs and symptoms of ureteral obstruction such as flank pain, fever, chills, nausea, or vomiting [12]. They may present with peritonitis, causing generalized abdominal pain and leukocytosis [13]. These postoperative symptoms are non-specific and can also be attributed to infection or abscess, bowel injury, ileus, or

bowel obstruction and must be placed into the correct clinical context.

If a ureteral injury is suspected, imaging is recommended with a renal ultrasound, triphasic computed tomography (CT) urogram with intravenous contrast, or magnetic resonance imaging (MRI) with contrast. If a ureteral obstruction is present, the imaging study will demonstrate hydronephrosis of the affected side with hydroureter down to the level of the lesion. If a urine leak is present, the CT or MRI may show a fluid collection or ascites. Once a ureteral injury is suspected, retrograde pyelogram or antegrade pyelogram can be used to confirm the diagnosis. A ureteral stent can be attempted at the time of retrograde pyelogram. If a ureteral injury is determined late (such as several months after the injury), a nuclear renal scan will aid in the evaluation of flow and function of the kidney,

Ureteral injuries are typically categorized by two variables: (1) location along the ureter and (2) length of the defect. The location of the defect is classified as either proximal, middle, or distal. Determining the location of the lesion is crucial as there are different management strategies to optimally treat each type of defect. The location can be diagnosed by performing a retrograde pyelogram, antegrade pyelogram, triphasic CT urogram study with IV contrast, or MRI with contrast. In some instances, a nuclear renal scan flow phase can reveal a distinct transition point that can signify the point of obstruction. The length of the injury is much more difficult to determine. If a complete ureteral obstruction is present, then the best way to diagnose the filling defect is to perform simultaneous antegrade and retrograde pyelograms. If a partial ureteral obstruction is present, many times the length of the defect can be measured by utilizing either a retrograde pyelogram or an antegrade pyelogram.

Management of a Ureteral Injury

Immediate Management

Once a ureteral injury is identified, the primary goal is to preserve renal function on the affected side by decompressing the kidney to allow for unobstructed flow of urine. This can be accomplished in several ways. If the injury is clearly identified intraoperatively, treatment options include (1) excision of the ureteral defect and primary anastomosis, (2) ureteral reimplantation, (3) cutaneous ureterostomy, or (4) ligation of the ureter and nephrostomy tube placement. Ureteral ligation and nephrostomy is reserved for unstable patients or in a trauma situation where other major injuries need to be addressed. If ureteral injury is suspected but not easily identified, as in the case of a ureteral contusion or thermal injury, then a ureterogram followed by antegrade or retrograde ureteral stenting is a reasonable option (Fig. 14.1).

If there is a delay in diagnosis or intraoperative management at the time of injury is unsuccessful, then percutaneous nephrostomy with or without antegrade stenting is the treatment of choice in the immediate setting. Many times, the degree of ureteral injury is not evident at the time it occurs, especially in the case of thermal injuries, as devitalized tissue may take several days to demarcate and weeks to stricture. Therefore,

many patients are managed with nephrostomy drainage to allow the injury to fully mature before definitive treatment.

Delayed/Definitive Management

Definitive management of ureteral injuries can be performed either ureteroscopically or by formal surgery. Ureteroscopic management is typically reserved for partial obstruction in a stented ureter. Techniques include use of the holmium laser, cold knife, hot knife, and balloon dilation. Robotic-assisted laparoscopic surgical techniques are utilized to definitively manage mature ureteral injuries and can be used in all settings traditionally managed with an open technique. Longer defects may require the use of a psoas hitch with or without a Boari flap or even ileal ureter interposition. The remainder of this chapter will focus on a discussion of those techniques with step-by-step instructions on how to perform a robotic-assisted laparoscopic ureteral reimplantation (ureteroneocystostomy).

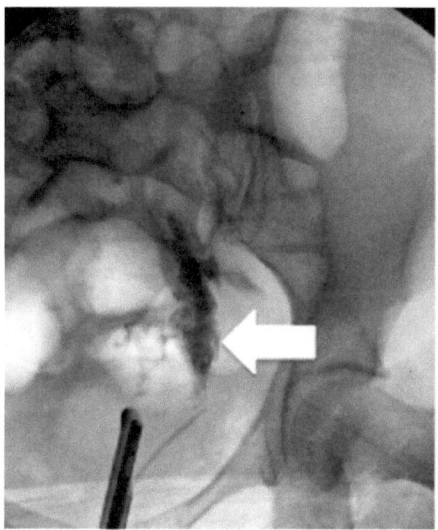
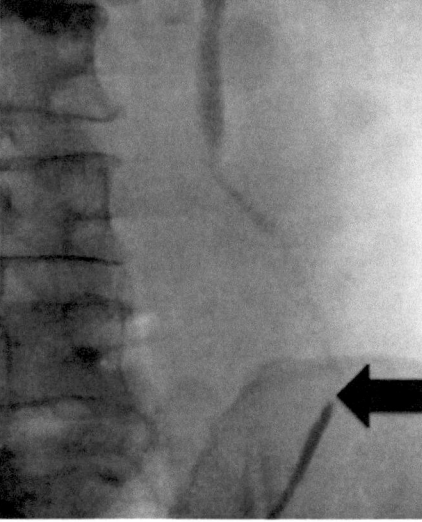
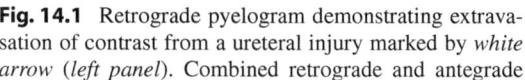

Fig. 14.1 Retrograde pyelogram demonstrating extravasation of contrast from a ureteral injury marked by *white arrow* (*left panel*). Combined retrograde and antegrade pyelogram demonstrating filling defect of the ureter marked by *black arrow* (*right panel*)

Robotic-Assisted Laparoscopic Ureteral Reimplantation

Preoperative Preparation

A urine culture is typically obtained preoperatively as these patients are at increased risk of either active urinary tract infection or asymptomatic bacteriuria given obstruction and presence of either a nephrostomy tube or ureteral stent. Culture-specific antibiotics should be given for at least three to five days before surgery. Additionally, a bowel preparation to decompress the colon is often used. An example of a regimen would be two doses of magnesium citrate in the afternoon and evening before surgery followed by a Fleet's enema before bedtime. Lastly, most ureteral injuries secondary to previous pelvic surgery occur in the distal third of the ureter; therefore, the following discussion will include a step-by-step approach to robotically reimplanting the ureter in a patient with a distal ureteral injury.

Patient Positioning, Trocar Placement, and Robot Docking

The patient is positioned in dorsal lithotomy position using Allen stirrups on the operating room table with the arms adducted using sleds (plastic upper extremity limb holders). The operating room table is then placed in maximum Trendelenburg position. The abdomen is shaved, prepped, and draped in a standard sterile fashion. A urinary catheter is inserted per urethra into the bladder and placed to gravity drainage. Pneumoperitoneum is obtained in a standard fashion through any variety of techniques. Typically, the anterior abdominal wall is elevated manually, and a Veress needle is introduced into the abdominal cavity in the right upper quadrant. Low initial pressures of 0–5 mmHg on insufflation at approximately 2 L per minute confirm proper Veress needle position. The abdomen is insufflated to approximately 15 mmHg pressure, where it should remain for the remainder of the laparoscopic portion of the procedure.

The camera trocar is placed just above the umbilicus. Three robotic trocars are placed: two are pararectus median trocars placed approximately 10 cm off the midline and 17 cm from the symphysis pubis bilaterally and the third is placed laterally, approximately two fingerbreadths off the anterior iliac crest, on the side opposite from the ureteral injury. Assistant trocars can be placed on the same side of the ureteral injury. All trocars should be placed under direct vision, if possible. A 30° down or 0° camera lens is ideal, depending on surgeon preference. The robot is now docked between the patient's legs. Typically, the surgeon will use monopolar scissors in the right hand, any type of bipolar graspers in the left hand, and an athermal grasper in the fourth arm. Figure 14.2 diagrams the standard trocar locations.

Colon Mobilization and Identifying the Ureter

The goal of the next phase of the surgery is to expose the ureter and ensure that it has adequate length to reach the dome of the bladder in a

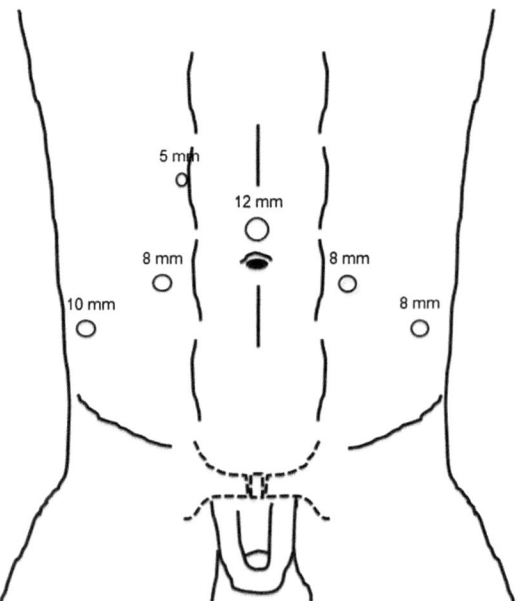

Fig. 14.2 Schematic of trocar sites for a right robotic-assisted ureteral reimplant. Note that two robotic 8mm trocars are positioned on the contralateral side of the intended side of surgery

tension-free fashion. All peritoneal adhesions blocking access to the ureter and colon should be taken down sharply with care to avoid bowel injury. The posterolateral peritoneum can be opened near the white line of Toldt to expose the ureter as it crosses the iliac vessels. To allow more distal exposure of the ureter, the bladder can be mobilized. This can be performed by incising the peritoneum just lateral to the medial umbilical ligaments and then dividing the urachus. The dissection is carried down towards the pelvis using a combination of sharp and blunt dissection to peel these structures off the anterior abdominal wall. This will mobilize the bladder and allow access to the bladder pedicles. Now the ureter is divided proximal to the injury and the distal end is ligated. Ligation can be performed with any number of materials including absorbable or non-absorbable sutures (such as Vicryl or silk suture) or clips (metal or synthetic polymer). It is our preference to use the Weck® Hem-o-lok® Polymer Locking Ligation System. The dissection of the ureter is continued proximally until the ureter is mobile enough to reach the dome of the bladder.

Ureteral Reimplantation

The bladder is filled with 200–300 mL of saline. The dome of the bladder is located and a 3–4 cm detrusorotomy is created, leaving the mucosa intact (the mucosa will bulge if this is done properly). Next, the ureter is spatulated, ensuring that there is healthy, non-strictured ureter present. Next, a 1–1.5 cm cystotomy at the end of the detrusorotomy is made and the corners of the spatulated ureter are anchored at 6'o clock and 12'o clock using two separate 4-0 absorbable (we prefer Monocryl) sutures. One of the Monocryl sutures is run to complete half of the anastomosis. Alternatively, interrupted sutures can be placed to complete half the anastomosis, based on surgeon preference. This provides sufficient strength to prevent tissue from tearing while placing a double-J stent. A double-J ureteral stent loaded over a wire is passed into the proximal ureter and renal pelvis using a standard stent

pusher. The robotic instruments allow the wire and stent to be easily manipulated. The wire is removed, and the distal end of the double-J stent is placed through the cystotomy into the bladder using robotic graspers. The second Monocryl suture is now placed in a running (or interrupted) fashion to complete the implant. The bladder is filled to determine the integrity of the anastomosis. If leakage is present, interrupted Monocryl sutures can be used to close any defects. Interrupted Vicryl sutures are used to close the detrusorotomy. A drain should be introduced through one of the ports and placed in a dependent portion of the pelvis.

Alternatively, in patients with a thin bladder wall, a full thickness opening can be made in the bladder. The anastamotic sutures can incorporate full thickness bites of the bladder wall and ureter. If a Foley catheter is to be left in place for several days postoperatively, an intraperitoneal drain is not always necessary.

Undocking and Closure

The robot is undocked and all trocar sites are closed in an appropriate fashion at the discretion of the surgeon. The drain is secured, and the bulb placed to suction. A urinary catheter is left in the bladder and placed to gravity drainage. If a nephrostomy tube is present, it can either be removed or capped. The patient is extubated and transferred to the recovery area.

Psoas Hitch and Boari Flap

In some situations, dissection of the ureter alone will not provide adequate length to perform a tension-free ureteral reimplantation. When this situation occurs, bridging the gap between the ureter and bladder can be achieved by performing a psoas hitch (Fig. 14.3) with or without a Boari flap. To perform a psoas hitch, the contralateral superior vesical pedicles can be ligated and divided to allow the dome of the bladder to move closer towards the ureter. The bladder is then tacked down to the ipsilateral psoas muscle using

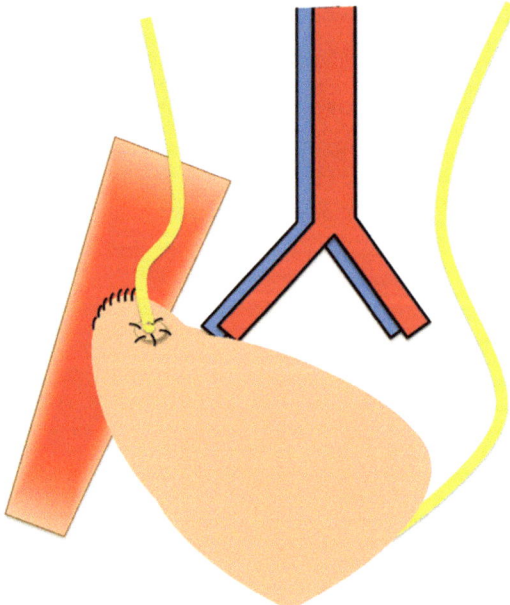

Fig. 14.3 Illustration of a right psoas hitch. The contralateral vascular bladder pedicle has been ligated, and the bladder is lateralized and tacked down to the right psoas muscle. The psoas hitch sutures are parallel to psoas muscle fibers

interrupted Vicryl suture. To avoid injury to the genitofemoral nerve, the sutures should always be placed vertically, in line with the muscle fibers. If the gap between the bladder and ureter is adequately bridged, then the ureter should be reimplanted as previously described.

If a psoas hitch does not provide adequate length to bridge the gap between the ureter and the bladder, then a Boari flap can be used (Fig. 14.4a). The base of the Boari flap should be at least 4 cm with a distal tip that is at least 2 cm. The flap is then tubularized. For added support, the Boari flap can be fixed to the psoas muscle, again with fixation sutures in line with the fibers of the psoas muscle. The ureter is then spatulated and reimplanted into the Boari flap. The posterior half of the anastomosis is completed first, the bladder flap is tubularized over a ureteral stent, and then the anterior anastomosis is completed (Fig. 14.4b). The cystotomy is closed in a watertight fashion in two or three layers using Vicryl suture (Fig. 14.4c). A urinary catheter should be left in place for at least seven to ten days to allow

adequate decompression and healing of the bladder. Some surgeons leave a suprapubic tube in place to maximally decompress the bladder when a Boari flap is performed. Robotic Assistance in creation of a Boari flap has been reported to shorten the duration of catheterization, to lower blood loss, and to lower complication rates [14].

Postoperative Management

The most important element of the postoperative care of the patient is to ensure adequate bladder drainage to prevent over-distention and risk of damage to the anastomosis. Gentle irrigation of blood clots that form in the bladder is the typical management of a poorly draining catheter. The intraperitoneal drain can typically be removed one to three days after surgery when output has decreased to less than 50–60 mL per day and urine in the catheter is clear. Elevation of the patient's serum creatinine postoperatively can signify a urine leak, and the drain fluid should be sent for creatinine. Assuming a normal and routine postoperative course, the urinary catheter can be removed five to six days after surgery. The indwelling ureteral stent is left in place four to six weeks and removed endoscopically in the office as an outpatient procedure.

Prevention of Ureteral Injuries

While there is no way to completely eliminate the risk of ureteral injury during pelvic surgery, there is no substitute for good surgical technique. Many injuries are associated with blind dissection and liberal use of monopolar electrocautery. Careful and meticulous dissection is the best method to avoid ureteral injuries. When extensive dissection is required in the area of the ureter, identifying and marking the ureter with vessel loops can be helpful.

Some patients may be at higher risk of ureteral injury because of peritoneal adhesions or inflamed tissues, especially those patients who have had previous abdominal surgery, pelvic radiation, or other inflammatory bowel, bladder,

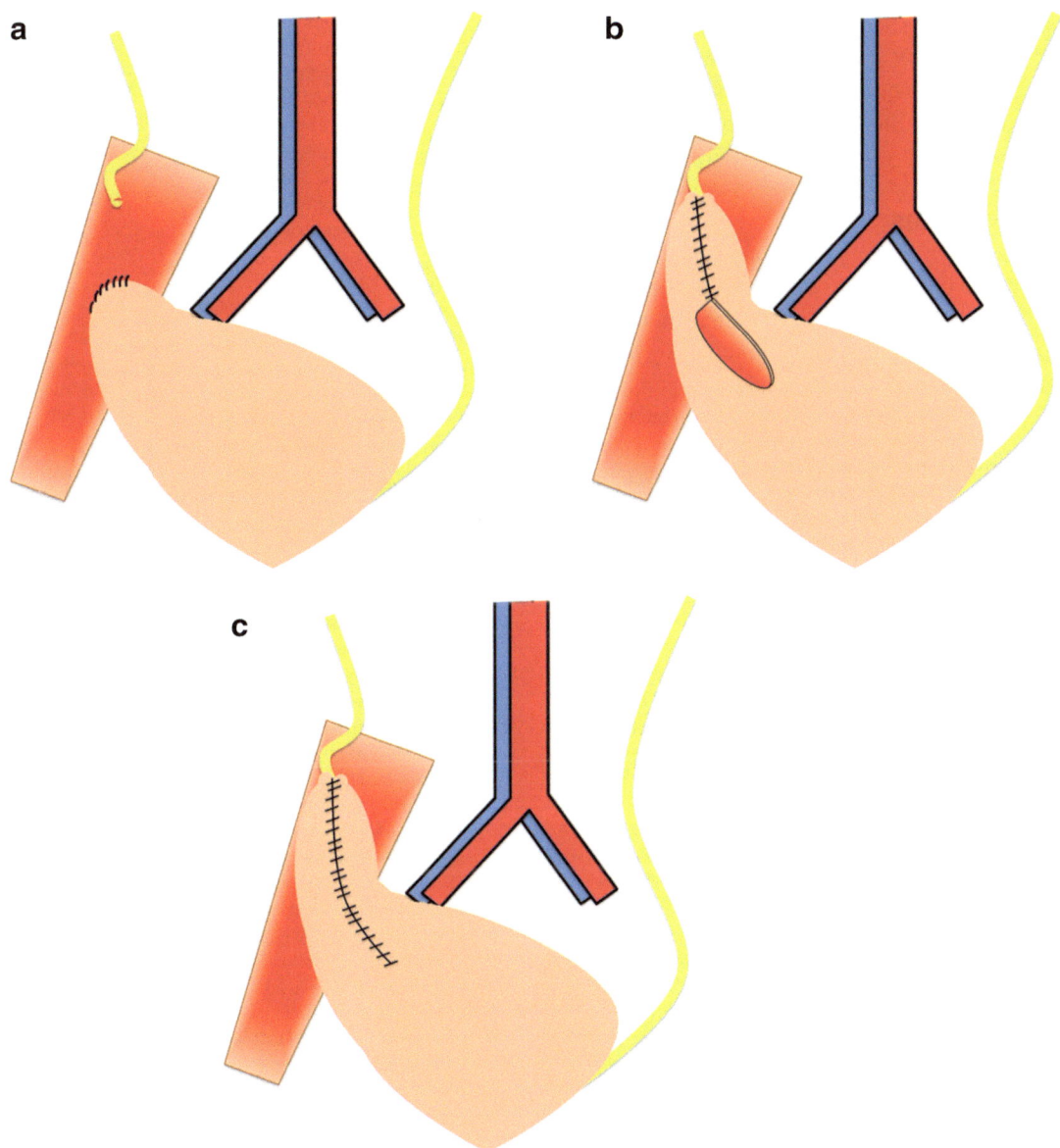

Fig. 14.4 Illustration of a right psoas hitch and Boari flap. A psoas hitch does not cover the ureteral defect (**a**). The flap created and tubularized (**b**). Completion of clo-sure of the bladder; the ureter is reimplanted at the apex of the Boari flap (**c**)

or gynecological conditions. A patient with an enlarged uterus, endometriosis, and clinically significant pelvic organ prolapse may also be at increased risk for ureteral injury [15, 16]. The primary surgeon may consult a urologist to place ureteral stents preoperatively to aid in the identification of the ureters intraoperatively. There are several stent types used (open-ended ureteral access catheters, double-J ureteral stents, lighted ureteral stents, and whistle-tip stents). And while use of preoperative stents may not reduce the risk of ureteral injury, they do aid in the identification of intraoperative ureteral injuries so that they can be repaired at the time of surgery [17, 18]. Whenever ureteral integrity is in question intraoperatively (and preoperative stents were not placed), one can always give IV dye (in the form of fluorescein, methylene blue, or indigo carmine) and visualize ureteral efflux cystoscopically.

Conclusions

Ureteral injuries are a known complication of pelvic surgery. Immediate management should focus on maintaining renal function by providing urinary drainage into the bladder or percutaneous nephrostomy. Robotic-assisted laparoscopic ureteral reimplantation is an excellent way to repair a distal ureteral defect once the ureteral injury has had time to mature.

References

1. Park J. Normal development of the genitourinary tract, Chap 111. In: Wein AJ, Kavoussi LR, Novick AC, Partin AW, Peters CA, editors. Campbell-Walsh urology. 10th ed. Philadelphia: Elsevier Saunders; 2012. p. 2975–3001.
2. Palmer LS, Trachtman H. Renal functional development and diseases in children, Chap 112. In: Wein AJ, Kavoussi LR, Novick AC, Partin AW, Peters CA, editors. Campbell-Walsh urology. 10th ed. Philadelphia: Elsevier Saunders; 2012. p. 3002–27.
3. Anderson JK, Cadeddu JA. Surgical anatomy of the retroperitoneum, adrenals, kidneys, and ureters, Chap 1. In: Wein AJ, Kavoussi LR, Novick AC, Partin AW, Peters CA, editors. Campbell-Walsh urology. 10th ed. Philadelphia: Elsevier Saunders; 2012. p. 3–32.
4. Chung BI, Sommer G, Brooks JD. Anatomy of the lower urinary tract and male genitalia, Chap 2. In: Wein AJ, Kavoussi LR, Novick AC, Partin AW, Peters CA, editors. Campbell-Walsh urology. 10th ed. Philadelphia: Elsevier Saunders; 2012. p. 33–70.
5. Gilmour DT, Das S, Flowerdew G. Rates of urinary tract injury from gynecologic surgery and the role of intraoperative cystoscopy. Obstet Gynecol. 2006;107(6):1366–72.
6. Tamussino KF, Lang PF, Breinl E. Ureteral complications with operative gynecologic laparoscopy. Am J Obstet Gynecol. 1998;178:967–70.
7. Saidi MH, Sadler RK, Vancaillie TG, et al. Diagnosis and management of serious urinary complications after major operative laparoscopy. Obstet Gynecol. 1996;87:272–6.
8. Baumann H, Jaeger P, Huch A. Ureteral injury after laparoscopic tubal sterilization by bipolar electrocoagulation. Obstet Gynecol. 1988;71(3 Pt 2):483–5.
9. Poffenberger RJ. Laparoscopic repair of intraperitoneal bladder injury: a simple new technique. Urology. 1996;47(2):248–9.
10. Ostrzenski A, Ostrzenska KM. Bladder injury during laparoscopic surgery. Obstet Gynecol Surv. 1998;53(3):175–80.
11. Manoucheri E, Cohen SL, Sandberg EM, Kibel AS, Einarsson J. Ureteral injury in laparoscopic gynecologic surgery. Rev Obstet Gynecol. 2012;5(2):106–11.
12. Grainger DA, Soderstrom RM, Schiff SF, Glickman MG, DeCherney AH, Diamond MP. Ureteral injuries at laparoscopy: insights into diagnosis, management, and prevention. Obstet Gynecol. 1990;75(5):839–43.
13. Liu CH, Wang PH, Liu WM, Yuan CC. Ureteral injury after laparoscopic surgery. J Am Assoc Gynecol Laparosc. 1997;4(4):503–6.
14. Do M, Kallidonis P, Qazi H, et al. Robot-assisted technique for boari flap ureteral reimplantation: is robot assistance beneficial? J Endourol. 2014;28(6):679–85.
15. Elliot SP, McAninch JW. Ureteral injuries: external and iatrogenic. Urol Clin North Am. 2006;33(1):55–66.
16. Vakili B, Chesson RR, Kyle BL, et al. The incidence of urinary tract injury during hysterectomy: a prospective analysis based on universal cystoscopy. Am J Obstet Gynecol. 2005;192(5):1599–604.
17. Kyzer S, Gordon PH. The prophylactic use of ureteral catheters during colorectal operations. Am Surg. 1994;60(3):212–6.
18. Merritt AJ, Crosbie EJ, Charova J, et al. Prophylactic pre-operative bilateral ureteric catheters for major gynaecological surgery. Arch Gynecol Obstet. 2013;288(5):1061–6.

Complications of Robotic Urologic Surgery

Kathleen C. Kobashi

Introduction

Urinary incontinence and pelvic organ prolapse are prevalent conditions that affect millions of women worldwide. Approximately 23.7% of women report at least one pelvic floor disorder (PFD) [1], and it has been estimated that 10% of women undergo surgery for urinary incontinence or pelvic prolapse in their lifetime [2]. However, with the increased awareness of PFDs, these numbers likely represent an underestimate.

As more attention has been placed on PFDs and their treatment, newer techniques have been introduced into the armamentarium of therapeutic options. Among the newer approaches that have been implemented are minimally invasive techniques, including robotic surgery, which have become a mainstay of reconstructive therapy. Given this evolution, it is imperative for surgeons to be familiar with the risks, benefits, and alternatives of these newer procedures. While robotic surgery provides many advantages, including increased visibility due to magnification, ease of performance over laparoscopic surgery, shorter hospital stays, and decreased postoperative pain and recovery time, complica-

tions related to the approach can occur. This chapter will focus on complications of robotic surgery and prevention strategies that can be applied to several techniques performed robotically to treat PFDs.

Types of Complications

Though robotic surgery is considered to be a minimally invasive approach, complications may occur—some that are similar to the risks of open surgery and others that are unique to robotic and laparoscopic surgery. Laparoscopy in urologic surgery has a reported complication rate of up to 13% [3] and a mortality rate of 0.2–0.97% [3, 4]. The rate of conversion from laparoscopy to an open procedure in a series of a variety of laparoscopic urological cases was 1.2–1.5% in two large single-institution series [3, 5]. Regarding pelvic floor reconstruction specifically, a meta-analysis of robotic sacrocolpopexy revealed an intraoperative and serious postoperative complication rate of 3% (range 0–19%) and 2% (range 0–8%), respectively [6]. Patients should be thoroughly and carefully counseled on the potential complications that include, but are not limited to, hemorrhage, infection, neurovascular or visceral injury (that may occur outside of the field of view and therefore be missed), failure to progress, necessity to convert to an open procedure, cardiopulmonary events, and complications specific to

K.C. Kobashi, M.D., F.A.C.S. (✉)
Virginia Mason Medical Center,
1100 Ninth Ave, Seattle, WA 98101, USA
e-mail: kathleen.kobashi@virginiamason.org

© Springer International Publishing AG 2018
J.T. Anger, K.S. Eilber (eds.), *The Use of Robotic Technology in Female Pelvic Floor Reconstruction*, DOI 10.1007/978-3-319-59611-2_15

the robotic approach, including mechanical problems and issues related to trocar placement and insufflation. Failure of the surgery to progress can occur when there are dense adhesions or other anatomic or technical issues that prevent the surgery from advancing toward the goal.

Minimizing the Risk of Complications

Patient Selection

The main keys to minimizing complications in robotic surgery are careful patient selection and surgeon preparedness. Surgeons should anticipate the potential risks as they pertain to each individual patient, with meticulous attention to detail and, whenever possible, minimize avoidable pitfalls. Past medical and surgical history and a careful physical examination should be performed, keeping in mind the numerous factors that can have specific implications in robotic surgery. Contraindications to robotic and laparoscopic surgery include coagulopathy, active bowel obstruction, hemoperitoneum or hemoretroperitoneum, intra-abdominal or abdominal wall infection, and suspected malignant ascites [7]. It is imperative to keep patients informed about all the known risks, benefits, and alternatives of treatment for their condition.

History

A history of chronic obstructive pulmonary disease (COPD) places patients at risk for hypercarbia due to the pneumoperitoneum. Elevated carbon dioxide (CO_2) levels can be arrhythmogenic due to the effects of CO_2 on the myocardium. Accordingly, patients with COPD should be evaluated with preoperative arterial blood gas and pulmonary function tests, and patients with cardiac arrhythmia should be treated preoperatively.

Prior abdominal or pelvic surgery or history of peritonitis can result in challenges with safe entry into the abdomen. Other concerning history would include benign ascites, abdominal hernia, and aortic or iliac arterial aneurysms.

Physical Examination

Overall performance status should be considered, particularly in the case of elective surgery such as that related to the treatment of pelvic floor dysfunction. Morbid obesity can render robotic surgery difficult due to the need for longer instruments, limited range of motion of the instruments, and challenges with obtaining and maintaining pneumoperitoneum. Morbid obesity can also result in elevated airway pressures that result in the need for abandonment of laparoscopy. Surgical scars may offer insight into the potential difficulty of trocar placement, and it has been suggested that when intra-abdominal adhesions are a concern, the abdomen is best entered subcostally at the left midclavicular line.

Abdominal wall hernias, organomegaly, or a pulsatile mass suggestive of an abdominal aortic aneurysm should be investigated preoperatively to ensure the safest route of entry for the patient.

Perioperative Preparation

Equipment Failure

Complications related to equipment malfunction are largely preventable with meticulous attention to detail. One series of 8,240 robotic surgeries at eleven institutions reported an equipment malfunction rate requiring cancellation of the case at 0.4%, with malfunction of the robotic arms or optics as the most commonly reported reason [8]. Proper training of the surgeon and operating room staff to familiarize the team with the equipment, including its capabilities and limitations, is imperative. Knowledge of troubleshooting techniques and partnership with the technical assist team are also important in order to minimize complications related to the equipment failure.

Patient Positioning

Proper positioning and padding of pressure points are critical to ensure safety in robotic surgery. Generally, in pelvic floor reconstruction, patients are placed in the lithotomy or low lithotomy position. Care must be taken to avoid excessive flexion of the hips or outward rotation of the legs, the latter of which can cause stretching of the femoral nerve. For pelvic floor surgery, the arms may be tucked by the patient's sides, and the hands and wrists should be placed in neutral position and pronated to avoid brachial plexus injury. Compressions stockings and sequential compression devices should be placed on the lower extremities to minimize the risk of deep vein thrombosis. All pressure points and bony prominences, including elbows, heels, and calves, should be padded to minimize the risk of rhabdomyolsis, compartment syndrome [9], or venous thrombotic events. The patient should be secured to the table using well-padded safety belts or tape across the chest, particularly given the frequent use of the extreme Trendelenberg position in pelvic floor reconstructive cases. Shoulder braces should not be used in this circumstance due to the risk of brachial plexus injury. Gel pads or beanbags can be helpful in preventing cephalad migration of the patient.

Neurologic complications may not be recognized until the postoperative period when the patient has difficulty with ambulation or describes sensory changes. Careful neurologic examination should be performed, and a neurologic consultation obtained. While nerve palsies can resolve within the first few postoperative days, recovery can also be slow, requiring prolonged physical therapy.

Intraoperative Complications

Complications During Abdominal Access

Complications related to entry into the abdomen are critical to understand. Irrespective of whether access is obtained via insertion of a Veress needle or open Hassan technique, injury to viscera or vasculature can occur during this step or during the subsequent insertion of the trocars.

Veress Needle Insertion

Improper positioning of the Veress needle into the abdominal wall can initially be difficult to detect. In fact, 1–2 L of carbon dioxide (CO_2) can be instilled with misleading abdominal distention and tympany that appear normal before incorrect placement is realized. However, if initial pressures exceed 10 mmHg, one should consider the possibility that the Veress needle is not located intra-abdominally. Assymetric abdominal distention or a sudden rise in insufflation pressure should also alert the surgeon to malposition of the needle. If incorrect needle placement is suspected, the Veress needle must be repositioned. In the event of multiple unsuccessful needle placement attempts, CO_2 evacuation and conversion to the Hasson technique should be considered.

Incorrect Veress needle placement can be avoided by confirmation of proper placement of the Veress needle prior to insufflation of the abdomen using the "aspiration, irrigation, aspiration", or "drop" technique as well as confirming that the needle can be easily advanced 0.5–1.0 cm without resistance. Upon entry into the abdomen, *aspiration* should not return blood, urine, or bowel contents; *irrigation* with sterile fluid should pass easily without resistance; repeat *aspiration* should return nothing; removal of the syringe should result in a prompt "*drop*" of the fluid level.

Hasson Technique

The rate of complications related to entry via the open technique is rare compared with that using the Veress technique, though the complications are generally similar. Bowel that is adherent to the underside of the abdominal wall can present a problem during access.

Vascular or Visceral Injury

When aspiration though the Veress needle returns blood, urine, or bowel contents, entry into a vessel, the bladder, or bowel, respectively, should be suspected. Typically, the needle can simply be removed, but once proper entry into the abdomen has been accomplished, the area of concern should be carefully inspected for hemostasis and integrity of the viscera. When initial insufflation pressures are elevated, consideration of entry into a solid organ or the abdominal wall should be considered, the latter described in the section above.

For vascular injuries, application of pressure to the area of concern can facilitate hemostasis. If hemodynamic instability ensues, a general surgery or vascular consultation should be obtained. The risk of vascular complications can be minimized by entry into the abdomen in avascular areas such as subcostally at the midclavicular line or supero-medial to the anterior superior iliac spine. When entering at the umbilicus, the needle should be pointed toward the pelvis. Making a small incision through which the fascia can be grasped, pulled up, and stabilized can also facilitate safe entry.

Complications involving the bladder can be minimized with Foley catheter placement prior to abdominal entry. Similarly, a nasogastric tube can be inserted to decompress the bowel. Entry into the lumen of the bowel can be heralded by asymmetric distention of the abdomen. Emanation of malodorous gas from the Veress needle can suggest intralumenal placement. The needle can be withdrawn and replaced at a different site, or an open Hassan technique can be utilized. When injury with the small Veress needle occurs, some authors advocate that formal repair of the injury is not necessary [10]. Indeed, it is thought that minor insufflation needle injuries of the bowel likely occur more frequently than recognized. Larger injuries, such as that which can occur due to injuries from trocar placement, should be repaired to avoid postoperative complications [11].

Complications Related to Insufflation

Surgeons should be knowledgeable about potential complications related to insufflation, how to detect them, and how to address them.

Subcutaneous Emphysema
Superficial placement of the Veress needle, peri-port leakage due to large port incisions, elevated intra-abdominal pressures, or prolonged surgical time can result in subcutaneous emphysema, indicated by crepitus over the abdomen or thorax. It is important that insufflation be stopped if there is any doubt about proper placement of the needle. In this situation, conversion to open technique should be considered. If a port site leak is suspected, a pursestring stitch or Vaseline gauze can be placed around the trocar. Care to direct the trocar toward the surgical field can decrease torque on the site that pulls the incision open. When a persistent leak is encountered, conversion to a larger trocar or a balloon trocar can be considered. Decreased pressure settings can also be helpful in the case of port leaks and subcutaneous emphysema.

Barotrauma
Elevated intra-abdominal pressures can result in barotrauma that, if unrecognized, can lead to more serious complications. Barotrauma is defined as physical injury or damage to body tissues due to pressure related to gas within a space; in the case of laparoscopy or robotic surgery, the abdomen. Initial signs of barotrauma may include increased ventilation pressure requirements, hypotension due to decreased venous return, and consequent impaired cardiac output. Causes of barotrauma can include malfunction of the insufflator or use of other pressure-producing devices such as an argon beam coagulator, which is rarely, if ever, utilized in pelvic floor reconstruction. Nevertheless, when an argon beam coagulator is utilized, a port valve should be opened to minimize the pressure effect.

When any of the above signs occur, the abdomen should be desufflated until hemodynamics return to normal. An attempt should be made such that re-insufflation does not exceed 10 mmHg.

Pneumothorax, Pneumomediastinum, Pneumopericardium
In rare instances, serious complications including pneumothorax, pneuomediastinum, or pneumopericardium can occur as a result of increased pressures or leakage of gas along natural openings in the diaphragm. Pneumothorax can present with subcutaneous emphysema, decreased breath

sounds, and/or hypertension or hypotension. A large bore needle should be placed through the chest followed by placement of a chest tube. Pneumopericardium, which has an estimated incidence of 0.8%, may have no signs or may affect cardiac function. If hemodynamic decompensation occurs, the abdomen should be desufflated and pericardiocentesis should be considered.

Hypercarbia

Hypercarbia is one of the most common causes of cardiac dysrhythmia during laparoscopic surgery. Patients with underlying pulmonary disease (e.g., advanced COPD) are at particularly high risk of developing hypercarbia intraoperatively. If hypercarbia occurs, first steps include decreasing insufflation pressures to <10 mmHg or desufflation of the abdomen, hyperventilation, and increasing tidal volume or positive end expiratory pressures. If these maneuvers are not successful in correcting the elevated CO_2 levels, a rare occurrence, changing the insufflant to helium has been suggested. However, complications related to helium have also been described [12, 13].

CO_2 Embolism

Insufflation directly into vasculature can lead to the devastating complication of a CO_2 embolism. This fortunately rare occurrence can occur shortly following insufflation or from direct injection of CO_2 into a large vessel or organ that can result in blockage of the right ventricle or pulmonary artery. As with most of the complications discussed up to this point, this can be avoided by use of proper technique to confirm placement of the Veress needle. A CO_2 embolus can be heralded by acute cardiovascular collapse, cardiac arrhythmia, cyanosis, or pulmonary edema. There may be an abrupt increase in end tidal CO_2 and hypoxia noted by the anesthesia team. The first response is desufflation and placement of the patient in the Trendelenberg and left-side down position (left lateral decubitus) to allow the gas bubbles to rise to the apex of the right atrium and prevent entry into the pulmonary artery. Hyperventilation with 100% oxygen should be performed and aspiration of the right heart via central line considered.

Injury Related to Trocar Placement

Clearly, the highest risk trocar placement is the first blind trocar that is placed following insufflation. A visual obturator can be utilized to mitigate the risk of vascular or visceral injury. Subsequent trocars can be placed under some visualization, though adhesions can still render secondary trocar placement challenging.

Visceral Injury

Injury to the bladder during port placement can be avoided by first ensuring an empty bladder with Foley placement. If bladder injury is suspected, the bladder can be filled to identify the site of injury and the defect should be formally repaired. This is then followed by Foley catheter drainage.

Bowel injury with a trocar should also be formally repaired, and a general surgery consultation should be considered, based on one's comfort level. It should be noted that bowel injury can be a complete transection (through both walls), or through just one wall into the lumen of the bowel. The latter can be detected by visualization of the mucosa of the bowel. Through-and-through injury can be harder to detect and may not be noted until secondary trocars are passed, allowing for visualization of other trocar entry sites.

Vascular Injury

Bleeding at any trocar site can result in dripping from the abdominal wall around the trocar. This complication can be minimized by the use of blunt trocars and transillumination of the abdominal wall to identify the inferior epigastric vessels prior to trocar passage. Should trocar site bleeding occur, this can be addressed using electrocautery applied through an opposite port. Direct pressure on the skin around the port can be helpful to tamponade the bleeding vessel. Alternatively, the trocar can be systematically torqued in different directions to identify the site of bleeding, and the vessel can be oversewn. Landman et al. [7] suggest the passage of a Keith needle along one side of the trocar. The needle is then brought back up through the abdominal wall on the contralateral side of the trocar to tamponade the bleeding vessel. A bolster made of several folded up gauze sponges can be secured down onto the skin using a #1 nylon suture to provide further pressure.

Injury to the great vessels upon placement of the trocars is a rare but serious complication that can be signaled by sudden hypotension and hemodynamic instability. If profuse bleeding is noted, the vascular or trauma team should be called, the abdomen opened, and proximal and distal control of the vessel obtained. If the trocar is still in place, it should be left in place to provide some tamponade and to facilitate identification of the injury.

Thermal and Mechanical Injuries

Thermal injury can occur as a result of several mechanisms including direct application of electrocautery, coupling, and failure of insulation. Direct injury via monopolar cautery can create a larger injury, while bipolar injuries are more focused and require direct handling of the tissue to occur. Coupling essentially involves conduction of thermal energy through contact of metal instruments with each other and surrounding tissues. Faulty insulation can result in the same outcome.

Thermal injuries to the bowel can appear as a small, blanched area on the serosa. Because the injury can be subtle and because injury can occur outside of the field of vision, it may go unrecognized for up to several weeks postoperatively. Patients may present with fevers, chills, nausea, vomiting, abdominal or trocar site pain, and/or signs of peritonitis. Bowel injury should be considered in any patient who presents as such within the first several weeks postoperatively. Patients may have leukocytosis with or without a left shift. Due to the intraoperative pneumoperitoneum, air under the diaphragm on abdominal imaging is not a reliable finding.

Small injuries discovered late in the postoperative period can be managed expectantly with observation and antibiotics; however, if the patient is ill, abdominal exploration should be performed. It is important to differentiate between a seroma, which many patients will have following laparoscopic or robotic surgery, and an abscess. Seromas will resolve spontaneously and should not be aspirated due to the risk of introducing infection into a self-limited collection.

Because thermal injuries that occur as a result of monopolar energy result in larger injuries, wide excision of tissue surrounding the injury should be performed. Conversely, bipolar injuries can be managed with a more localized excision.

This risk of thermal injury can be minimized by confirmation of intact insulation of instruments, direct visualization of the entire metal area of instruments prior to applying electrocautery, meticulous isolation of the area to be cauterized from surrounding tissues, establishing that the surgeon is the only individual who controls the cautery, and avoidance of leaving unattended cautery instruments in the abdomen.

Even with careful attention to detail, direct injury to bowel or vasculature can occur. These are more often immediately recognized than are thermal injuries and can be addressed promptly. If superficial injury to the serosa of the bowel is noted, it can be oversewn. If entry into the lumen occurs, resection versus primary repair can be performed with irrigation of the abdominal cavity with copious amounts of antibiotic solution. Dependent upon the skill level of the surgeon, bowel injuries can be addressed robotically; however, many require laparotomy. If the bowel injury is not suspected until the postoperative period, a CT scan with oral contrast can confirm the diagnosis and the need for immediate return to the operating room to definitively address the injury.

In pelvic floor reconstruction, specifically sacrocolpopexy, the most common potential site of bleeding is at the anterior sacral space during exposure of the anterior longitudinal ligament at the sacral promontory. This region is rich in vasculature, with the pelvic plexus and the middle sacral vein and artery being located between the common iliac vessels. If bleeding is encountered in this region, direct pressure can be placed on the area, the insufflation pressure temporarily increased, and thrombogenic products and tacks may be utilized [14].

Postoperative Complications

Postoperative complications are not unique to robotic surgery. However, there are several issues of which the minimally invasive surgeon should be aware in order to promptly address any potential issues of concern.

Bowel Herniation and Incisional Hernia

Herniation of bowel into the port site incisions can occur. Patients may present with abdominal pain, nausea/vomiting, or pain at a specific port site in the early postoperative period. This situation requires surgical attention, but is best avoided by direct visualization upon removal of the trocars at the end of surgery and visual inspection of each of the port sites to ensure that no omentum or bowel has been entrapped. The fascia of bladed trocar sites >10 mm should be formally closed. Some authors support the non-closure of non-midline port sites placed with bladeless, radially dilating muscle-splitting trocars of up to 12 mm [15]. When return to the operating room is necessary, pneumoperitoneum can be reestablished and the affected loop of bowel or omentum gently removed with atraumatic graspers intra-abdominally combined with manual reduction through the port site. The bowel should be carefully inspected to ensure viability, and if there is any concern, resection of the compromised segment should be performed.

Bowel Injury

As discussed previously in this chapter, bowel injury may not be detected intraoperatively, particularly if it is due to a thermal injury. Any patient who presents postoperatively with abdominal pain, fevers, leukocytosis, or signs of peritonitis should have bowel injury in the differential diagnosis.

Deep Vein Thrombosis and Pulmonary Embolism

Deep vein thrombosis (DVT) and pulmonary embolus (PE) are potential complications of any surgery, with risk that increases with increased length of operative time. Although studies have not demonstrated an elevated risk of DVT with laparoscopic surgery, the theoretical effects of decreased venous return related to the increased intra-abdominal pressure created by the pneumoperitoneum should be considered. Best practice recommendations for DVT prophylaxis should be referenced, and appropriate prophylaxis, such as pneumatic compression stockings and in some patients, low molecular weight heparin, should be implemented [15, 16].

Rhabdomyolysis and Compartment Syndrome

Rhabdomyolysis and compartment syndrome are rare complications following long-duration minimally invasive surgery [7, 9, 17]. In urology, rhabdomyolysis has most frequently been reported in patients with high BMI who have undergone renal surgery requiring the lateral position with a kidney rest placed under the body. The flank pressure resulting from the flexed position compounded by the kidney rest has resulted in this serious complication. Compartment syndrome has been reported in prolonged gynecological procedures related to the lithotomy position and resultant pressures on the lower extremities. Although these complications are fortunately rare, surgeons should be aware of their possibility and consider this condition in patients who present with severe pain in the lower extremities following long pelvic floor reconstructive surgeries. When rhabdomyolysis is suspected, serum creatinine kinase should be checked. Normal CK levels range from 45 to 200 U/L. With rhabdomyolysis, CK levels can rise to 10,000–200,000 U/L or more. For compartment syndrome, evaluation of compartment pressures and/or orthopedic or general surgery consultation can be obtained.

Ocular Complications

Ocular complications are rare complications in laparoscopic surgery [18]. Corneal abrasions, which are not unique to minimally invasive surgery, will generally resolve without lasting sequelae. Corneal abrasions can occur due to direct trauma to the open eye from facemasks or other objects, exposure that causes drying of the eye, and chemical injury from, for example, solutions such as betadine. A devastating but rare complication thought to be associated with increased ocular pressures related to prolonged steep Trendelenberg position, is ischemic optic neuropathy that can lead to permanent loss of vision. Both the surgical and anesthesia teams should be aware of these potential complications and take measures to minimize these risks.

Conclusions

Over the past few decades, laparoscopic and robotic surgery have become major components of urologic and urogynecologic surgery. Indeed, robotic surgery has become a mainstay in female pelvic floor reconstruction. Procedures that once required sizeable incisions and extended periods of convalescence can now be performed with greatly improved comfort and shorter recovery times. The ability to provide a minimally invasive approach for patients with pelvic floor disorders desiring to address issues that affect their quality of life has been satisfying for patients and surgeons alike. That said, it is imperative that clinicians be aware of the potential complications that can occur with robotic surgery and be prepared to address them and be proficient at doing so. Arming oneself with knowledge prepares one to provide the best possible care for patients.

References

1. Nygaard I, Barber MD, Burgio KL, et al. Prevalence of symptomatic pelvic floor disorders in US women. JAMA. 2008;300(11):1311–6.
2. Olsen AL, Smith VJ, Bergstrom JO, et al. Epidemiology of surgically managed pelvic organ prolapse and urinary incontinence. Obstet Gynecol. 1997;89(4):501–6.
3. Parsons JK, Varkarakis I, Rha KH, et al. Complications of abdominal urologic laparoscopy: longitudinal five-year analysis. Urology. 2004;63(1):27–42.
4. Salman M, Bell T, Martin J, et al. Use, cost, complications, and mortality of robotic versus non-robotic general surgery procedures based on a nationwide database. Am Surg. 2013;79(6):553–60.
5. Vallencien G, Cathelineau X, Baumert M, et al. Complications of transperitoneal laparoscopic surgery in urology: review of 1311 procedures at a single institution. J Urol. 2002;168(2):23–6.
6. Serati M, Bogani G, Sorice P, et al. Robotic assisted sacrocolpopexy for pelvic organ prolapse: a systematic review and meta-analysis of comparative studies. Eur Urol. 2014;66(2):303–18.
7. Ordon M, Eichel L, Landman J. Fundamentals of laparoscopic and robotic urologic surgery. In: Wein AJ, Kavoussi LR, Partin AW, Peters CA, editors. Campbell-Walsh urology. 11th ed. Philadelphia: Elsevier; 2016. p. 195–224.
8. Lavery HJ, Thaly R, Albala D, et al. Robotic equipment malfunction during robotic prostatectomy: a multi-institutional summary. J Endourol. 2008;22(9):2165–8.
9. Bauer EC, Koch N, Janni W, et al. Compartment syndrome after gynecologic operations: evidence from case reports and reviews. Eur J Obstet Gynecol Reprod Biol. 2014;173:712.
10. Neuberger TJ, Adrus CH, Wittgen CM, et al. Prospective comparison of helium versus carbon dioxide pneumoperitoneum. Gastrointest Endosc. 1996;43:38–41.
11. Schwartz MH, Falena I, Cinman N, et al. Laparoscopic bowel injury in retroperitoneal surgery: current incidence and outcomes. J Urol. 2010;184(2):589–94.
12. Bongard FS, Pianim NA, Leighton TA, et al. Helium insufflation for laparoscopic operation. Surg Gynecol Obstet. 1993;177:140–6.
13. Clifton MM, Pizarro-Berdichevsky J, Goldman HR. Robotic female pelvic floor reconstruction: a review. Urology. 2016;91:33–40.
14. Kang DI, Woo SH, Lee DH, Kim IY. Incidence of port-site hernias after robot assisted radical prostatectomy with the fascial closure of only the midline 12 mm port site. J Endourol. 2012;28(7):848–51.
15. Forrest JB, Clemens JQ, Finamore P, et al. AUA best practice statement for the prevention of deep vein thrombosis in patients undergoing urologic surgery. J Urol. 2009;181(3):1120–7.
16. Violette PD, Cartwright R, Briel M, et al. Guidelines of guidelines: thromboprophylaxis for urologic surgery. BJI Int. 2016;118:351–8.
17. Sukhu T, Krupski KL. Patient positioning and prevention of injuries in patients undergoing laparoscopic and robotic-assisted urologic procedures. Curr Urol Rep. 2014;15(4):398.
18. Kan KM, Brown SE, Gainsberg DM. Ocular complications in robotic-assisted prostatectomy: a review of pathophysiology and prevention. Minerva Anesthesiol. 2015;81(5):57–66.

Index

© Springer International Publishing AG 2018
J.T. Anger, K.S. Eilber (eds.), *The Use of Robotic Technology in Female
Pelvic Floor Reconstruction*, DOI 10.1007/978-3-319-59611-2